P9-CDI-390

Eating By Design

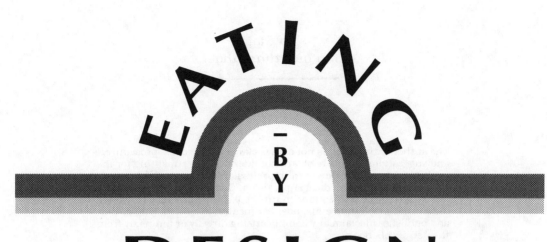

EATING
-BY-
DESIGN

The Individualized Food Personality Type Nutrition Plan

Carrie Latt Wiatt

POCKET BOOKS
New York   London   Toronto   Sydney   Tokyo   Singapore

to Cigi
my guardian angel

The author of this book is not a physician and the ideas, procedures, and suggestions in this book are not intended as a substitute for the medical advice of a trained health professional. All matters regarding your health require medical supervision. Consult your physician before adopting the suggestions in this book, as well as about any condition that may require diagnosis or medical attention. The author and publisher disclaim any liability arising directly or indirectly from the use of this book.

POCKET BOOKS, a division of Simon & Schuster Inc.
1230 Avenue of the Americas, New York, NY 10020

Copyright © 1995 by Carrie Latt Wiatt

All rights reserved, including the right to reproduce
this book or portions thereof in any form whatsoever.
For information address Pocket Books, 1230 Avenue
of the Americas, New York, NY 10020

Library of Congress Cataloging-in-Publication Data

Wiatt, Carrie Latt.
    Eating by design : The Individualized Food Personality Type
Nutrition Plan / Carrie Latt Wiatt.
        p.   cm.
    Includes bibliographical references.
    ISBN 0-671-89811-6
    1. Eating disorders—Popular works.   2. Food habits—Psychological
aspects.   3. Diet—Psychological aspects.   4. Personality.
I. Title.
RC552.E18W53   1995
    613.2′01′9—dc20   95-10958
                                                                   CIP

First Pocket Books hardcover printing August 1995

10 9 8 7 6 5 4 3 2 1

POCKET and colophon are registered trademarks of
Simon & Schuster Inc.

Text design by Stanley S. Drate/Folio Graphics Co., Inc.

Printed in the U.S.A.

ACKNOWLEDGMENTS

To my clients:
You're the foundation of Diet Designs. I applaud your courage, dedication, and willingness to put your best selves forward. Thank you for all the wonderful experiences—I will treasure them always.

To my parents, Mimi and Arron, who taught me to follow my heart and my head, to pursue a life with purpose and meaning.

To my sister Andi and my brother-in-law Stuart:
Your laughter and joy of life are with me always.

To my wonderful team at Diet Designs:
For your commitment, I am grateful.

To Elizabeth Miles:
For the talent, energy, and love you put into this book. I will always cherish you.

To Tom Miller:
My editor and friend, you are a tireless perfectionist. I've learned so much. Thank you from the bottom of my heart.

To Amanda Urban:
Thanks for believing in me.

To Dr. Diana Donner and Dr. Enid Zaslow:
Your contributions to this book were invaluable.

To Jim:
Thank you for everything.

CONTENTS

III

PERSONAL PRESCRIPTION FOR YOUR FOOD PERSONALITY TYPE

IV

THE DIET DESIGNS KITCHEN

INTRODUCTION

YOU EAT WHO YOU ARE

If the old maxim "you are what you eat" were true, a week on a diet of steamed vegetables, dry wheat toast, and plain tuna fish would permanently transform you into a paragon of health and virtue. But we all know by experience that this is not the case. Most diets are eventually derailed by a simple psychological fact: You have a distinct, **individual food personality type** that drives you to eat *who* you are. All the diets in the world can't change your innate personality traits.

Eating By Design is about working with your own personality profile to harmonize your mind and body with your eating habits. It focuses on what is *right* for you, not what is wrong, and it capitalizes on your inborn strengths. This book can free you from the diet syndrome forever! *Eating By Design* is a comprehensive, lifetime plan that works with your food personality type to achieve your personal best.

I grew up as one of the first generation of children with two working parents. Just as I entered my teenage years and began to worry about my body image, my mother began a new career as a lawyer and left me adrift in a diet of prepared convenience foods. The breakup of my family table struck a deep chord of fear in me.

I inherited a love of cooking from my grandmother, who was famous for her pot roast. But without a role model for how to relate to food, I was afraid of being fat. I wanted to offer the same love and care to my fragmented family that my grandmother had offered to me—but without the high fat content that would make my worst nightmares come true. I became a healthy cook to make my family functional again.

When I began Diet Designs, my Hollywood nutrition practice, I knew that with many celebrities among my clientele, I would be working with personalities—but all my training in nutrition and cooking hadn't prepared me for just how different people's personality types can be when it comes to food. Diet Designs gave me a hands-on education.

My personality-based approach has proven so effective that some of the fittest physiques in Hollywood now rely on it to manage their weight and health. After a decade of perfecting Eating By Design, I'm thrilled to share it beyond my circle of clients in an easy-to-use blueprint for lifelong fitness.

This book gives you the tools to determine your food personality type. It will mobilize your self-acceptance and self-awareness, giving you the key to unlock your inner power and set your healthy self free.

While Americans are getting fatter and fatter, my clients have lost their weight and kept it off. In the past decade, the overweight sector of the population has risen from 58 percent to 66 percent—*two out of every three people in the nation.** Weight loss success rates have plummeted to the point where about 90 percent of people who lose weight on a diet gain it all back again, prompting many to give up their dreams of health and self-esteem in despair. My clients, on the other hand, are fit, well fed, and at peace with themselves. Why is Eating By Design succeeding where other diets are so dramatically failing?

Diets don't work for Americans because most diets prescribe the same solution for all different kinds of problems, leaving you stuck in a destructive pattern of food conformity that fights your individuality. The problem is compounded by social, cultural, and family norms that place a high value on rich communal meals and shared food, which can encourage you to eat according to other people's needs instead of your own.

You know you think, feel, and act differently from others. So why would you expect to eat like everybody else? Though you might sit down to eat with other people, remember, you're always alone when you swallow. And it's usually you who's lifting the fork to your mouth.

The framework for *Eating By Design* developed the way my practice did. I intuitively identified a variety of personality-based eating styles. Curious to know more, I consulted with psychologists to achieve a scientific understanding of why different types of people eat the way they do.

What I found is that central attributes of our personalities are genetically programmed at birth. More and more, researchers are corroborating evidence of the biological basis to personality. The implications for weight management are crucial: Fighting your basic self with superficial diets that don't fit is futile. The inevitable outcome is failure.

Of course, your experiences and relationships further influence and refine your basic traits. Ultimately you are a product of what you bring to your environment and what it brings to you. So while you can't change your food person-

---

*1983 to 1993, National Health and Nutrition Examination Survey III.

ality type, you can *modify your relationship* with food to take advantage of your strengths.

At Diet Designs, I've used personalized techniques and recipes to help hundreds of people lose weight permanently. I work as a relationship counselor, helping each person inject understanding and respect into his or her relationship with food. From dynamic Hollywood executives who take my meals to power lunches at expensive restaurants . . . to movie stars perfecting their bodies, or even going significantly underweight to play special roles . . . to reclusive writers and artists who overeat in their private creative space . . . to kids, the elderly, and entire families . . . to pregnant and nursing mothers . . . to former celebrities who have slipped from the public eye and are pulling it together for a comeback . . . to all kinds of busy people, from Supermoms to Type-A superachievers—everyone has a different personality type with different needs. I treat each client as the unique individual she or he is. Perhaps you'll recognize yourself in these food personality types:

- If you commit to caring and providing for others, you're a **Nurturer;**
- If you hide your emotions with a smile, you're an **Artful Dodger;**
- If you're in love with sensual pleasure, you're a **Passionflower;**
- If you never seem to get happy or full, you're the **Blue Rose;**
- If you were born with an abundance of high emotion and drama, you're a **Shooting Star;**
- If everything has to be in its place, you're a **Perfectionist;**
- If you're totally absorbed in your private projects, you're the **Soloist;**
- If you demand more from yourself than you can possibly give, you're a **Lotus Eater;**
- If you're prone to stress and pressure, you're the **Power Player;**
- If you're committed to enlightenment but are sometimes misled, you're a **Yin-Yang;**
- If you're always looking for an exotic adventure, you're the **Thrill-Seeker;**
- If your head is far in the clouds, you're a **Dreamer.**

In Part One, first you'll take a quiz to find out which food personality type you are. Then you'll read all about your food personality type—I tell revealing anecdotes about my clients, sometimes dramatic, sometimes funny, that illustrate what kind of tendencies you have and what your biggest healthy eating challenges are. In Part Two I explain my basic Eating By Design principles. To further personalize your prescription for Eating By Design, you'll determine your Eating Quotient, a calculation of your daily caloric needs based on your body composition and background. You'll take a quiz to assess your current eating habits. You'll learn special proportioning and timing techniques to keep your energy equation balanced. And you'll explore the world of gourmet low-fat cooking with recipes tailored to your own food personality type.

Then, in the same way that your doctor prescribes a treatment based on your medical history and current problems and goals, in Part Three I write you a Personal Prescription that takes the individual variables of your food personality type into account. The plan I prescribe for your type delivers maximum health, fitness, and satisfaction, acting like your own personal nutritional counselor to help you meet your health and weight management goals while staying true to your inner nature.

Of course, everyone is a mixture of food personality types; everyone contains each type to a greater or lesser degree. Life is a process, and each person contains a spectrum of types and colorations. But you'll soon see that you have one *dominant* food personality type and two or three subtypes. Read on and come up with your own personal interactive mixture.

Ultimately, this is a book about eating as a natural and joyous activity, an affirmation of self and well-being. It will serve as a complete user's manual to your personal eating style, teaching you to use food to maintain and enhance your health, please your palate and your personality, and fuel your energy and productivity. It's a long-term strategy for self-care, giving you confidence in your choices through all the trends and fads of the future. *Eating By Design* works with you as a whole—mind, body, and spirit—to let you be yourself as you partake of the pleasures of food that we are all blessed to share.

YOUR FOOD PERSONALITY TYPE

Eating By Design is a comprehensive manual for personalized nutrition, and I trust that you will eventually explore all its nooks and crannies. You don't need to read it in order. You might find yourself skipping around to areas that interest you the most. That's fine, and I wish you happy wandering. But if you want the most direct route to Eating By Design, I suggest you follow these steps:

- Take the quiz in this chapter to identify your food personality type and assess your current eating habits.
- Read the chapter in which you predominate first. Read the rest of Part One to meet each of the food personality types, focusing on your major two or three types.
- Read Part Two for an introduction to the Eating By Design program, including my nutritional principles and fat-burning agenda. Take the quizzes there to assess your current eating habits and knowledge, and to determine your Eating Quotient, a personalized calorie count for weight loss or maintenance.
- Continue on to Part Three and read the Personal Prescription for your food personality type and subtypes. Study this chapter carefully, experimenting with the meal plan and following your Eating Quotient to start to realize the healthy benefits of Eating By Design.
- Read the Master Lists and Guidelines for shopping and snack lists, restaurant and travel tips, then consult the Master Exercise Plan for your personal fitness level—all of which will help you put your Personal Prescription into action.

- Scan Part Four, the Eating By Design Kitchen, for the low-fat cooking techniques and recipes (specially tailored to your food personality type) that have made my program such a hit. Read this part for years to come—and enjoy the food!
- Read through the remaining Personal Prescriptions at your leisure for further insight on why we all eat the way we do.

✳

Identify Your Food Personality Type

You can identify your major food personality type by assessing the feelings, behaviors, and tendencies that shape the way you eat. You'll notice in taking the Food Personality Type Quiz that the questions are about *you*, not your eating habits. This is because the Eating By Design premise begins with personality—the inner, psychological workings that drive you to eat the way you do.

The twelve food personality types are based on a combination of personality categories that psychologists use in their work, with the observations from my ten years of research at Diet Designs. Never before has eating behavior been systematized in this way. I'm thrilled to be able to share my personal consultation experience with you in this format.

Food Personality Type Quiz

For each question below, circle the number that most accurately represents how you generally feel. Answer the questions as honestly and precisely as you can, focusing on how you are now rather than how you were in the past or wish to be in the future. Don't spend too long on any one question.

1. I tend not to ask for help because it makes me feel guilty and selfish.

   ALMOST ALWAYS ⑤   OFTEN ④   SOMETIMES ③   RARELY ②   NEVER ①

2. I feel that people criticize me more than I deserve.

   ALMOST ALWAYS ⑤   OFTEN ④   SOMETIMES ③   RARELY ②   NEVER ①

3. "Eat, drink, and be merry!" is my motto—I live in the here and now.

   ALMOST ALWAYS ⑤   OFTEN ④   SOMETIMES ③   RARELY ②   NEVER ①

4. I feel fragile and vulnerable, and I am easily hurt.

   ALMOST ALWAYS ⑤   OFTEN ④   SOMETIMES ③   RARELY ②   NEVER ①

5. I don't like it when other people set limits or boundaries on my behavior.

ALMOST ALWAYS ⑤ OFTEN ④ SOMETIMES ③ RARELY ② NEVER ①

6. I like to have a sense of order in my life, so I keep myself organized with schedules, routines, and lists.

ALMOST ALWAYS ⑤ OFTEN ④ SOMETIMES ③ RARELY ② NEVER ①

7. I feel like an outsider at work, at school, or in social situations because I don't seem to know the right things to say or do.

ALMOST ALWAYS ⑤ OFTEN ④ SOMETIMES ③ RARELY ② NEVER ①

8. Once I start to eat, drink, smoke, etc., it's hard for me to stop.

ALMOST ALWAYS ⑤ OFTEN ④ SOMETIMES ③ RARELY ② NEVER ①

9. I have a very busy schedule, but I feel that I can always stretch myself a little further.

ALMOST ALWAYS ⑤ OFTEN ④ SOMETIMES ③ RARELY ② NEVER ①

10. I believe that there are spiritual and mystical aspects of life that science doesn't adequately describe.

ALMOST ALWAYS ⑤ OFTEN ④ SOMETIMES ③ RARELY ② NEVER ①

11. I would rather strike out on my own than be confined to a boring routine.

ALMOST ALWAYS ⑤ OFTEN ④ SOMETIMES ③ RARELY ② NEVER ①

12. I believe that someday all my hopes and dreams will come true. I wish someone would love and take care of me forever.

ALMOST ALWAYS ⑤ OFTEN ④ SOMETIMES ③ RARELY ② NEVER ①

13. I help people when I see they need it, often without waiting to be asked.

ALMOST ALWAYS ⑤ OFTEN ④ SOMETIMES ③ RARELY ② NEVER ①

14. I procrastinate and put things off to the very last minute.

ALMOST ALWAYS ⑤ OFTEN ④ SOMETIMES ③ RARELY ② NEVER ①

15. I look to people, things, or substances to give me pleasure.

ALMOST ALWAYS ⑤ OFTEN ④ SOMETIMES ③ RARELY ② NEVER ①

16. Though I may look successful on the outside, I feel sad inside.

ALMOST ALWAYS ⑤   OFTEN ④   SOMETIMES ③   RARELY ②   NEVER ①

17. I enjoy being the center of attention. The more eyes and ears that are focused on me, the better I feel.

ALMOST ALWAYS ⑤   OFTEN ④   SOMETIMES ③   RARELY ②   NEVER ①

18. I fall short of my own high standards and expect more of myself.

ALMOST ALWAYS ⑤   OFTEN ④   SOMETIMES ③   RARELY ②   NEVER ①

19. I feel most fulfilled and happy in my own space.

ALMOST ALWAYS ⑤   OFTEN ④   SOMETIMES ③   RARELY ②   NEVER ①

20. I obsess about how much I eat and exercise, and how thin or fat I am.

ALMOST ALWAYS ⑤   OFTEN ④   SOMETIMES ③   RARELY ②   NEVER ①

21. I like to be at the helm, guiding the project and making it happen.

ALMOST ALWAYS ⑤   OFTEN ④   SOMETIMES ③   RARELY ②   NEVER ①

22. It's important to me to be very closely attuned to my inner self and the spirits of people around me.

ALMOST ALWAYS ⑤   OFTEN ④   SOMETIMES ③   RARELY ②   NEVER ①

23. I tackle new situations with high energy, confidence, and without fear of mistakes or danger.

ALMOST ALWAYS ⑤   OFTEN ④   SOMETIMES ③   RARELY ②   NEVER ①

24. I feel that a loving partner would give me all the happiness and fulfillment I could ever want.

ALMOST ALWAYS ⑤   OFTEN ④   SOMETIMES ③   RARELY ②   NEVER ①

25. I get more joy from helping others than helping myself. But I have a hard time accepting help from others in return.

ALMOST ALWAYS ⑤   OFTEN ④   SOMETIMES ③   RARELY ②   NEVER ①

26. I don't like it when people make unrealistic demands of me, and I might respond by not cooperating.

ALMOST ALWAYS ⑤   OFTEN ④   SOMETIMES ③   RARELY ②   NEVER ①

27. I crave a variety of new sensations and pleasurable experiences.

ALMOST ALWAYS ⑤   OFTEN ④   SOMETIMES ③   RARELY ②   NEVER ①

28. I'd rather not get involved with other people because they may expect more than I can give.

ALMOST ALWAYS ⑤   OFTEN ④   SOMETIMES ③   RARELY ②   NEVER ①

29. When I feel bored or empty, I look for distractions and diversions to liven things up.

ALMOST ALWAYS ⑤   OFTEN ④   SOMETIMES ③   RARELY ②   NEVER ①

30. I feel most secure when I do the job myself, so I can be sure that it's done right.

ALMOST ALWAYS ⑤   OFTEN ④   SOMETIMES ③   RARELY ②   NEVER ①

31. I'm most comfortable when surrounded by my closest friends and family. I would rather be with them than meet new people.

ALMOST ALWAYS ⑤   OFTEN ④   SOMETIMES ③   RARELY ②   NEVER ①

32. I eat far beyond the point of hunger or pleasure.

ALMOST ALWAYS ⑤   OFTEN ④   SOMETIMES ③   RARELY ②   NEVER ①

33. My work needs to come before my private life, social events, and fun.

ALMOST ALWAYS ⑤   OFTEN ④   SOMETIMES ③   RARELY ②   NEVER ①

34. I look for words like "pure," "organic," "natural," and "environmentally friendly" when selecting products and services.

ALMOST ALWAYS ⑤   OFTEN ④   SOMETIMES ③   RARELY ②   NEVER ①

35. Whatever I'm doing, I like to push the limits and take risks.

ALMOST ALWAYS ⑤   OFTEN ④   SOMETIMES ③   RARELY ②   NEVER ①

36. I'd rather let other people make decisions than make them myself.

ALMOST ALWAYS ⑤   OFTEN ④   SOMETIMES ③   RARELY ②   NEVER ①

37. I put my energy and ideas to work more for others than for myself.

ALMOST ALWAYS ⑤   OFTEN ④   SOMETIMES ③   RARELY ②   NEVER ①

38. I don't show my anger directly, but somehow it seems to come out in other, subtle ways.

ALMOST ALWAYS ⑤   OFTEN ④   SOMETIMES ③   RARELY ②   NEVER ①

39. I live for the pleasure, flavors, and total experience of good food.

ALMOST ALWAYS ⑤   OFTEN ④   SOMETIMES ③   RARELY ②   NEVER ①

40. I feel unhappy about the things I've handled poorly and the mistakes I've made.

ALMOST ALWAYS ⑤   OFTEN ④   SOMETIMES ③   RARELY ②   NEVER ①

41. I show my feelings easily, and they can run from hot to cold in a matter of minutes.

ALMOST ALWAYS ⑤   OFTEN ④   SOMETIMES ③   RARELY ②   NEVER ①

42. I tend to be more rational and logical than emotional.

ALMOST ALWAYS ⑤   OFTEN ④   SOMETIMES ③   RARELY ②   NEVER ①

43. I prefer solitary activities or sports to teamwork.

ALMOST ALWAYS ⑤   OFTEN ④   SOMETIMES ③   RARELY ②   NEVER ①

44. I self-medicate to calm down, escape from pain and pressure, or keep my emotions and anxieties under control.

ALMOST ALWAYS ⑤   OFTEN ④   SOMETIMES ③   RARELY ②   NEVER ①

45. The more I achieve, the better I feel.

ALMOST ALWAYS ⑤   OFTEN ④   SOMETIMES ③   RARELY ②   NEVER ①

46. My curiosity about alternative approaches to life can leave me confused and undecided.

ALMOST ALWAYS ⑤   OFTEN ④   SOMETIMES ③   RARELY ②   NEVER ①

47. I would rather drive fast than obey the speed limit in all areas of life.

ALMOST ALWAYS ⑤   OFTEN ④   SOMETIMES ③   RARELY ②   NEVER ①

48. I believe my soulmate is out there somewhere, and we will find each other one day if we haven't already.

ALMOST ALWAYS ⑤   OFTEN ④   SOMETIMES ③   RARELY ②   NEVER ①

49. I have a high tolerance for emotional and physical hardship.

ALMOST ALWAYS ⑤   OFTEN ④   SOMETIMES ③   RARELY ②   NEVER ①

50. When someone asks me to do something I don't want to do, I put it off or do a bad job.

ALMOST ALWAYS ⑤   OFTEN ④   SOMETIMES ③   RARELY ②   NEVER ①

51. I indulge my sensual self.

ALMOST ALWAYS ⑤   OFTEN ④   SOMETIMES ③   RARELY ②   NEVER ①

52. I feel unmotivated and uninterested in my daily tasks.

ALMOST ALWAYS ⑤   OFTEN ④   SOMETIMES ③   RARELY ②   NEVER ①

53. I have trouble waiting for things; I do what I want when the spirit moves me.

ALMOST ALWAYS ⑤   OFTEN ④   SOMETIMES ③   RARELY ②   NEVER ①

54. I consider every decision very carefully to be sure that I don't make a mistake.

ALMOST ALWAYS ⑤   OFTEN ④   SOMETIMES ③   RARELY ②   NEVER ①

55. I am polite and courteous to everyone, but I tend to avoid close contact with people.

ALMOST ALWAYS ⑤   OFTEN ④   SOMETIMES ③   RARELY ②   NEVER ①

56. I remember my past with pain and regret.

ALMOST ALWAYS ⑤   OFTEN ④   SOMETIMES ③   RARELY ②   NEVER ①

57. I establish rules and take charge of situations to make sure that I am successful and reach my goals.

ALMOST ALWAYS ⑤   OFTEN ④   SOMETIMES ③   RARELY ②   NEVER ①

58. I worry about the physical and spiritual health of the planet.

ALMOST ALWAYS ⑤   OFTEN ④   (SOMETIMES) ③   RARELY ②   NEVER ①

59. I thrive on the natural high that comes from challenging experiences and new situations.

ALMOST ALWAYS ⑤   OFTEN ④   SOMETIMES ③   (RARELY) ②   NEVER ①

60. I like movies or novels that have happy endings; I don't like sad endings.

(ALMOST ALWAYS) ⑤   OFTEN ④   SOMETIMES ③   RARELY ②   NEVER ①

Now fill in your score for each question in the appropriate box below. Add the numbers in each column to get your rating (5–25) for each personality type.

1	2	3	4	5	6	7	8	9	10	11	12
1	2	3	4	4	4	2	3	3	3	4	2
13	14	15	16	17	18	19	20	21	22	23	24
4	3	4	2	2	4	4	4	4	5	2	2
25	26	27	28	29	30	31	32	33	34	35	36
4	4	2	2	5	5	5	5	3	3	1	2
37	38	39	40	41	42	43	44	45	46	47	48
4	1	2	3	4	2	2	1	4	1	1	1
49	50	51	52	53	54	55	56	57	58	59	60
2	3	3	2	3	4	1	3	4	3	2	5
TOTALS 15	13	14	13	16	19	13	16	18	15	10	12
Your rating for personality style: #1	#2	#3	#4	#5	#6	#7	#8	#9	#10	#11	#12
Nurturer	Artful Dodger	Passionflower	Blue Rose	Shooting Star	Perfectionist	Soloist	Lotus Eater	Power Player	Yin-Yang	Thrill-Seeker	Dreamer

9

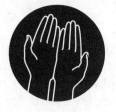

1

THE NURTURER

"Cleaning your house while the kids are still growing is like shoveling the walk before it stops snowing."

—PHYLLIS DILLER

I dreamed I was in my kitchen, putting together yet another perfect meal for my family. Suddenly I looked out the window and there, floating in the sky, larger than life, was my mother. She was thrusting something at me—a boiled chicken, yellow with congealed fat and dripping schmalz from the wings. "Eat, eat," she was saying, and with every pronouncement of the word, she grew. She kept waving the chicken, screeching "Eat!" in increasingly desperate tones, until she was so big she filled the sky and blocked out the sun. My God, I thought, I've become my mother! It wasn't until I woke up that I realized I'd just been watching too much late-night Woody Allen.

—CONFESSIONS OF A NURTURER

✳

Sophie was a supermom. I could practically see the big varsity letter "S" on her chest when she walked into my office lugging a ten-gallon purse and trailing an unhappy-looking eight-year-old in headgear. "Straight from the orthodontist," I thought, "And now she's going to try to focus on her personal eating issues while half her mind is committing her son's headgear schedule to memory." I foisted Jimmy off on my long-suffering assistant so I could meet with Sophie alone. I wanted to be the only caretaker in the room.

Sophie was devoted to taking care of her husband, four active children, two dogs and a cat, and a large house, along with charity work and volunteer efforts for school and community issues. She grew up in a close family with a loving mother who made three home-cooked meals and ironed her husband's shirt every single day of the year. Sophie pursued her own dreams of helping people by earning a degree in speech pathology. When she married Gene, a resident at Cedars-Sinai Hospital where she worked, she had no question what her next move would be: start a family and work hard to make it every bit as wonderful as hers was.

But somewhere between marriage to the doctor of her dreams and creation of the perfect family, Sophie got fat. I could see the forty pounds of unconscious eating as plain as day on her body, the selfless by-product of sampling her own cooking, nibbling on the kids' cupcakes, and portioning her own plate for the appetite of an adolescent boy. I was about to reassure her of the magic ability of the Diet Designs program, with its prepared, preportioned meals, to eliminate unconscious eating—when, all of a sudden, Sophie told me that she had not come in for herself at all!

Sophie said she needed my help because her sixteen-year-old daughter Kelly had recently begun to act strangely about food, refusing to eat at dinner, picking and moving her food around on the plate. Though she wouldn't eat with her family, Kelly would plow through bags of cookies and freezerfuls of pizza with her friends, then go on group crash diets in a dangerous form of adolescent bonding. Sophie didn't know what to say to Kelly to draw her back to the family table, so she had come to me for coaching.

This was a red light for me. Sophie obviously had her own food issues to confront, which she couldn't see through the smokescreen of concern for her daughter. I questioned her gently about her own weight, but met a blank brick wall.

It was as if her very visible problem were made invisible by her attention to others. My only hope for helping Sophie was to treat her dilemma with Kelly, then show her how caring for her family could translate into caring for herself, and help her set a good example for her children. Her healthy eating solution had to be shared at the communal dinner table.

Unfortunately, Sophie's schedule was a hectic one of erratic eating before she sank down, exhausted, in her chair at the head of that dinner table. She was up at six thirty every morning getting her husband off to work and the kids off to school. Days were full of shopping, cooking, and cleaning; errands for the house, church, neighbors, and relatives; and complicated patterns of kid shuttling worthy of an air traffic controller. She rarely took time to sit down to a meal, but instead picked and nibbled throughout the day from the endless stream of nourishment she provided to others. By the time she dished up the last supper plate she was completely drained, ate ravenously and polished off potential leftovers during cleanup. After a heavy dinner, it was all she could do to keep her eyes open long enough to supervise her kids' homework and trundle everyone off to bed. She often fell asleep on the couch, the newspaper on her lap still turned to the front page.

What Sophie needed before she could embark on any effort for Kelly was an energy-maximizing plan to fuel herself through the demands of her day and leave a little spunk to spare for her family's healthy eating education. I told Sophie I would give her a plan for the whole group, working with her to trace the process from the shopping cart to the kitchen to the table—if she would promise to commit to the project first. This meant scheduling and portioning her own meals regardless of what the rest of the family was doing or eating, managing her energy flow, and paring off excess fat to keep up with her family's frantic pace and to show Kelly what it meant to have a healthy approach to her diet and body. She agreed.

My first trip to Sophie's house was an eye-opener—I had forgotten what teenagers can eat. The cupboards, refrigerator, and freezer were packed with infinite varieties of sugar-sweetened cereals, snack cakes, doughnuts, chips, canned and packaged spaghetti and noodle dishes, condensed canned soup, crackers, cookies, caramel corn, salted nuts, instant breakfast drinks, industrial-sized tubs of mayonnaise and peanut butter, four different bottles of creamy salad dressing ("each kid likes a different kind," said Sophie), sliced lunch meats, processed cheeses, jugs of soda, canisters filled with chocolate chip cookies and mini candy bars, Popsicles, ice cream, and pizza three different ways: frozen, refrigerated, and in a mix.

"Wow," I said in amazement. "It looks like the pantry of a hotel restaurant in here! Who eats all this?" I could have given Sophie the frightening statistics about the fat, salt, and sugar content of her kitchen, but I didn't want her to feel that she'd been slowly killing the family she was trying to feed. Instead, I handed her a supermarket list to stock up on healthy foods for the whole family, and recipes for an oil-free marinara sauce to last all week and turkey meat loaf, mashed potatoes, and apple cobbler for the family's inaugural low-fat dinner.

I called Sophie the next day for a report on how the new dishes were received. Kelly had pronounced the dinner gross, but everybody else loved it. And instead of finishing off the meat loaf during cleanup, Sophie saved it for a sandwich for Gene's lunch. He was pleasantly surprised to have an alternative to greasy hospital cafeteria food. I knew we had cleared the first hurdle.

But Kelly was not so easily won over. She continued to resist Sophie's efforts, saying it was all gross and she was "not into health food." I asked Sophie if she could convince Kelly to do a session in the kitchen with me. Mother finally struck a bargain with daughter—an hour of her time in exchange for an extra night out with the car. I was overjoyed. If I could just get to Kelly, Sophie's soft spot, I knew I would have full family support for my mission.

In a private conversation with Kelly, I determined that her rejection of family dining wasn't indicative of a disorder—it was just normal teenage rebellion and concern for her changing body image. I was happy to have the opportunity to help at this crucial stage of her adolescence. Armed to the teeth with recipes and statistics, I compared fat and calorie counts between my version and the originals for barbequed chicken pizza, enchiladas, layered bean-and-cheese dip, burgers, Chinese chicken salad, fudge brownies, and hot fudge sundaes, comparing the number of servings Kelly would have to eat of each to gain a pound. I described how dietary fat turns into body fat and aggravates skin problems—two teenage phobias. Then I asked her if she'd like to learn to make any of my recipes. "Yes, please," she said. "The pizza, layered bean dip, burgers, and brownies."

I invited Sophie into the kitchen to join us in whipping up the dishes, and soon the three of us were chatting and giggling over a pan of brownies. Minutes later, Kelly was on the phone to a friend saying, "I'm telling you, you can have three of these brownies for the calories of one regular one. It is *so cool*." I confided to Sophie that if she added some fresh fruit and vegetables, Kelly could essentially live on this diet until she decided to do otherwise. I was happy to see that Sophie, even as she dug into the stack of dirty dishes, was smiling.

Sophie went on a three-month cooking marathon, adapting the favorite family recipes with low-fat cooking techniques, testing the new versions out on the gang, and perfecting every last detail of her redesigned dishes. She was up late at night portioning and freezing the products of the day, and was awake extra early in the morning to pack lunches for everyone instead of leaving them at the mercy of the school and hospital cafeterias as before.

I kept expecting Sophie to drop from exhaustion, but with lots of encouragement from me that this was the best possible example she could set for Kelly, she developed her own schedule of interval eating and portion control that trimmed off twenty pounds and doubled her energy. We held our consultations in her kitchen while she cooked up her latest low-fat wonder, quizzing me on further fat corners to cut from their favorite dishes.

Kelly lived happily on my versions of pizza and brownies and served them to her friends. The rest of the kids and Gene hardly noticed the transition to a low-fat diet, though Gene finally complimented Sophie on her appearance and asked if she'd been on a diet. "What about you?" she replied. "You're barely holding your pants up!"

Gene hopped on the scale to discover that he'd lost ten pounds without even trying. This was Sophie's greatest triumph—to peel off her husband's extra weight without making him suffer. I told Sophie that it was great about Gene, but not to overlook that she herself had lost twenty pounds. What an achievement that was!

Ever the Nurturer, Sophie had to help others to help herself. That was okay with me. All that mattered was that *I* had helped *Sophie*.

The truth is, I chose a career in nutrition because, like a mom, I wanted to devote my life to helping others. You see, I am a Nurturer too.

✳

Nurturers specialize in putting the needs of others before their own, whether at home or on the job. They're never happier than when they're caring and shouldering the burden of other people's crises and daily needs. Not all Nurturers are parents. I've worked with those in many walks of life, but we all have one thing in common: an instinct for caring. Whether serving family, friends, co-workers, or community members, Nurturers are generous, with willing ears and helping hands. They are the best friend, the warm hearth, the steady hand, the organizer of birthday parties. Unselfish, altruistic, and strong and steady as a rock, Nurturers provide stability to society. I'm always happy to have Nurturer clients—we bond instantly in our concern for caring, our instinct to provide. And if anyone deserves the care of a program like Eating By Design, Nurturers do.

Unfortunately, it's often hard to persuade Nurturers to accept this kind of care. Their constant coping on behalf of others can conceal their own problems and needs. Personal issues tend to simmer away on the back burner while those of the rest of the world are at full boil on the front. As often as not, this includes their diet.

As a Nurturer, you're probably an excellent culinary provider to everyone but yourself. While you offer food to those around you as necessary nourishment and a symbol of love, your own food choices, mealtimes, and portion sizes are all subjugated to theirs. This self-sacrificing practice can lead to erratic eating, poor nutritional quality, and the substitution of food for thanks and relaxation, all of which can sap your energy and good health—making you, ultimately, less of a help to those around you than you could be.

My Nurturer clients repeat a common theme: "So much to do, so little time. . . . So many needs, so few of them mine." Caretaking is a basic human

NURTURER STYLE

CARING CHARACTERISTICS	CROSSFIRE
+ You are strong, supportive, and a self-sacrificing savior of those in need.	**—** It's hard to make a sandwich when you're nailed to the cross.
+ You are a generous provider and stoker of the home fires.	**—** Your generosity can turn you into the local food pusher.
+ You campaign tirelessly for all causes, worthy and otherwise.	**—** You're overworked and underpaid.
+ You forgive and forget.	**—** You can be so forgiving that you enable unhealthy habits in the name of people-pleasing.

instinct, and few of us could make it without nurturing from others. But as one who more often offers than asks for support, you need to ask yourself, who's taking care of the caretaker?

Eating By Design is a handbook to help you give the gift of health and a joyful approach to eating well to the ones you love. But it's also a gift to *yourself,* as you relax and allow *me,* in a sense, to take care of *you.* How's that for a switch?

✳

Self-Sacrificing Starvation

Remember that airline safety instructions always tell you to put on your own oxygen mask first and then attend to your child? The idea is that no matter how caring your instinct, you can't help anybody if you're not breathing. Nurturers tend to be so busy sacrificing themselves that they starve all day and make up for lost calories at the dinner table, after everyone else has been attended to. Heavy, end-of-day dining topples you into bed full and exhausted, to wake to the onslaught of a busy new day feeling sluggish; then you skip breakfast out of disinterest and time pressure, and so on, in a repetitive cycle of fatigue and caloric catch-up. Caring for others is a high-energy sport, and you of all people need to be stoked up for the many emergencies, large and small, that come your way. Your Personal Prescription in Part Three will show you how.

✳

The Nurturer as Food Pusher

The Pusher and the Junkie

Your first interaction with the world is through your mouth, sucking on the life-giving nipple provided by your mother. This is the one time in life when you can eat as much as and whenever you want—you need only yell, and your family is there to tend to your needs. That basic association between being cared for and being fed is deeply embedded in your subconscious.

We are socially conditioned to equate food with love. The food of your family table can symbolize love, stability, and safety throughout your life. For the Nurturer, food is a primal way of caring for other people, providing the glue to fix what is—or isn't—broken. To feed is to love; to be fed is to be loved; to clean your plate is an achievement and a bid for approval. Feeding is a natural Nurturer instinct reinforced by family patterns across generations. But you can take feeding too far. There's a fine line between feeding hungry people and pushing to junkies.

Food pushing can take many forms: constant and repeated offers or presentations, insistence upon second helpings, comments about how much trouble or expense went into the dish, declarations of the dish's inadequacy that beg to be disproven, solicitous remarks about the recipient's health or body weight, and a multitude of variations on the classic caretaking themes: "Just a little bit; it's a special occasion; it's so good; I made it just for you." Pushing food on people shapes destructive eating habits. No matter how much love is vested in the food you serve, your need to see it eaten can lead to weight control issues for those you feed, and inappropriate emotional attachments to eating.

Everyone who's cooked a meal has indulged in food pushing at one time or another. But repeated invocation of the food pusher's mantras can create food addicts. The next time you offer without being asked, remember that the mother doesn't offer her breast until the baby cries. Your Personal Prescription will encourage you to portion food according to *real* needs.

Your Child's Future Fat

In fact, looking for hunger signals when feeding your child is important from infancy onward, because body fat patterns are established in the earliest stages of life. We speak jokingly of "baby fat" as a cute aberration automatically corrected by Mother Nature, but only babies under age two need a layer of fat to support their rapid growth and physiological development, and even infants can carry more fat than they need. Every fat cell in your body is laid down for life. And all these fat cells are created early: during the last trimester in the womb, in the first year of life, and at adolescence. You can't diet fat cells away at any time of life; the best you can do is try to empty them of their corpulent cargo. But an empty fat cell is hungry, eager to convert any passing calorie into body fat. The more fat cells you have, the greater your lifelong tendency toward the storage of body fat. So a fat baby is cellularly programmed to become a fat child, and a fat teenager to become a fat adult.

COMMON FUTURE FAT TRAPS

Here are some of the fat traps that parents unknowingly set for their children. Eating By Design will help you avoid these behaviors when feeding your flock to insure their healthy future:

- Overfeeding.
- Offering high-fat, high-salt, and high-sugar foods.
- Promoting the clean plate club.
- Using food as a reward or expression of love.
- Presenting a negative role model in your own relationship with food or your body.

Codependence in the Kitchen

Prolonged food pushing can lead to a cycle of mutually reinforcing destructive behavior that is often called codependence. I ran into an old client with his new bride at a party a few months after their wedding. June was lovingly hand-feeding Thomas a wedge of Brie baked in puff pastry. I marched up and said hello; Thomas choked, wiped his mouth, flashed a brilliant smile, and introduced me to his new wife. "June, this is Carrie. She haunts me at all the high-calorie Hollywood parties." I tried not to stare at his encroaching double chin.

Soon after, Thomas and June were in my office, describing their newlywed eating habits in a kind of point-counterpoint. Thomas's side of the story sounded like June was shoving food down his throat; June's version sounded like he was begging for richer, grander meals. Both genuinely felt they were serving each other's needs. Both were gaining weight. Both were unhappy.

At the center of this cycle of codependence in the kitchen was June's habit of creating wonderful concoctions *just in case* Thomas wanted something when he got home, woke up, finished reading his script, etc. June hoped to please Thomas with her surprise, Thomas hoped to please June by eating it, and both felt close to each other when they shared the moment and the food. They ate whether or not they were hungry because June had *anticipated* a potential need without *asking* whether it was real.

I asked June to make a new rule for herself: Ask, don't anticipate. Every time she contemplated making something for Thomas, she had to ask him in advance if he actually wanted it. Thomas, in turn, was required to answer honestly, not out of his desire to make June feel accepted and needed.

After a few tough weeks, June accepted the truth: Many of her unsolicited offerings were extraneous, more food than Thomas wanted or needed. Thomas also had to face the fact that he had a very difficult time saying no. He was afraid of hurting or offending June by rejecting her offers of food. Both Thomas and June were caught in a cycle of pleasing without needing.

The dynamics of feeding other people can be very complex. While June was trying to please Thomas by feeding him his favorite foods, she was also subconsciously keeping him "safe" in their relationship by making sure he carried a few extra pounds. Thomas was pleasing June by eating what she fixed for him, and colluding in her efforts to keep the relationship safe by not questioning the food's fat content, even though his previous experience with Diet Designs made him wise enough to know better.

Declare Yourselves a Lean Team

Though codependence in the kitchen can unravel your healthy resolve, cooperation in Eating By Design can strengthen your commitment. You can let your family know that sharing a healthy diet is an expression of your love for each other, and the strength of cooperation will help make it stick. Lean Teams work together to nourish each other's soul, sanity, and self-esteem. Imagine the following scenarios:

- You are a loving wife. Part of your personal identity is bound up in feeding your husband, whom you adore and wish to surround with all the warmth and security the world can provide. When he phones with news of a personal triumph or tragedy at work, you consider cooking up a thick steak with herb butter and pan-fried potatoes to celebrate or commiserate. But then, you stop and consider what happens to your husband's heart when he eats the butter-drenched steak. You resolve: Tonight, I will grill the best-quality free-range chicken breast, smother it with yummy onions and herbs, and share a very special moment with my husband. He deserves total care.

- You are a loving husband. You know your wife loves to go out to dinner as a welcome break in her busy schedule. You decide to offer her the ultimate luxury by taking her to your favorite French restaurant for a rich meal, because you love her and she is being celebrated. Then, you stop and think: My wife is happiest when she feels good about herself and her food choices. Tonight, I will choose a new restaurant, call ahead, investigate the preparations, and choose something healthy for us to eat that will energize us and enhance the moment.

- You are the *best* best friend in the world. Your buddy has just phoned you in a suicidal frenzy because her boyfriend has told her it isn't working out. Your first instinct is the Total Care Package: A large pizza, two pints of premium ice cream, spoons, napkins, and a shoulder to cry on. Then, you stop and consider the consequences. Tomorrow, your best friend will wake up feeling abandoned, rejected, *and* bloated. In addition to her emotional weight, she will bear the heaviness of ice cream, pizza, and self-hatred. You reconsider. You go to her house armed with baked tortilla chips and salsa, frozen yogurt, and the personal ads.

Your Personal Prescription in Part Three contains many specific suggestions for providing healthy food that truly nourishes the people around you, to make you all a Lean Team together.

Nurture Without Nourishing

There are many ways to cure or care for someone who isn't hungry. You can deepen your nurturing relationships with others by developing ways to care without calories:

- Go for a walk together.
- Send flowers, fine bath products, a favorite CD or book, or a gift certificate for spa services.
- Tell a story, play a game, or sing a song.
- Talk.
- Rent a movie and watch it together.
- Offer to run an errand or take care of a household task.
- Go on a special excursion.
- Hug, kiss, have sex.
- Teach.
- Volunteer for those in need, such as the homeless, hungry, illiterate, battered children, etc.
- Work for arts, community, church, or youth groups.

Your commitment to the human race is a vital thread in our social fabric. Serving others without food will feed your own self-esteem and help you serve humanity even better.

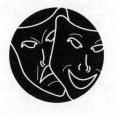

2

THE ARTFUL DODGER

"I'll think about it tomorrow."

—SCARLETT O'HARA

❋

Annette came to me at age thirty-eight ready to try for her first pregnancy—provided, she said, she could shed thirty pounds first. With all the stress and hormone treatments of a late-in-life pregnancy, she didn't want to be weighed down with extra body fat. I was impressed that Annette understood the dangers of carrying extra weight at conception for both the mother and the baby, and took her on gladly, unaware that I was stepping into a hornet's nest.

It seemed that Annette had put off having children all this time in the name of her career. She worked as an assistant vice president in the finance department of the family business, a national retail empire. It struck me as a strangely obscure position, at age thirty-eight, for the boss's daughter, and not demanding enough to prevent her from having children if she had truly wanted them. Indeed, it quickly became clear that Annette was ambivalent about her commitment to her career, making this long postponement of motherhood all the more mysterious.

"I was supposed to be the shining star of the business, a fashion retail mogul," said Annette bitterly. "All my life, my father pushed me to be a business whiz, and my mother tried to mold me into a glamor queen. Finally, when I flunked out of business school, they got the message that this was not my destiny. My father offered me a position in the finance department, still hoping that I would work my way up the ranks. I took the job to spite him, and to show the company that I was a real person despite being my father's daughter.

"Throughout my thirties, my father kept nudging me, saying I would surely be promoted to vice president if I would just put in a little overtime, contribute that extra something. But the harder he pushed, the less I wanted to advance. When he told me my next financing proposal was the big one that could shoot

21

me to stardom, I developed a distaste for the project and turned it in late with sloppy interest rate projections. He finally gave up, and we developed a comfortable routine: I do my job, earning a moderate income and maintaining my standing in the family, and he slips me fat checks every birthday and Christmas—in case my husband's outrageous salary isn't adequate to insure a trust fund for his unborn grandchildren, the family's last great shining hopes. I smile politely, then use the money to spend the summer in Europe, where I think I personally support the pastry-making business."

This was Annette's first mention of food, so I took advantage of the moment to ask about her background in terms of eating. "Oh, I had a miserable childhood. My mother had me on a constant diet from age eight on. She is permanently thin and beautiful and was determined I would be the same. She always told me I was lucky; her only motivation for staying thin was her social life, while I had the promise of a high-profile career to keep me on track. I did a million diet plans, had angel food cakes with saccharine-sweetened fruit sauce for my birthdays, and was sent to a fat farm masquerading as a summer camp at age twelve. My mother watched every morsel of food that went into my mouth—at least publicly.

"I learned early on to keep a private stash of treats in my room, to which I retreated after every loathsome low-cal meal. Once I was a teenager and going out with friends, my mother's attempts to make me diet became a joke. I would dutifully share a grapefruit and a plate of green beans with her for dinner, then go out and have pizza, hamburgers, and ice cream.

"To this day, my mother serves me less than everybody else when we have dinner at their house; she incessantly invites me on spa vacations; and she gives me designer clothes a size too small 'as incentive.' I still love decadent desserts and other rich foods."

Annette declared herself a diet "lifer," always on one plan or another but never actually reaching her weight loss goal. This time, though, she said, she had to take off every last one of those thirty pounds before she would try to conceive. If she couldn't reach a simple weight loss goal, she surely wasn't fit to be a mother. I wondered where Annette had gotten the idea that control over your weight correlates with good motherhood, but she was defensive and adamant on the point, so I decided not to push. The pressure on me was intense. If Annette doesn't get this weight off, I thought, I'll be responsible for a baby not being born. Please, let this be the plan to change her life!

Soon after Annette left my office, I had a phone call from her husband, Mark, asking how he could help. He told me that Diet Designs would be the latest in a string of diet programs for Annette, none of which had provided any lasting success. This was the most comprehensive—and expensive—to date, and it was his gift to Annette for as long as she wanted it. "We want this to work so badly," he said. "Annette really feels she needs to do it before we can go forward with this pregnancy, and that's our number one priority right now. Children would make Annette so happy." I wished I could agree.

Mark worried that he hadn't been much of a help to Annette's dieting efforts in the past. Whenever he offered advice or help, she seemed to think that he was criticizing her; when he kept his distance from the issue, she felt alone and abandoned. Mark said he felt stuck between a rock and a hard place, but he truly wanted to help Annette prepare her body to have a baby.

Annette was cautiously optimistic about the first week of Diet Designs food. She had never actually enjoyed eating anything on a diet—until now. Her curiosity was piqued—how did we make such rich, thick sauces? But when she got on the scale and hadn't lost a pound, her curiosity turned to suspicion. Why was I calling this diet food when it so obviously wasn't? It didn't taste like it, and it didn't work!

I apologized to Annette for the disappointment, explaining that there are many factors involved in weight loss and one week was really too short a time to accurately judge progress. Then I asked if she had stuck strictly to her eating and exercise plan all week. She hemmed and hawed. After half an hour of gentle prodding, Annette's sad story emerged.

Early in the week, Annette had been reprimanded by her manager in a meeting, in front of the company's bankers, for failing to pull together the numbers for an important credit proposal. She said it was a misunderstanding, but the vice president publicly embarrassed her, berating her oversight and sarcastically remarking in front of everybody that maybe she thought her father's pockets were so deep that he didn't need bankers. She left the meeting smiling but infuriated, fed her Diet Designs lunch to a stray dog on the street, and went to her favorite wine bar for a plate of paté and sausage, a glass of red wine, and a tart tatin.

I smiled, wondering aloud how the dog had liked the penne with wild mushrooms and goat cheese. Annette, surprised at the joke, laughed and said, "Just fine—probably a lot more than I did my paté."

In the middle of the week, Annette's mother had stopped by just before dinner, exclaiming over how she had heard about Annette's new diet plan from Mark, how exciting it was, and how much they were looking forward to being grandparents. Annette resented this intrusion on her new effort; the last thing she needed was her mother breathing down her neck. As she ushered her out of the house, she felt anger building against both Mark and her mother, coconspirators. Alone, Annette made a quick peanut butter and mayonnaise sandwich and vengefully wolfed it down. That night, she served Mark and herself steak and cream puffs for dinner, declaring that her mother had spoiled her appetite for Diet Designs.

Then on Sunday night, Mark, as was his habit, was talking about his goals for the work week. He went on to ask Annette, "How's the new diet going? Have you set some goals and objectives?"

"Of course," she responded dryly, "to lose fifty pounds by tomorrow. Here, why don't you finish my fish?" After Mark went to bed, Annette weighed in. With the week's slipups and a day of food and water in her body, Annette was actually heavier than her prediet weight, which she had taken in the morning. She wrote off the week as wasted and ate a pint of ice cream.

I'm accustomed to discussing obstacles to healthy eating with my clients, but Annette's life was a virtual minefield. "I can see you have to face a lot of issues in this process," I began. "That must be quite exhausting."

She sighed. "I know I sound pathetic. It's just that I've been at this so long, I feel like I can't win. I don't know why everybody has to meddle in my affairs."

It did sound like Annette was doing Diet Designs by committee, and I knew that too much outside encouragement could sap her of her personal commitment. "It sounds like you have a difficult history with your mother. But it doesn't really matter what everyone else thinks. Is losing this weight something that you want?"

"Of course!" retorted Annette. "I've told you, I need to do it so I can get pregnant. How much more could I possibly want it?"

Defenses, defenses, I thought. But I said, "Bravo! You should only do it to please yourself!"

Unfortunately, eating was one of Annette's primary ways of pleasing herself. Hunger reminded her of childhood deprivation, of leaving her mother's dinner table starving and furious at having been served an apple for dessert while her brother had chocolate chip cookies. Maybe if her mother had lightened up and allowed a treat here and there, Annette wouldn't have kept a pile of candy bars in her room.

Likewise, I sensed that the adult Annette needed a little freedom and TLC. I offered her three "legal cheats" to choose from when she was angry or frustrated, including a low-fat version of the forbidden chocolate chip cookies. I also made her an appointment with a trainer specializing in aerobic boxing. I thought a session with the punching bag would do her good.

Annette's progress on the program was gradual, but I emphasized that I was there to see her through every hitch and hindrance. We had to jump over several stumbling blocks. First, Annette complained I was starving her to death. When I responded by giving her additional snacks, she claimed the extra granola bars were preventing her from losing weight. Next, she said she was tempted to cheat while cooking dinner for Mark. She resisted when I suggested that she let him cook for himself. "But I've always cooked for Mark!" she exclaimed. We compromised by sending him double portions of Diet Designs meals. Then she claimed that the fertility treatment she took was bloating her—true, but I had to convince her that water weight was temporary, and no excuse to abandon her efforts to lose body fat.

Just when things were starting to go better, I received a call from an agitated Annette. She was going to her mother's house for a formal dinner, where she feared that the usual slights of being singled out for small portions and no dessert would drive her to angry eating. I advised Annette to select the most delectable dishes from her Diet Designs meals to take to her mother's house, and have them served especially to her.

I also recommended to Annette that she take some time to think about her dynamic with her mother vis-à-vis food. I suspected that her anger at feeling deprived by her mother's injunctions to diet was coming between Annette and her goal. Dodging the issue by swallowing the anger in the form of "cheat" foods was sabotaging her best efforts.

The early part of the evening was a great success, Annette reported, with her mother leaning over throughout the meal to inspect her plate. What is that, black bean soup? All those carbohydrates while you're on a diet? . . . Barbequed chicken pizza? And could that be chocolate cheesecake? You are obviously being led down the garden path with this so-called diet program!

"And I just kept smiling and eating with glee, announcing at the end of the meal that, indeed, I had lost five pounds on this so-called diet program," said Annette. "You know, I think she was actually jealous! Suddenly, the prospect of getting thin while eating things of which my mother disapproved seemed very appealing."

Nevertheless, Annette's resentment toward her mother for her constant meddling in her personal eating habits brewed right alongside the coffee, and while the guests sipped nightcaps in the living room, the two of them had it out in the kitchen. In a rare moment of assertiveness, Annette told her mother how angry she got when she told her what to eat, how to look, and who to be. She told her that a lifetime of resisting her mother's efforts to control her had left her incapable of making good decisions for herself. And she told her that she couldn't possibly bring herself to have a child while she was feeling so much anger toward her own mother.

Then Annette went home, told Mark she didn't want a baby, trashed all the Diet Designs food in the refrigerator, and took a long walk by herself. Annette couldn't describe exactly what happened during the course of that walk, but she came to me the next day and said she wanted to start over, this time for herself.

Unburdened of the baby plan and some of her anger toward her mother, Annette started to lose weight consistently, and her complaints and excuses all but dried up. With my encouragement, she continued to talk with her mother and Mark about her issues with them. We agreed that twenty-five pounds was a more realistic goal than thirty, and decided to reassess things when she got there.

✳

Self-perpetuating obstacles to healthy eating like Annette's—temptations, frustrations, and ambivalence about how and why we should become fit in the first place—can undermine the best-laid diet plans. Artful Dodgers always have the best intentions, sometimes more good intentions than any single person can possibly handle. But you tend to get tripped up along the way by circumstances, events, and your ability to dodge the issue at hand.

The "art" of the Artful Dodger is your ability to appear easygoing, cheerful, and relaxed on the outside, appealing qualities that draw people to you and make them think you have everything under control. But things seem to happen to you, booby traps that interrupt your progress toward success or completion in work and personal projects. Naturally, these impediments can make you angry. But in keeping with your laid-back style, you are unlikely to express your anger directly. You might find other ways to do it: missing deadlines, forgetting to do things—or perhaps eating too much.

Many Artful Dodgers have an uneasy relationship with their weight because the society in which they want to get along and be comfortable carries mixed messages about body image and food. Though on the one hand each body is considered the autonomous territory of the person—an important defense for you—on the other hand, media images, cultural mores, and perhaps even individuals in your life state or imply a certain standard for appearance to which you are expected to measure up, regardless of your own feelings or opinions. The way you choose to eat is also subject to scrutiny and criticism. If these contradictions and invasions of your independence make you angry, you are not alone. And if you express that anger by subconsciously sabotaging your attempts at dieting, you are also not alone. You, like Annette, are responding to a very real hurt with a tangible, if self-defeating, strategy.

If you encumber your healthy eating efforts with unexpressed anger and too much beating around the bush, you can sabotage yourself and end up with less than you deserve—less health, happiness, control, and autonomy. Your anger will whip back at you like a boomerang, chipping away at your self-esteem and undermining your good intentions. Before you take on another unrealistic self-improvement plan destined for failure, perhaps it's time to stop and assess what health and well-being mean to you, and develop a personalized approach to self-care that makes you truly comfortable and content, poised to dodge no more.

ARTFUL DODGER STYLE

THE ART	THE DODGE
+ You are easygoing, sweet, and optimistic.	− Your unexploded anger can be as lethal as a buried landmine.
+ You wear a happy face.	− You are a master of disguise.
+ You never refuse.	− You often resist.
+ You don't make waves.	− You can disrupt your own natural rhythms.

Eating By Design helps you to discover what you want from your food and ease into healthier eating habits with a few easy steps:

- Find your motivation.
- Embrace the enterprise with an open mind.
- Map out your usual dodges and commit to a steady course.
- Design your own diet, so you've got nothing to dodge around.

Your Personal Prescription in Part Three walks you through each of these steps. Soon, you'll be a master of the art of eating well.

※

Decide for Yourself

Annette's life was more a negation of what others wanted for her than an affirmation of what she wanted for herself. Thus, she was ambivalent about getting fit, a goal with connotations of childhood hurt and manipulation. She used failure to defend herself against complying with the demands of others. But when Annette finally admitted that she did want to be thin, she insisted less on the reasons why she couldn't be. Once she found a desire that came from within instead of without, many of her barriers melted away.

Ironically, it was when Annette realized that she could enjoy eating in a way forbidden by her mother and still become thin that she made the commitment to do it. She mobilized her anger in her favor. Not everyone can do this; many people have to let their anger go to make the decision for self-care. But I applauded Annette's resourcefulness. She confirmed the validity of my antisabotage strategy: Make your own decision to take care of yourself, and then find the process that works for you.

Chances are that you have some inner conflicts of your own about how eating well and losing extra body fat should fit into your life. I find it helps to sort out the sources of your motivation before undertaking a commitment to a new way of life, so that you only embrace changes that address your own interests. Your Personal Prescription helps you decide why and how you want to take care of your health and well-being.

While others or even you might have thought or said you "should" lose weight or eat less fat, the truth is that you *deserve* the best food, the best body, and the best health. These are basic human rights that no one can deny you. But they are also attained by a personal process that no one else can enter into on your behalf. Others can direct and assist you, but ultimately, you are responsible for your own success.

Many diet plans offer less than you deserve. They forbid foods, promise unrealistic results, dictate what you eat, and tell you how fast or slow you must go. They seem like punishment for a crime you didn't commit. They ask for sacrifices and penance, trying to control how you live your daily life. It's no wonder that rigid diet plans bring out the rebellious streak in you. They are not your just desserts.

Eating By Design offers all the fun, nourishing foods and fat-burning results you deserve.

Slide out of Sabotage

To be a healthy eater, you don't have to make a big change today, or resolve that you will succeed by next month. You are already a success. And you are changing every moment, by living, talking, listening, breathing, reading this book. Just as you might have slid into eating habits you don't like, you can slide into new ones that offer more, little by little, step by step. The smaller your resolutions and declarations, the smaller your obstacles will be.

Your Personal Prescription asks you to keep doing what you already do: Eat. Sleep. Move. Breathe. Work. Play. As you do these things, you inevitably make choices, day in and day out. Starting today, try to make choices that bring you the fit and healthy life you deserve. Ignore the eyes looking over your shoulder and the world breathing down your neck. Accept and appreciate every little success, in the present moment. Your Personal Prescription helps you to slide out of sabotage and into your healthy self.

※

Steer a Clear Course

Shed Your Suspicions

You may have been misled or misunderstood in the past. Once you've been disappointed, it's natural to protect yourself against further hurt with a healthy dose of suspicion. But beware: Suspicion can be hazardous to your health.

- Suspicion eats away at your insides, emptying your center and making you hungry for security. Because suspicion locks security out, many people satisfy that hunger with food.
- Suspicion raises your stress levels, which can increase your risk of diseases such as hypertension, stroke, and gastric disorder as well as your rate of anxious eating.
- Suspicion paralyzes you, preventing you from taking the first step toward a better way of being. Suspicion falsely tells you that every step is dangerous and irrevocable. Suspicion is healthy fear run amok.

Second-guessing your own ability to deal with contingencies as they arise slows you down. But if you know in advance what obstacles you might encounter and trust your own ability to work your way through them, you can proceed with your Personal Prescription as freely as a well-greased wheel. Stay tuned for suspicion-banishing strategies.

False Failures

When Annette got on the scale at the end of the week and found she had gained weight, she was devastated by her failure. But Annette's gain was a false failure. First of all, she had changed her weigh-in time from morning to night, and was carrying a natural accumulation of food and fluids in the evening that wasn't there in the morning. Secondly, she knew she had significantly strayed from her plan twice that week, and weight loss was unlikely. In addition, she used the artificial boundary of the week to excuse her subsequent ice cream binge, pretending that past "failure" justified further bingeing as long as it was within the seven-day timeframe.

The search for false failures is a classic dodge. False failures are a license to fail further, a passive rejection of the undertaking. But you have already decided that health and fitness are what you want and deserve. To you, false failures are false friends.

Remember, you are successful already and changing in every moment. Try to judge yourself less and reward yourself more. Your false failure mirages will evaporate into thin air.

Yell and Tell

If Annette had confronted her boss about his sarcastic and humiliating comment, told her mother to butt out, and explained to her husband that setting goals made her afraid of failure, she probably wouldn't have needed to act out her anger in mute consumption. She needed to yell when she was angry and tell people what was on her mind. Eating just buried her anger deep inside and enveloped it in fat.

Of course, this is easier said than done. Perhaps you hold similar monologues all the time, telling people exactly what you think inside, but never getting it out.

Anger is a natural by-product of living. When someone cuts you off on the freeway; when your spouse makes social plans without consulting you; when your boss belittles your contribution to a project; when you're committed to so many responsibilities that the whole world seems to be loudly demanding your time, the natural response is anger. When constructively expressed or diffused, anger is perfectly healthy. When bottled up, it can be lethal.

Changing your mode of expression and interaction with the world is a big project beyond the scope of this book. The good news is that you can take small steps to release your anger that will support your healthy eating efforts. Here are some expressive outlets that can help free your emotions to undertake Eating By Design with a clean slate:

- Write your feelings down in a letter directed to the person who is making you angry. Keep the letter for awhile as a reference, a reminder of why you feel the way you do. When the feelings have passed, throw the letter away.
- Take up a vigorous sport. Express a grievance every time you hit or kick or slap the ball. Go ahead! Get it out!
- Take an assertiveness training course.
- Do primal scream therapy.
- Practice small, mild expressions of what you want and need with someone you trust.

Anger is an emotion that wants to get out. Eating By Design means that you won't stuff it back inside with your supper.

Don't Weigh

After Annette's first weigh-in disaster, I made a request that she found very hard to grant: to throw away her scale. She was so accustomed to measuring herself and coming up short that the process provided a strange comfort, a confirmation of her failure. "I would rather know I failed than not know at all," she moaned.

But as soon as Annette stopped hopping on the scale, she had no excuse to stray from her eating plan. She learned to appreciate eating well for the experience itself, the way it made her feel good and in control. When her mother inquired about her "progress," Annette simply responded, "I'm a healthy eater, and I don't know how many pounds my bones, muscle mass, bodily fluids, and fat weigh at this moment." ("Ooh, I love saying that to her," Annette exclaimed to me). Her mother thought she'd been abducted by some strange cult, but couldn't deny that Annette seemed healthier, happier—and thinner.

Once every three months, Annette weighed herself on the scale at my office, to confirm that, indeed, this new process was working a positive transformation. Her loss was slow but steady. For the first time in her life, reported Annette, failures didn't multiply themselves.

I recommend that you begin Eating By Design by reducing your reliance on "failure creators": scales, tape measures, skin calipers. Start by doubling your normal interval between weigh-ins, measurements, etc. If you normally weigh yourself every morning, switch to every other day; if once a week, aim for once every two weeks. Keep extending the time until you get to once a month. Then use your monthly check-ins to see how the numbers reflect what you already know: You are continually becoming a healthier you.

Just Say Yes

Many messages in our society encourage us to resist. Don't take drugs; don't endure harassment; don't cheat, lie, or steal. Question authority. Doubt your god. Amid so many injunctions of what not to do or believe, it's no wonder that we resist the evidence that eating low-fat foods in controlled amounts will make us thinner and prevent life-threatening disease.

I suggest you embrace the promise and positive impact of eating well.

Yes, I Can

- Feel good.
- Look good.
- Make good eating choices.
- Live in the body I want.

I can, and I will. Starting today. Starting right now. The only trick to a healthy eating plan is keeping it perpetually in the present, in the moment of reading this sentence. The past is past. Future mistakes can be corrected. Take action now. Read your Personal Prescription.

3

THE PASSIONFLOWER

"Whenever you see food beautifully arranged on a plate, you know someone's fingers have been all over it."

—JULIA CHILD

✳

An ancient Roman banquet was truly a feast for the senses, a tribute to human passions. You began by bathing, then donning a robe especially for dining, which you could change at any time during dinner should the effort of eating leave you soaked in sweat. After annointing yourself with scented oils and putting on a fragrant wreath, you entered the banquet hall and reclined on your own private couch. As you tied one napkin around your neck to catch any spills and kept a second one on hand for wiping sticky or greasy fingers, you listened to the host describe the foods and wines at length, including their origin, freshness, and method of preparation.

Then the eating began. Should your stomach get full before your palate had its fill of pleasure, you had the perfectly polite option of using a peacock feather to tickle the back of your throat and "clear some space" for more. You ate as long as you liked; in fact, to clear a guest's plate before he was finished was so serious an act as to be considered an omen of sudden death.

Of course, the Roman Empire fell. Perhaps all that dining slowed them down.

✳

Melissa was a perfume magnate, a poor girl from Brooklyn who had made good in the elegant world of fine scents. A street-smart child grown into a sophisticated woman, Melissa built her fortune by providing olfactory pleasure and devoted her spare time to the remaining senses, including her taste buds. "When I was a kid we were very poor," she told me in our first meeting. "Food was a succession of stews, soups, and casseroles that all looked and tasted the same. I used to save up money from my paper route just to buy a slice of pizza; that was a special treat. Dining in high style was a slice of pepperoni, extra cheese."

Now Melissa ate thin-crusted pizzas in fancy restaurants, covered with imported smoked salmon and caviar, made by the highest-paid chefs in the world—just as an appetizer. Melissa the Brooklyn kid had eaten pepperoni pizza out of hunger. Melissa the grown-up millionaire ate out of appetite.

In fact, as a true Passionflower, Melissa did just about everything out of appetite, which was finally catching up with her just before her fortieth birthday. She came to me, not because of the recent news from her doctor that her cholesterol levels had hit the roof at 290, but because she felt that her thighs were flapping in the wind.

Melissa was a charmer and a challenge. She subscribed to the richer-is-better theory, summing it up for me as follows: "Why have plain steak when you can top it with foie gras and a Port wine sauce? Why add just cognac when you also have cream in the refrigerator? And if a tablespoon of butter is good, isn't two tablespoons better? I hate doing things halfway!" Constantly roaming the globe on business, she sought out the finest restaurants and treated clients to lavish feasts during which she was so attuned to the epicurean proceedings that one of her guests finally asked her "Are you a CEO—or a chef?"

More important, from my standpoint, was her doctor's complaint about her cholesterol levels. But Passionflowers are more concerned with pleasure in the present than danger in the future. That's where I come in. Of course, I love the pleasure of good food, but I've found ways to enjoy it without endangering my future.

But how could I help a woman who had deliberately devoted a lifetime to acquiring a taste for the richest foods the planet has to offer? Melissa expected to suffer terribly on the Diet Designs program, deprived of the pleasures of the palate. But, she reasoned, she had been faithful to her husband for the entire year they were married; she should be able to give up gourmet food for the six weeks or so it would take to lose ten pounds.

Melissa didn't know my sensual secret: that she could eat low-fat in high style. I tantalized her with a bit of the Diet Designs menu for the coming week: Seared fresh ahi tuna with a Dijon shallot sauce; sun-dried tomato and goat cheese pizza with a thin, crisp crust; fettuccine with wild mushroom sauce.

"Is that one meal?" asked Melissa. "I might survive this ordeal after all."

"No, Melissa, those are three separate meals. But one step at a time."

Melissa was enthusiastic about her first delivery of food, complimenting the use of fresh herbs, baby vegetables, top-quality chicken and seafood, flavorful sauces. But there was a hitch. "I want to try it all now! I want to know what the Pesto Lasagna tastes like, and the Thai Coconut Chicken with basmati rice. Please let me take bites!" I told her that was fine. There's no denying a

Passionflower a moment of pleasure. But Melissa thwarted me. She sampled everything, pronounced it delicious—and then went out to dinner.

At one of L.A.'s best restaurants, Melissa ate every bite of a five-course meal, each with an accompanying glass of wine, amounting to a couple of days' worth of calories. I summed up the situation and faxed Melissa an emergency copy of my restaurant guidelines, telling her that next time this happened—which was likely to be that very night—she should order according to those instructions. Since she was already on a first-name basis with many of L.A.'s finest chefs, I suggested to Melissa that she show them the guidelines and ask them to create some healthy delicacies that would satisfy her discriminating tastes. Three chefs out of ten told Melissa to stay home while she was on a diet; I promptly stopped recommending those restaurants to any of my clients. The remaining seven said they would be happy to turn their talents to Melissa's requests.

Melissa had a mild case of fat withdrawal at first. She was so accustomed to ultrarich foods that she wasn't prepared for the cleaner, more direct flavors of low-fat cuisine. She pouted, stole forkfuls off her companion's plate, and popped chocolate truffles when she couldn't live another minute without feeling her mouth coated with a film of fat. But she maintained an enthusiastic spirit, and soon she embarked on an odyssey of taste exploration, exclaiming that she had a new understanding of the sweet nuances of fresh fish, the smoky intensity of grilled chicken, the woodsy darkness of wild mushrooms when they weren't masked with butter, oil, and cream.

Melissa took off her extra weight in six weeks, just in time for a business trip to Italy. At our final meeting, she sported a new and impeccably tailored Armani suit. "Thank you so much for helping me depart on this journey in style. And now I am free to fly across the ocean and dive into a plate of glistening green olive oil, the kind you find only in Italy."

"Melissa, in my business, I don't like to encourage repeat customers," I replied, fearful of losing my latest success story to a Roman orgy. "Why don't you have tiny bites of everything you love in Italy, but use what you've learned over the past weeks to have fun without getting fat. Concentrate on the pastas and grilled meats and seafood, and take it easy on the olive oil. I want to see you back here looking just as sharp as you do now, ready to tell me all about your food adventures abroad."

Melissa came back with several new distribution deals and the same physique she had left with. Yes, she had nibbled on beef carpaccio, tiramisu, and country bread dunked in fresh olive oil, but she had also discovered new favorites— pasta with bitter greens and lemon, calamari on the grill, and intensely flavored fruit ices.

✳

I love to work with Passionflowers because they tend to be fun-loving, exuberant, and caring. They are also in many ways already committed to eating well. As a Passionflower, you may feel that eating and other sensually gratifying activities are as important as breathing—as personal, as organic, and as essential to life.

Passionflowers are discerning consumers, willing to invest time and energy in the all-engrossing experience of food. The drive to satisfy your sensory receptors gives you a heightened appreciation of the taste, smell, texture, and sight of food. You are willing to search long and hard for the best, the unusual, the exotic gourmet ingredient. Every meal is a banquet, a taste experience, a defining moment for your sensual self.

This enthusiasm and discrimination can be your ally in eating for health and fitness. But it can also be your mortal enemy. Your appreciation can become so focused in the present moment that you overindulge, choosing rich foods and eating beyond the limits of satiety. The effect of eating too much and too richly is inevitable: hangovers and upset stomachs in the short term, and excess body fat soon thereafter. Fat in your diet and on your body is implicated in deadly disease, which could cut short your appreciation of the pleasures of this planet. And in addition to the health risks it poses, extra body fat is not very sensually pleasing. Why not pursue a way of eating that satisfies the passion of both your palate and your physique?

PASSIONFLOWER STYLE

PASSIONS	PROBLEMS
+ You appreciate the moment to the fullest.	− A moment on the lips is a lifetime on the hips.
+ You are intimately in touch with your sensual self.	− You lose touch with your willpower and boundaries at the drop of a truffle.
+ You possess discriminating tastes.	− You equate fine food with the taste of fat.
+ You are warm and welcoming, a consummate host and guest.	− You just can't say no.

✳

Eat Low-Fat in High Style

Many of the foods we commonly call "gourmet," including the dishes served at fine restaurants, are full of saturated fat in the form of butter, cream, and rich meats. This full-fat aesthetic stems largely from a particular style of French cooking popularized in this country early in the century as "fancy" food. Our enthusiastic adoption of this cooking style predated scientific understanding of the huge health risks of dietary fat and obesity.

Fortunately, we're in the midst of a flavor revolution that recognizes that some of the most intense gustatory experience comes from the natural flavors of vegetables, fruits, herbs, and spices. Reductions of broth and wine, flavored vinegars, aromatic vegetables, and fresh herbs all enhance and add flavor to food, while fat acts to coat the palate and mask taste sensation. By replacing reliance on fat with a complete appreciation of food's natural aromas, textures, and tastes, you can gratify your senses without feeding your fat cells.

Don't worry, you won't suffer—at least not for long. Scientific studies show that you can, indeed, reduce your taste for fat by eating less of it. The trick is to go gradually, slowly reprogramming your palate to a new level of taste discrimination. And remember, you've probably done it before—when you acquired a taste for coffee, olives, wine . . .

Your Personal Prescription in Part Three walks you through reprogramming your Passionflower palate while opening a new world of low-fat taste sensation.

✳

The Slow, Sensual Road to Eating By Design

I never ask a Passionflower to stop enjoying *food so much*. I do ask you to stop enjoying *so much food*. You are likely to overeat out of the most innocent glee, the most unconscious rapture. To prevent this, your Personal Prescription teaches you to bring your pleasure to the forefront of your consciousness, along with a plan for how much to eat and when to stop.

I've found that when people are eating for pleasure, the easiest way to keep control is to slow down, and remember that you will eat again in the future. These principles are important for two reasons:

- It's sensually displeasing to be uncomfortably full. The feeling of oversatiation interferes with other sensual pleasures, including a basic sense of well-being. Generally, the theory of maximizing pleasure requires you to stop eating when you're full. After all, sex isn't much fun when you're stuffed.

   Unfortunately, the body is slow to send messages of satisfaction to the brain. It takes about fifteen minutes for a full stomach to get word to the hypothalamus, your mental hunger center. In the meantime, you are in eating ecstasy, feeding a hunger that you don't yet know is history. If you surrender to pleasure and repeatedly fill the fifteen-minute time lag with food, your stomach stretches, requiring more and more input to send the signal of satisfaction. The trick is to anticipate the hypothalamus by looking for other signals of satisfaction. Your Personal Prescription tunes in to these signals.

- Though you're probably not a conscious overeater, your sensual self lives in fear of being hungry. This is partly because it's easy for your senses to confuse the distinction between hunger—the biochemical cues that flag your body's need for fuel—and appetite, a pleasure-seeking desire. An unsatisfied appetite is equivalent to pleasure deprivation, the ultimate horror. Every meal feels like the last, especially if something special is being served. "Who knows when we'll get this Beluga caviar again?" is essentially a grown-up version of "When am I going to eat again?" If you're sure you can eat more wonderful food when hunger strikes again, the drive to overdo diminishes.

The Symbolism of Sophisticated Eating

Sometimes sophisticated food is as gratifying for its symbolism as for its sensory qualities. Melissa did a lot of elaborate entertaining, staging exquisite dinner parties with the best caviars, patés, meats, wines, rich sauces, and sumptuous desserts for all of her friends. Even after beginning my program, Melissa insisted on entertaining in this manner, often serving herself a separate, low-fat meal. Eventually, I realized that for Melissa, the rich food was a symbol of her acquired prosperity and discrimination, and served as tangible evidence of her place in society. Sharing fancy meals made her feel whole, accepted, and privileged.

I challenged Melissa to serve the "formal" menu I had devised for her meal plan at a dinner party, and to tell her guests that she had spared no expense to prepare a special low-fat gourmet feast. I also advised Melissa to focus on the occasion and her companions as much as the luxurious repast, feeding both her sensual appetite and her sense of belonging to a special set of people.

Your Personal Prescription provides gourmet dishes you can proudly serve to your most discerning guests—*and* share with them in perfect health.

✳

Assess Your Physical Aesthetic

If you're having any doubts about the pleasures of Eating By Design try the following exercise:

> Strip naked. Take a good look at yourself in the mirror. Now have a little self-appreciation session. Tell yourself this affirmation.
>
> *I am a person of discriminating tastes. I love the beauty of wonderful foods, high art, and the human body. My body is a beautiful example of form and grace, with lovely angles and curves and an overall feeling of fitness and firmness. I love living in this body, and I want to continue to appreciate its beauty far into the future.*

If you should discover that your body is less beautiful in its composition than you would like, don't fear. Just read on to your Personal Prescription to shave off your extra fat while still enjoying all the sensual pleasures of eating well. You'll love yourself all the more for it. And if there's one thing that makes a Passionflower bloom, it's love.

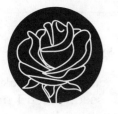

4

THE BLUE ROSE

"Blue . . . songs are like tattoos
You know, I've been to sea before . . ."

—JONI MITCHELL, "BLUE"

✳

Danielle was a creative young screenwriter who had just scored her first big success—a hit film with the top writing credit. Five years ago she had come to Los Angeles from New York to pursue her life's dream of writing movies, and after hard work and paying her dues, Danielle had by all appearances truly made it. She should have been feeling on top of the world.

"But I really don't feel anything except blank and fat," Danielle told me in our first meeting. "My writing bores me, my body disgusts me, and I'm completely paralyzed at the prospect of starting a whole new project. I haven't written a word in a week. I can't seem to do anything but eat."

The whole movie industry waited and watched Danielle's next move. She was in the enviable position of having a reputation to live up to. Doubting her own ability to do so, Danielle stopped working—and started eating with a vengeance.

An intervening friend brought Danielle to me, concerned about this manifestation of pain in what should have been a moment of victory. Because Danielle had made many sad and self-deprecating comments about being fat, her friend thought a weight loss program might spark Danielle's will to get back to work and realize her promise.

I've been working in weight management long enough to know that forty pounds of body fat alone is rarely the sole difference between a sad and a happy person, but I hoped I could at least help Danielle out of the habit of turning her blues into body fat. Meanwhile, I knew that Danielle's long-term health depended on working on the root sources of her sadness. With the support of her friend, I gently persuaded her to seek professional psychological help. I explained that she need only go as far as she wanted to, but any work she did on her emotional situation could only help her weight loss efforts. Reluctantly, she agreed.

The preliminary diagnosis by Danielle's therapist was a complete shock to the patient, though not to me: Danielle was clinically depressed. When I next saw Danielle, she was confused, resentful, and grappling with what, if anything, to do about the diagnosis.

Danielle said she had always been moody, experiencing bouts of sadness and sleep marathons for weeks at a time. Her thoughts had always been permeated by a desire to eat, and sometimes that was all that got her out of bed. "Constant cravings," she called it. Before this latest film, the many jobs she had held down while waiting for a script to sell had kept her busy and out of the house, distracting her somewhat from incessant hunger. But a day off at home could mean an extended session in front of the soaps with an array of snacks. She was always canceling her social plans; she just didn't seem to have the energy, and it was hard to really connect with people in L.A. This gave her even more time with television and her favorite snacks—her most intimate friends.

Since her success and the transition to full-time writing at home, Danielle's mood swings had gotten more intense, and her eating had started to edge upward. "I go through days when I'm like a zombie in front of the computer, feeling heavy and hopeless and with nothing to say. When I can't get a sentence out, I turn to food to try to start a spark. A Pop-Tart might provide a moment of inspiration to get through a patch of dialogue or a tricky transition. But as soon as that good feeling wears off, I'm back to the kitchen for more, and so on all day long until I'm disgusted by my body and hopeless about ever being a thin person. But something about eating seems to lift the heaviness from my head, at least for a while. It gives me something to do when I don't want to do anything else."

The diagnosis of clinical depression made it very clear to me what Danielle was going through. She was self-medicating her sadness with junk food. Along the way, she was taking in far too much fat and, frankly, far too much food.

Though she agreed to try Diet Designs at the encouragement of her friend, Danielle was not an enthusiastic client. She couldn't see making her joyless days even more barren by depriving herself of food, and she was pessimistic about her ability to change her eating habits and her body over the long haul. "I've always eaten when I don't know what else to do," she said. "And now, with this depression thing, I don't know what's going to happen. Maybe it's just not the right time to diet." But it was *exactly* the right time for Danielle to diet— with a mood-enhancing, energizing meal plan, in conjunction with professional therapy to help her make some decisions about handling her depression.

Despite her resistance, I sent Danielle home with a week's worth of Diet Designs food and a meal plan, asking her simply to try it out, even if just for a day. When you're depressed, action speaks louder than words. She agreed while at my office. But back at home, the meals sat untouched in Danielle's refrigerator. Her boyfriend was doing an excellent job of talking her out of trying it. He was afraid a "diet" would be too much pressure on Danielle in this vulnerable time of her life, one more thing that might go wrong. This was an understandable concern from a loved one confronting an unexpected psychiatric diagnosis, but of no help to Danielle. She needed to take action, not freeze up, and I told her so. I recommended that she continue with therapy and let me help her formulate a healthy eating lifestyle to alleviate her constant cravings and improve her mood. The result would be a happier relationship with her body. The alternative—living with her ever-present hunger for junk food— was bound to pressure her even more.

Danielle responded that she was hesitant to spend a lot of time and money on therapy to treat her "emotional weakness," and she didn't see the relationship between her depression and her "gluttony." She was convinced that this whole mess was a result of her failings, and she agreed with her boyfriend that this was no time to be adding to that list.

Finally I convinced Danielle to try one small thing: a small fat-free carbohydrate breakfast for a natural mood boost first thing in the morning. I didn't care what she did the rest of the day. Danielle was a confirmed junk food devotee accustomed to skipping breakfast, then snacking on Pop-Tarts and doughnuts as the cravings struck—a practice that just seemed to make her hungrier and less focused on her work. But by beginning the day with a bagel or a bowl of cereal, Danielle was able to attack her work with less anxiety, and go a couple of hours hunger-free. Hm, she said. We seem to have something here. I was elated—a little happiness would go a long way toward staving off Danielle's hunger.

Next I added four more carbohydrate mini-meals to Danielle's day, in addition to lunch and dinner, which I left up to her. When she told me that she finished each one feeling calm, focused, and ready to move on to the next task; that she was getting a lot more writing done; and that the craving for constant food input was diminishing, I asked her to take the next step: a full-time meal plan. She agreed.

The complete meal plan, which added more carbohydrates and a moderate amount of protein at dinner to her current schedule, made Danielle happy and satisfied. She also felt good about her therapy, and at her doctor's advice, started taking the antidepressant drug Prozac. The drug, like the diet, made the world a brighter place for Danielle, enabling her to get down to work, get out of the house for necessary meetings, and get on with the business of living.

But all was not sunshine and happiness for Danielle. In fact, she had a particularly hard time after the sun went down, feeling empty and pessimistic as she reviewed the day's work and wondered whether this script was going to live up to the last one, or catapult her back into oblivion. Her moods were hard to face down in the darkness, and sometimes a package of cookies was sacrificed to Danielle's sadness. That empty package made her really feel hopeless, thinking, "This diet is the one concrete, constructive thing you're doing right now, and you can't even get that right? You are truly a loser."

I reassured Danielle that she'd come a long way from where she began, and I could tell she was just steps away from fine-tuning her diet to her moods. I suggested she make those steps literal, by walking out of her apartment every day and going over to the gym. A midafternoon workout would boost her mood and jump-start her metabolism. I asked her to pick a time and go every day, even if she didn't stay long.

This was just the action Danielle needed to embrace Diet Designs as a lifestyle, not a doomed effort at self-deprivation. She finished the day feeling lighter and more energetic, strong enough to stand up to her nightly self-assessments. The exercise seemed to control her cravings, so when her stomach said "full," her brain believed it. And after a week of moderate daily workouts, Danielle had lost two pounds. "I'm actually doing it!" she said. "This feels good."

Within a month, Danielle had taken off ten of the forty pounds she wanted to lose. She was writing, eating normally, feeling "pretty much fine all the time," increasing the intensity of her workouts, and cautiously expressing optimism for both her new script and her healthy lifestyle. "These seem like simple accomplishments, but I'm counting my blessings," she told me. "I get up every morning. I work every day. And I eat good food for a good mood."

Let Hollywood wait for Danielle's next work of genius. What mattered was that she had successfully transformed food from a foe to an emotionally positive force, and was making the basic moves every day that add up to a healthy life.

That made my own spirits soar.

✳

Food and mood are intimately connected. Nearly every one of my clients reports having eaten out of a "mood" or a "feeling" of being bored, burned out, alone, hopeless, unfocused, or inadequate. To experience these feelings occasionally as a bout of the blues is perfectly normal, and there are some good physiological and psychological reasons to crave certain comfort foods to soothe yourself back to equilibrium.

But if you feel chronically down, you are a Blue Rose—and you *might* be clinically depressed, a biochemical condition with implications for your desire for food. Researchers are discovering that clinical depression is much more widespread than had been realized—eleven million Americans suffer each year, with the number rising. There might be several types of depression that stem from different chemical imbalances in the body.

In my practice, I've encountered intense and recurring feelings of sadness and inadequacy in even the highest achievers, the most beautiful, and the famous. In fact, high achievers are particularly susceptible to depression. Though many people keep these feelings locked away in their daily lives, they might soothe themselves with food on a continual basis. The Blue Rose is especially susceptible to chronic cravings.

The Blue Rose isn't weak-willed or a natural glutton. Depressed people are caught in a spiral of sadness, chemically induced cravings, and weight gain that deepens their despair. Clients often come to me with the chicken or the egg question: I don't know if I gained the weight because I'm depressed, or if I'm depressed because I gained weight, but now I'm miserable and eating all the time.

Fortunately, the Eating By Design Personal Prescription can help the Blue Rose, both in controlling your intake and boosting your mood with a meal plan specially tailored to your psychological profile. Though your melancholy may seem large and unmanageable, small steps toward healthy eating offer hope.

BLUE ROSE STYLE

SUNSHINE	SHADOW
+ You are sensitive and delicate as a rose.	− Your emotional aura is tinged with blue.
+ You are emotionally attuned and sympathetic.	− You can become overwhelmed by the tragedies and traumas of life on earth.
+ You are modest and self-effacing.	− You can slide into self-loathing at the drop of a handerkerchief.
+ You are creative and complex.	− You can be paralyzed by the complexities of the world.

✳

Feeling Better Through Food Chemistry

Constant Cravings

Reaching for the cookie jar when you're upset is a classic mood control move. Our bodies may know what research is only beginning to discover: Eating carbohydrates stimulates the brain's release of serotonin, a neurotransmitter that soothes you, lifts your mood, and signals satiety to your brain. Reaching for food may be a physiologically functional reaction to feeling depressed.

Current research in depression, mood, and temperament is exploring the role of several neurotransmitters and biochemical processes in feelings and behavior. Though the biochemistry of depression is complex, findings continue to focus on the importance of serotonin, which is shown to be deficient in depressed people. The popular antidepressant drug Prozac works by enhancing serotonin levels, smoothing out mood swings and making you more mellow. The discovery that drugs such as Prozac also seemed to assist in weight control suggested tantalizing possibilities about the link between biochemistry and appetite.

In addition to its mood effect, serotonin is instrumental in signaling a sense of satisfaction to your appetite center. It makes intuitive sense, then, that people with low levels of serotonin, like many Blue Roses, would experience less satisfaction and fullness from food than nature intended. This weak link in the satiety chain could induce you to eat more than your body actually needs.

Working on the assumption that misfired messages to eat can cause chemically driven overeating in some people, a 1980s study tested the serotonin-enhancing drug Pondimin on obese patients and found it to assist in weight loss with minimal side effects. Subjects reported that the drug freed them from food obsession. Since then, some doctors have begun to prescribe the medication to obese patients. Meanwhile, the FDA has approved the use of Prozac for the treatment of bulimia, and is considering other obesity applications for antidepressant drugs.

Danger in the Drug Culture

Though some patients swear by the mood- and food-mediating effects of antidepressant medication, many medical and nutritional professionals, myself included, have deep reservations about drug-induced weight control. First, pills are a quick and temporary fix. Like fad diets, they do nothing to cure the underlying condition of eating too much of the wrong foods. While medication might help to control cravings, it doesn't educate the patient on the components and workings of a healthy diet. No pill can provide the nutritional know-how that goes into nourishing a healthy body.

Secondly, antidepressants can produce side effects ranging from disorientation to a disturbing alteration in your daily behaviors. Many antidepressant users report not feeling "there," not caring enough about important issues, or feeling fuzzy around the edges. I believe that in the coming decade, we'll find ourselves evaluating more closely the pros and cons of regulating biochemistry through prescriptions, scrutinizing the potentially revolutionary repercussions for human nature and society.

Thirdly, antidepressants are expensive, presenting a tough economic choice and a disincentive to continue treatment.

Fortunately, prescription drugs might not be the only route to better brain chemistry and craving control for the Blue Rose. As with other ailments originally treated with intrusive and expensive drugs, such as hypertension and high cholesterol, a much more organic solution lies close at hand in the simple daily practice of a healthy diet.

Good Food for a Good Mood

Even before enthusiasm grew for antidepressant drugs as treatment for depression or obesity, researchers were exploring the role of food in mood and biochemistry. Husband and wife team Richard and Judith Wurtman, brain and nutrition researchers, respectively, pioneered studies in the 1970s linking depression, diet, and serotonin. Following the discovery that eating high-carbohydrate biscuits improved obese patients' moods, and that premenstrual women and smokers trying to quit tended to eat more carbohydrates than the general population, they traced the route between carbohydrate consumption and serotonin production. They concluded that glucose in the bloodstream stimulates serotonin release in the brain. Eating sweet or bready things that easily break down into glucose improves your mood.

The Wurtmans interpreted this discovery to mean that serotonin-deficient people were eating to feed their chemical imbalance. The research jury is still out on whether a craving for carbohydrates is the body's natural self-medication for depression—that is, a physiological response to psychological distress—or a function of the faulty satiety signals caused by low serotonin levels. In either case, the evidence is compelling that a carefully proportioned plan of carbohydrate mini-meals can enhance serotonin production to improve your mood and keep you satisfied, while fueling a healthy, leaner body. Your Personal Prescription is based on biochemical reactions to give you more satisfaction and energy with less food, letting your mind and body work together toward happiness and health.

✳

Upward Mobility

It's hard to commit to anything, most of all to yourself, when you're down or disappointed. Danielle's depression completely immobilized her, sapping her motivation to reach out from her living room to real life. The bottom of the pit is dark, making it hard to envision digging your way back out to the light, and a healthier, happier you. It's easier to despise your lack of resolution than to do anything about it.

Your Personal Prescription for Eating By Design provides a seven-day ministep plan for getting your healthy-eating program in gear, along with food and nonfood ways to cope with your changing moods. With a little careful tending, the Blue Rose can flower into happiness and health.

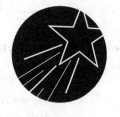

5

THE SHOOTING STAR

"If you've got it, flaunt it."

—MEL BROOKS, *THE PRODUCERS*

✳

A shooting star is actually a supercharged meteor fragment, burning a bright flame as it skims through the atmosphere at thousands of miles per hour. While shooting stars are radiant, fast, and a brilliant pleasure to behold, they can burn out. You don't have to.

✳

Elise was a hugely successful real estate agent for fabulously expensive properties in Bel Air, Beverly Hills, and Malibu. Her name was constantly in the paper in connection with the sale of some celebrity home. Elise called me on her return from one of the top spas in the Southwest, portraying her experience as a total disaster—her favorite chef was on vacation, so she spent the week drinking margaritas at the local Mexican restaurant. She came home to find her husband entertaining French friends who persisted in ordering meat and cream sauces at every meal—tempting Elise to follow suit. Finally, she had stumbled on a rugged outdoor path while showing a house in Malibu, hurting her knee and sidelining her from her workout routine. "Can you return me to a vestige of my former self?" she asked. "And the sooner the better!" Of course I said yes.

Never have I met a woman to whom so many things happened. From carjacking to mudslides, Elise always had a startling excuse for blowing her diet, missing a consultation, or exercising erratically. Nevertheless, Elise was an enthusiastic client who loved the food and approached the program wholeheartedly—as if she were playing a very amusing game. She lost six pounds in two weeks, and sailed out my office singing, "Gorgeousness lies just around the corner!" She was full of plans for shopping sprees and celebrations when she reached her goal.

But there was a hitch in the script, a devastating miscue that arrested Elise in her careening course toward fitness. Elise hit a plateau when she went a week without dropping a single, solitary pound. She was horrified and swore not to eat another bite until she'd lost two pounds.

I had to pull out all the stops to convince Elise that plateaus are natural and healthy, that fasting is not, and that if she just stuck to the program and her workout routine, she would continue to lose weight. She pouted, she posed, she gestured wildly; but finally, lured by the promise of shopping for the high-fashion clothes she liked, beach vacations in the south of France, and occupying center stage at social events without self-consciousness, Elise agreed to try again.

She jumped off the scale in my office, flung her scarf around her neck, grabbed her shoes, ran stocking-footed to her convertible, and sped off to her health club—where she joined a step class in the middle without warming up, used two blocks instead of her usual one, and wrenched her back so badly that she fell victim to an incurable hunger for chocolate. Many rich pastries later, Elise called me from her invalid's position on the couch, feeling fat, miserable and disillusioned with dieting.

"Elise," I said, "remember that you create you own destiny. Your body is a living organism, and it gets very angry when you treat it like an inanimate object, stressing and straining it because you are too impatient to let it develop in its own time. Now, can you slow down long enough to let your new lifestyle take effect?"

I told Elise to get up off her couch, get dressed, and come meet me at a big charity event where many of my famous clients were guests. I pointed out the most glamorous ones, a living portfolio of Diet Designs success stories, all dressed up in their evening best. Elise was indeed awed and decided to try again.

I altered Elise's meal plan to suit her dramatic personality and served up an endlessly varied succession of searingly spicy food. I changed our consultations from weekly to monthly to prevent any plateau crises, and I asked her to take the half hour on our weeks off to do something else for herself—a manicure, haircut or color, facial, shopping—a rotating menu of self-improvement projects, always changing, but at the same time on the same day. Eventually Elise began to see her healthy diet as part of pampering herself—something she couldn't *possibly* live without.

Six months later, Elise had lost her weight, and had gone through three different hair colors and two styles, numerous reinventions of her nail and makeup color scheme, and enough spa treatments to turn her bones to jelly.

When she hit her goal, we celebrated with a very festive salad-and-mineral-water party at her office, where we took pictures and paraded Elise around for admiration and congratulations. Then I immediately sent her out to buy a stunning new swimsuit.

✳

Shooting Stars are larger than life, intense in their feelings, actions, and perceptions. Their very presence can electrify and warm a room, captivate companions, and leave a lasting impression. They are easily enticed, eager to embrace and explore a world of fascinating people and events. Working in Los Angeles, I have *lots* of Shooting Star clients—actors, actresses, producers, and a constellation of other shining personalities.

Shooting Stars are *fast*—quick to adopt and quick to abandon, rejoicing one minute and despairing the next. When you're happy, you are very happy; when you're sad, you're inconsolable. The life of a Shooting Star is large, full of victory and defeat, adventures and misadventures. You are inspired and improvisational, living the moment without a long-range plan. Shooting Stars are always in a rush to perfect their bodies, because when it comes down to it, they're attention-getters who like to *look good.*

As a Shooting Star, you can be doubly troubled by weight management concerns—while your love of the spotlight magnifies the importance of a few pounds gained or lost, you're also prone to extremist thoughts that make any long-term commitment to healthy eating difficult. You might find that though feeling the least bit fat can be a source of intense despair, food provides instant solace when tragedy is crashing down around your ears. For many Shooting Stars, this leads to a cycle of weight loss and regain as dramatic and changeable

SHOOTING STAR STYLE

BRIGHT FLAME	BURNOUT
+ You move in a burning blur of energy, excitement, and emotion.	— You can forget to properly fuel the fire and crash dramatically to earth.
+ You enthusiastically embrace new enterprises.	— You abruptly abandon projects at the first sign of boredom or delay.
+ You shine in the spotlight with the natural glow of generosity, passion, and self-confidence.	— The bright lights blind you to the details of an organized and careful life.
+ You present yourself with flair and fashion.	— You pay more attention to outer beauty than inner well-being.

as their emotional lives—but with increasingly troublesome and potentially cataclysmic physical consequences.

Though your unstoppable spirit might move from one episode to the next with energy and aplomb, you are only awarded one body to carry you through all the roles of a lifetime. To serve you well, that body needs a steady diet of wonderful things.

✳

Tales of a Dramatic Dieter

Shooting Stars tend to dash toward diet plans based on blind trust in schemes that promise swift and painless results. Perhaps you bought this book expecting it to be one of a series of temporary, unscientific solutions to your weight management problem, to be cast aside when it didn't work or you got bored. But temporary solutions based on unsubstantiated weight loss gimmicks will never make you permanently thin and healthy. Do any of these false promises look familiar?

FALSE	TRUE
Skipping meals helps you lose weight.	*Skipping meals slows your metabolism and predisposes you toward bingeing.*
Papaya or other enzyme-based treatments burn body fat.	*Body fat is burned by expending more energy than you consume. Period.*
Eating food in special combinations changes its calorie content.	*Calories are immune to the chemistry of combination.*
Body fat can be quickly lost.	*Water and muscle can be lost fairly quickly. You lose a pound of body fat when you burn 3,500 more calories than you take in—about seven hours of high-impact aerobic exercise with no increase in daily diet.*

It took a lot more experience, research, and testing on my part than it does the creators of irresponsible, ineffective weight loss treatments and plans, but I'm amply rewarded by the success of my clients. My only concern is that you never fall victim to false claims again, but use Eating By Design for a scientifically proven, permanent, and exciting way to attain the body and physical well-being you've always longed for.

✳

Create a Healthy Character to Last a Lifetime

Invent a Healthy Self

We create ourselves with everything we do—every word we speak, every gesture we make, every food we do or do not eat. With every action, we invent who we are today and who we will be tomorrow. To prepare yourself for Eating By Design, stop now to take the time to invent a healthy self, and hold on to that beautiful person as you read through this book. By the time you reach your Personal Prescription in Part Three, you'll be naturally prepared for what it offers—beauty, energy, and vitality.

The first step toward achieving your personal best is to create a healthy character in your mind's eye, then internalize it into your body and let it take over and eradicate any bad habits or personal issues that stand between you and perfect health.

First, pick a fit and healthy character whom you know and admire from television, screen, stage, politics, or private life. Imagine that character eating breakfast, lunch, and dinner, exercising, and sleeping. See how his or her healthy habits result in the beauty and appeal that drew you in.

Now, imagine the character that you want to play on your own personal stage, as fit and glamorous as the public person you admire—but you. Watch your healthy, beautiful self:

- *Enter a room.*
- *Converse with a group of admiring listeners.*
- *Accept an award.*
- *Eat a light breakfast in silk pajamas with sunlight streaming into the room. It feels great to fuel up for an exciting day with a perfectly sized portion of healthy food.*
- *Nibble on sushi at lunch with colleagues. You are so involved in the conversation that you eat just a bite at a time and leave half of it on your plate.*
- *Share dinner with friends at a bustling restaurant. You look at your heaping plate of pasta and protest, "All of that for little old me?" Your friends laugh; what a ridiculous idea! Ask the waiter for another plate, put half the pasta on it, and pass it to your friends.*
- *Walk down a sunny beach or street in shorts and halter top, sipping on a frozen cappuccino and enjoying the admiring looks you receive.*

Once you've created your healthy self in your mind, all you have to do is act the part to look the part—just stay in character and keep your perspective clear.

A Photographic Perspective on Your Personal Best

The camera lens adds ten pounds. The glare of the spotlight adds ten years. In a world where your appearance is constantly judged in the distorting gaze of others, how do you gain perspective on how you actually measure up?

Many of my Hollywood clients are literally in the business of being perfect. They are always in front of the camera, perhaps completely naked, representing an idealized vision of human beauty to an audience they don't know and will never meet. For many actors and entertainers, physical perfection is a full-time job. They work with me one-on-one, hire private chefs and personal trainers, and focus their full attention on their bodies for months at a time. When they're done, they are as close to perfect as human beings as we see on this planet. But the pressures and time requirements of this endeavor are tremendous. Only those who get paid for it can really manage it.

For the rest of us, the goal is not *perfection*, but *personal best* in health and beauty. We work not for the moment when the director calls "Roll 'em!," but for a lifelong process of looking and feeling good. This is the premise of Eating By Design, and in Part Two you'll find a unique way to assess your body composition and progress that gives you perspective on your personal best.

Meanwhile, why not take a trick from the book of the stars? Right now, take a snapshot of yourself, either nude or in your favorite outfit. Once a month, as you follow your Personal Prescription, take an updated photo. Build your self-portrait gallery as a personal portfolio of your progress in the process of living well. Make yourself your own star.

✳

All the World's A Stage

The Shooting Star loves to be onstage, basking in the glow of the spotlight, talking, laughing, acting, interacting—enjoying the attentions of other people. Simply put, the Shooting Star is a social animal.

But though social occasions might be your *raison d'etre*, the social whirl can lead to eating disorientation: What do I do with my hands and my mouth *now*? For mere mortals, the answer is often "seek food and eat." But you have another course to chart. The Shooting Star can seek people and talk.

To prepare your healthy self for the social whirl you live in, imagine who you're going to see today and why you're looking forward to seeing them. Picture yourself talking animatedly with others, looking great in your best clothes. Think of all the things you want to share with people you haven't seen in awhile. Think of who you want to meet. Ask yourself, was I invited here because

I'm such a good eater, or because my host thought that I would make sparkling conversation?

✳

Don't Eat for Drama

Though you might eat like a delicate bird when you're "on" and the eyes of the world are feeding your self-esteem, what happens when you're off, down, or devastated? The Shooting Star is likely to eat for drama.

Elise described the disasters that transpired when she got home exhausted after work, hungry from undereating at the previous meal and devastated that she hadn't closed a house sale: "I eat like a jungle creature, ripping, tearing, gulping. I've been known to scoop up ice cream with my bare hands, or pluck meat off the grill before it's quite done and pop it directly into my mouth."

When alone, Elise slipped out of her publicly controlled character and ate with the same exaggeration that marked her speech, movements, and emotions. Her animalistic appetite came from skipping meals and snacks, overplaying her "onstage" persona to the extent of starving herself, or from a burning need for excitement when she was bored. Food was like a prop in Elise's life, used to heighten the drama of the moment.

Food is *not* a prop. Food is fuel for your Shooting Star, able to stoke your flame with protein, carbohydrates, fats, vitamins, and minerals. Eating By Design will teach you how to choose the very best. The better you fuel your flame, the brighter you will shine.

✳

The impulsive eating typical of Shooting Stars is generally rooted in an old habit of trying to pull something off before being caught by an authority. Another form of this "rebellion by food" is a propensity to pick at other people's plates. Whether you believe in the magically enhancing force of your companions' culinary karma or simply think everyone else makes better food choices than you, food looting is a subconscious cry for someone to tell you no, stop, don't do that anymore, you may not! You are testing the limits, proving every time that no one can say no to you.

The next time you get the urge to rebel against an imaginary authority figure, stop and make that authority figure *you*. You're a grown-up now, and you can play any role you please. Choose the Eating By Design solution to make your character lean and trim.

Go back to the vision of your healthy self. Jump into character and reexperience how good it feels to be that beautiful person, shining in the spotlight. Now picture your character alone, exhausted, grieving over a lost love. Does this tragic figure have a bag of potato chips and a box of cupcakes by his or her side? No! The character sobs, listens to tumultuous music, burns a few letters, takes a walk in the rain, and goes on to the next scene, as beautiful as ever.

DRAMATIC EATING DANGERS

The following miscues might distract you from your healthy role. When you meet these diversions, stick resolutely to your script. You know your healthy role from the inside out, and no obstacle can prevent you from playing your part.

- Fad diets: pills, powders, fasts, food combining, timing, eliminating certain food groups, or any other strange eating behavior that promises instant results.
- Intensive weight loss experiences—spas, centers, etc.—that don't teach you to transfer your new habits to the real world.
- Excuses, including time constraints, illness, nerves, and dramatic life events.
- "Special" occasions featuring "special" foods.

The best self-indulgence is living well. A healthy eating plan has its own momentum, providing inspiration and energy to accelerate you into a dynamic future. Every small step you take toward Eating By Design is a great stride toward becoming your healthy self. Be patient with your body. It functions according to biological rules that can't be hastened by will or technology, and needs only your help to find its optimal form. Every good choice you make moves you closer to your personal best in beauty and health.

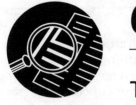

6

THE PERFECTIONIST

"A work of art is never finished; it is merely abandoned."
—PAUL VALÉRY

*

I recently went to a Mexican restaurant with my family to celebrate my mother's birthday. Surrounded by boisterous patrons downing margaritas and plates of cheesy beans, my father, a rather *particular* man, was wearing a grim and rigid face. Dad gets uncomfortable anytime he's asked to depart from his nightly dinner of broiled chicken, baked potato, and steamed vegetables. But to add insult to injury, a national nutritional group had just come out with the bad news about the high fat content of the average Mexican restaurant meal (well, it was news to *some* people). Dad glared angrily at the menu and announced he couldn't possibly eat anything. "Please, Arron, it's my *birthday*," murmured Mom. "Go to town. Have a veggie burrito."

Versed as I am in the eating habits of Perfectionists, I knew there was no way a burrito would pass this man's lips. Philosophically, I handed Mom a birthday margarita and braced for Dad's ordering ordeal: "I want plain grilled chicken, no sauce. Some steamed rice; plain white, not that spicy orange kind. No beans, I can't digest them. No lard, no cheese. Forget the tortillas; I prefer to eat with my knife and fork. You don't have Italian dressing? Then skip the salad. And no onions on anything. If I so much as see an onion on my plate, I'll send the whole thing back." And indeed, the plate went back three times before Dad pronounced it satisfactory, a naked chicken breast alongside a mound of plain rice. Our fajitas had long since lost their sizzle, and the waiter had almost lost his cool.

I've learned one thing from years of dining out with a Perfectionist: It's best to tip very generously.

❊

Amy ate the same thing every single day, thus staying absolutely stable at twenty pounds over her healthy weight. This was a big improvement on yo-yoing up and down through the same seventy-five pounds of body fat in a series of uncontrolled fasts and feasts, as she had seen her mother do while growing up. Organized, efficient, productive—perfect, really—in every other aspect of her life, Amy reasoned that though she was heavier than she'd like to be, at least the situation was somewhat under *control,* and that this departure from her mother's example of wild weight fluctuations and crazily changing diets was enough to make her happy. Or so she told me at first. By the end of the meeting Amy admitted that she knew she could do better. Deep down inside, she thought she really should be able to make her body . . . perfect.

I wanted to reach out and give Amy a hug and tell her that she was already perfect as a person and there's no such thing as a perfect body, but she seemed a bit too professional for this kind of emotional effusion on our very first meeting. Instead, I told her that I would be happy to work with her to transform her deep-set habits into healthy ones that would help her look and feel *better.* I avoided the "P" word. I know not to promise too much to Perfectionists. It just jacks up the pressure they put on themselves.

Amy was the indispensable assistant to one of the most powerful—not to mention demanding and hot-tempered—talent agents at CAA in Hollywood. Mike had hired Amy for her perfectionism and attention to detail, and though he paid her handsomely for her unsurpassable competence, he would just as easily fire her for the slightest slipup. The pressure to be perfect was constant. Every day, Amy performed superhuman organizational acts with Mike's phone calls, meetings, clients, and contracts with a concise system of lists, procedures, and computer databases. She brought order to chaos with repeated daily routines that she stuck to like religion—including her meals. Breakfast was always an oat bran mega-muffin from the vendor who came by at ten. At one she ordered lunch, an overstuffed tuna or chicken salad sandwich from the local deli. Then she looked forward to her usual four o'clock frozen yogurt—half chocolate, one quarter vanilla, and one quarter strawberry. She always ate pasta for dinner; at home, it was fresh cheese tortellini and pesto sauce from the refrigerator case of her local market, and Tofutti for dessert. She enjoyed always knowing what she was going to eat and looked forward to every meal as a predictable comfort in the disorder of her day.

Muffins, tuna, pasta, Tofutti—Amy thought she ate lightly. She wouldn't dream of touching fried food, staunchly avoided ice cream, never buttered her bread, and ate only at her scheduled times. Nevertheless, the hidden fats (the muffin was loaded with oil; the tuna salad full of mayonnaise; and the pesto sauce, tortellini filling, and Tofutti were all prime fat contenders) combined with the sheer quantity of her diet (from the mega-muffin to the plateful of pasta, each of her portions was about double what Amy needed) loaded her down with twenty perpetual extra pounds. And, though she didn't know it, some basic nutritional imbalances in Amy's diet were sapping her energy and threatening her long-term health.

I met Amy when her boss, Mike, joined the Diet Designs program, and she, assigned the task of administering him his meals, called me with a million questions about how to do it right. She was so inquisitive about how Diet Designs worked, what it cost, how long I'd been in business, my nutritional stance, and my opinion on food safety issues that I thought she was a potential competitor trying to get my operating details.

In fact, Amy was quite taken with the Diet Designs concept. "I love the way each meal is all wrapped up in its own container, and you know exactly what to eat, when. It's so *structured.*" When Mike lost five pounds in the first week, Amy signed on too. She was anxious—about not liking the food, being hungry, feeling weak, and, I intuited, losing the sole source of comfort in her very hard days—but she was committed and determined. Diet Designs looked like her ticket to perfection.

I knew that for Amy to succeed past the first week, the first thing we had to do was get all that Tofutti and pesto sauce out of her house. Old habits die hard and provide irresistible temptations to habit-bound people. I scheduled a personal visit to help Amy through the ordeal. Indeed, her kitchen was stocked exactly as expected: a refrigerator full of fresh pasta and sauce, a pantry stocked with nutty wheat bread, cans of tuna, ten jars of mayonnaise in the smallest size ("I don't like it to sit open in the refrigerator too long," said Amy. "Germs.") and a freezer neatly stacked with muffins, frozen yogurt, and cartons of Tofutti. There wasn't a fruit or vegetable in sight. Rarely have I cleaned out a kitchen with so little to salvage. "You can keep the tuna," I said. "Everything else must go." Amy looked pained, but dutifully took out a trash bag and me-thodically placed each offending item inside, carefully, as if saying good-bye. I assured Amy that she would like some of her new Diet Designs meals as much as her old favorites. "Whatever it takes to do it right," she told me. If only my other clients were so dedicated!

Amy followed the meal plans to the tee, complying with every instruction and often inventing ones I hadn't thought of. At work, she lived on the phone and fax, and I was soon inundated with telecommunications. Questions flowed in by phone: The bag was sitting at reception for fifteen minutes; is it possible the cooked chicken dish has gone bad? How many calories and grams of fat in tonight's dinner? Is it better to reheat with the top on or off? The meal plan says to accompany dinner with steamed vegetables, but doesn't say how much? Am I really allowed to eat these desserts? Wasn't the pizza slice bigger this week than last? How many pretzels in an ounce? The fax was filled with her daily food logs, neatly typed with notes requesting nutritional analyses of her intake.

Amy also worried about the nonfat yogurt I prescribed for breakfast, and the fat-free cheese on the Diet Designs pizzas. "My doctor tells me that I'm allergic to dairy, that milk is responsible for my nervous stomach." I explained that, first of all, she was more likely to suffer from lactose intolerance, which we could treat, than an allergy. And did her stomach get better when she cut out the dairy? "Well, no. The upset feeling seems to correlate pretty closely with stress on the job." She admitted that the yogurt seemed to sustain her through the morning, and her stomach felt better than before. When I explained the importance of dairy as a lowfat source of calcium, she agreed to accept it.

After a few weeks on the program, Amy had narrowed her menus down to the six dishes she liked best—not optimal for nutritional variety, but she had lost ten pounds, and the repetition seemed to work for her.

Then disaster struck, or so it seemed to Amy: For the first time, she went for a week without losing weight. I assured her that such a plateau is normal, especially after losing so quickly for the first few weeks. Like all things, weight loss plateaus will pass. But Amy was frantic and angry at herself for "blowing it." She skipped lunch, worked all afternoon, then went on an aerobics marathon at her health club that pushed her far beyond the limits of her endurance and low blood sugar level. Then, desperate with hunger and self-imposed stress, she polished off two large bags of rice cakes, her favorite snack. She called me on a carb overload, disgusted with her "binge" and ready to abandon the whole project. If she couldn't do it right, she didn't want to do it at all. It was back to muffins and Tofutti for her.

Since Amy was so desperate to reassert control over her weight loss, and since she was choosing unhealthy ways to do so, I agreed to shave 100 calories off her day by eliminating one snack, and to allow her to add an hour of extra aerobic exercise per week, to get that inverse relationship between intake and outgo working a little faster. She was enthusiastic, and took off her remaining ten pounds at 1,100 calories a day. I'm very cautious about lowering calories too far—you run the risks of nutritional deficiency and shutting down the body's metabolism—but I could almost hear "Perfection" calling to Amy from ten pounds away, and far be it from me to stand in her way. Those were 1,100 of the most carefully controlled calories ever, incorporating every single food on my usual program. I will take no shortcuts when it comes to nutritional balance.

Amy was ecstatic to reach her goal. The pleasure she took in the achievement seemed to come as much from finishing what she had set out to do as from joy in her slimmer physique. But now came the tricky part: Could Amy maintain her weight on her own, outside of the structure of Diet Designs? It's my favorite thing in the world to set a successful client free, but Amy didn't want to go. She fought me tooth and nail, content to eat Diet Designs food for the rest of her life—until I promised to show her how to cook her favorite Diet Designs dishes, and pointed out how much money she could save in a year. Perfectionists are no dummies.

✳

As a Perfectionist, you probably like to do things right. You tend to know what you like, from food to clothes to work, and you stick with your habits for years on end. Always thinking ahead, you counter every threat of chaos with plans, schedules, and scrutiny. Control, you reason, is within my reach.

When you turn your great analytical power upon yourself, you might find you come up short. With little patience for your own limitations, you constantly push yourself to be better, brighter, more prepared—more perfect.

Though Perfectionists prefer to have perfect health and perfect bodies, food is often one of your few rewards, a repetitive routine of favorite meals to mark off your busy, productive days. The trouble is, this routine might be nutritionally imbalanced and/or overloaded with calories; and beloved though it may be, it will ultimately bore you and be replaced by a new routine, with the same potential problems. So, though Perfectionists make excellent dieters in the short run, they often don't end up with the perfect health and bodies they expect from themselves in the long run. This is a source of great Perfectionist unhappiness.

Like eating, perfection is a process, not an end. Your best body and health begins with a happy and healthy feeling toward food, with just enough flexibility to keep the process vital.

PERFECTIONIST STYLE

PERFECTIONS	IN PROCESS
+ You do it and do it right.	− Others may see you as a control freak.
+ You always make the stitch in time to save nine.	− Your urge to control the future can turn you into a worrywart.
+ You are a paragon of self-control, structure, and order.	− You can seem like an emotional Vulcan to people who don't have your disciplined mind.
+ You spot the typographical error in every life event.	− You can't see the forest for the trees.

✳

Perfection Is a Process

Perfectionists have a tendency to take on the worries of the world. In your zeal to make everything go well, you heap concerns and responsibilities upon yourself without a sense of limits or boundaries. The idea that you can fix the world's imperfections can impel you to take them all on. The same instinct that causes you to overcommit can easily lead you to overeat. Anxiety and worry are enemies of a healthy eating plan.

Perfectionists often get overwhelmed by their dietary questions and concerns, which can paralyze their commitment to the process of eating well.

Let me reassure you that your concerns are normal. Like any new undertaking, a healthy eating plan takes a little getting used to. But your Personal Prescription emphasizes structure and planning to make you feel secure about Eating By Design, and if you follow it as best you can, I guarantee that it will prove itself to you. You will feel fit and energetic and reduce your risk of life-threatening disease.

You don't have to eat perfectly to be well. You just have to eat well most of the time. No single slipup will make you fat or clog your arteries. The only possible nutritional catastrophe is an *ongoing* disregard for healthy eating (and exercise) principles. It's healthy to worry about heart disease if you respond by eating a low-fat diet with plenty of broccoli (along with other vegetables and fruits). It is not, however, particularly constructive to worry about whether you're cooking the nutrients out of your broccoli.

(By the way, you do lose some, but not all, of the vitamins when you cook vegetables. No matter what, it's better to eat overcooked vegetables than no vegetables at all.)

Your health will be enhanced if you keep your life commitments manageable. You probably can't single-handedly solve all the problems presented by your workplace, your family, your friends, your community, the environment, the nation, or the culture. Letting go of the nonessential, the unsolvable, and the lower-priority tasks will make every self-improvement process, including healthy eating, more possible. Remember that perfection is a process, and what is unsolved today will probably be improved by tomorrow.

Never Cry Wolf

Special requests and advance planning are Perfectionist specialties and crucial to following a healthy eating plan. But sometimes the perennial questions of a Perfectionist can sound like the little boy of legend crying "Wolf!" Unlike the character in the story, Perfectionists sound the alarm not to toy with other people, but out of a genuine belief that the menacing creature is at their door. For that reason, Perfectionists make great watchdogs and advocates—but, like my father, they can make annoying dinner guests.

Many Perfectionist dieting attempts are sabotaged when your special requests and questions get so minutely detailed that the provider of your food can't figure out what your true priorities are. If you send back your oil-free vegetables because they're overcooked, the chef might send out a whole new plate that's lightly cooked but swathed in butter. If your lengthy list of eating requirements causes your host to mistakenly think you're vegetarian, you might be served an oily potato dish instead of the low-fat grilled chicken that the rest of the guests are eating. If you repeatedly reject the healthy cooking efforts of your spouse, friend, or family because some small detail displeases you, they will certainly give up trying to please you at all. And when you've complained about the air conditioning, the table's position, the unripe tomatoes, and the flabby rice, the waiter might dismiss you as impossible to please, and fail even to forward your request for oil-free fish to the chef.

Your Personal Prescription in Part Four will help you distinguish discrimination in your eating habits from overkill. It will provide enough structure and precision to let you lighten up. Laugh. Live a little.

Some of the details may slide, but that's all right. Perfection is a process.

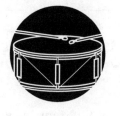

7

THE SOLOIST

"I want to be alone."
—GRETA GARBO

✳

The Lone Ranger was one of those guys who did his best work on his own. Boldly riding through the rugged and crime-ridden terrain of the Wild West, he fought evil, defended innocents, and generally brought good to a society in which he chose not to participate. In the corrupt social atmosphere of the frontier, the Lone Ranger's strength lay in his solitary style.

But the Lone Ranger's solo suppers by the campfire began with beef jerky and finished with tinned pork and beans. As he ate his unhealthy but convenient repast in the glow of the embers, the Lone Ranger set a precedent for solo dining that continues to this day: quick, easy, short on fresh fruit and vegetables, and full of fat and salt.

Who knows what finally became of the Lone Ranger? Did he end his days in a shoot-out, defending the virtue of a frontier belle? Did an unfriendly Indian put an arrow in his back? Or did he die a rather less than romantic death of cardiac arrest or stroke, alone and corpulent, out on the plains with vultures circling overhead?

✳

Jay was an invisible ghost client, a disembodied voice at the other end of the phone or the modem—ironic, given the very physical nature of my work. Jay's assistant initially called to express Jay's interest in the program, wondering if I could consult with him via electronic mail. I had to admit that my business was so people-oriented that I hadn't gone high-tech, and didn't have access to E-mail. Stymied, the assistant gave me Jay's "direct-dial" phone number and requested that I call him. The number was indeed direct—to an answering machine that picked up on the very first ring. I left several friendly messages, apologizing for my electronic inadequacy and suggesting we set up a meeting. I didn't realize that proposing a meeting with Jay was like suggesting that we move a mountain.

Jay is the wealthy and reclusive founder of a very successful computer software company, famous for rarely leaving his Bel Air retreat. I didn't know what this near-legend might want from me. I asked around. Amazingly, despite Jay's stature in the community, I couldn't find anyone who had actually met him. Jay was a mystery man.

When Jay finally phoned me, I felt as if I had a very skittish fish on the line that I had to play quite delicately to keep him from slipping the hook and swimming away. It turned out that Jay wanted what everybody else does: improved health and fitness through a higher-quality eating plan. Years of frozen junk food eaten on an erratic schedule in the glow of his computer terminal had left Jay feeling fat and sluggish. He was about to embark on some huge, top-secret new venture—rumor linked it to interactive media and Hollywood— and he wanted to recapture his health for greater endurance at the keyboard. Or so I gathered from the fifteen sentences or so that he spoke during our first conversation.

Despite having a public profile as president of a multinational corporation, Jay had been private all of his life. The only child of a single working mom, he used his long hours at home alone to read, work math problems, and build mechanical gadgets, and he was winning science fairs by age ten. His mother encouraged him, telling him she hoped his promising mind and self-discipline would make his future brighter than their current life.

Regular mealtimes and social occasions for eating were rare during Jay's childhood. His mother never seemed to notice what and when he ate, said Jay, and as a result, neither did he. So when he looked down one day to see that his body had spread out into the profile of a stout, sedentary, middle-aged man, he was surprised and dismayed. He had lost his father to heart disease and had horrible memories of the intrusive, public nature of his hospital care. He didn't want his fat ever to land him in a similar situation.

I sent my first delivery of Diet Designs meals to Jay, explaining that though his solitary ways made him a perfect client—he was far from the temptations of restaurants or parties, close to his refrigerator of Diet Designs food, and already accustomed to eating prepared meals—it would be best for us to meet in person to test his body fat and perhaps clean out his pantry and freezer. Not necessary, said Jay, and he was off the phone like lightning.

Jay continued on my meal plan for several weeks completely incommunicado. I like to keep track of my clients' progress, but my phone calls all ended in the black hole of his answering machine. So I was surprised when one day, for the first time since our initial consultation, *Jay* called *me*.

Jay cut off my eager inquiries abut his success with the program by saying, "It's really wonderful—but my favorite part is that I don't have to talk about it." He went on to tell me that he'd called because he had a business lunch coming up at a sushi restaurant, and he needed some advice on what to order, since he couldn't stand raw fish. Jay hated to do business in person, let alone over lunch. He had a terrible time keeping his creative head on straight while still managing to eat gracefully—without, as he put it, "drooling and blowing my iced tea out of my nose." Why, my goodness, I thought to myself. This brilliant man isn't just an eccentric recluse. Jay the computer genius and millionaire is *shy!*

I recommended plain grilled or steamed fish—any sushi restaurant could do it—with rice and cucumber salad. Jay thanked me, said he was "seeing results," and quickly hung up. I felt as if I'd spoken with a ghost.

My Christmas gift from Jay was completely unexpected: a computer modem with software that allowed me to network directly with him, so that we could have electronic conversations by typing at our keyboards. This opened up a whole new avenue of communication between us. Here, in his element, Jay was witty, forthcoming, and full of questions and comments. He shared his daily challenges, gave me a running log of his intake, performed pop nutritional analyses with his amazing head for numbers, and generally kept me amused and logged on. We had a great time on-line while Jay took his weight off.

I've had an electronic relationship with Jay for years now. He comes back to the program periodically, whenever he realizes that he's gone unconsciously off track while inventing a new technology. He treats me as a trusted old friend, a star in his small constellation of intimates. Though I always deal with him delicately, like the unhooked fish about to slip away, Jay calls me his "willpower of steel." This is one area in which this Lone Ranger doesn't mind a little help from a friend.

✳

Soloists are generally an independent lot, self-motivated and happy in their own company. Like the masked crusader of legend, Soloists are comfortable roving the frontier, often doing important and pioneering work, but they can feel closed in in a crowd. From Merlin the Magician, the famous hermit, to Greta Garbo, the prima donna of privacy, Soloists often make a great impact— but from a distance.

As a Soloist, you probably work more with your thoughts than your emotions, doing as you choose without asking permission or seeking validation from other people. Your ability to focus without distraction or drama makes you an unusually productive person, very much in touch with your projects if, perhaps, somewhat out of touch with the people around you.

But inside most Soloists is a sensitive person, open to bonds with others yet hesitant to become vulnerable. Their response is often to build thick walls within which they create a safe space for their intimate worlds. Within this world, they are deeply committed to their work and whomever they choose to let in. But outside, in strange contexts, Soloists can seem shy and standoffish.

Your Soloist-style independence probably means that you make your own decisions about when, where, and what to eat without undue concern for custom or how other people perceive your appearance. But the danger is that by depriving yourself of companionship and intimacy, you might fill up with unhealthy food, eating without regard for the primary resource of the Soloist: your personal health.

SOLOIST STYLE

INNER STRENGTHS	OUTER OBSTACLES
+ You are thoughtful, analytical, and blessed with a rich inner life.	– You are a beautiful butterfly wrapped up in a thick cocoon.
+ You march to the beat of a different drummer.	– Your stride looks out of synch to the rest of the world.
+ You are an independent and original thinker.	– You are slow to share talents and skills with others.
+ You have relationships as deep as the deep blue sea in the safety of your inner world.	– You are at sea without a life preserver in the social whirl of the outside world.

✳

Declare Your Independence Through Eating By Design

Out of the Clutches of Caretakers

Autonomy and independence are basic human rights—until something goes wrong with your health, jeopardizing your ability to care for yourself. No one is more dependent than a sick person. Stroke, heart disease, diabetes, and cancer—all associated with high-fat diets and excess body weight—can bring an abrupt end to your independent lifestyle, depriving you of privacy and making you personally and financially reliant on others.

The best way to maintain your freedom is to stay healthy and strong—nourishing yourself with good food, exercising, balancing leisure and work, and warding off disease before it strikes. Declare your independence by breaking your bonds with self-destructive eating habits. Follow your Personal Prescription for choosing low-fat, low-sodium, low-sugar foods, and free yourself from:

- Fear of diet-related disease.
- The impositions of rigid diet plans.
- The energy-sapping effects of digesting dietary fat.

✳

Come out of Your Cocoon

Unwrap Yourself

As I got to know Jay better by E-mail, I came to understand that he genuinely liked to feel intimately connected to other people. What made him a little different from the rest of the world was that he only needed a few trusted confidantes, good friends who formed a backbone of safety and security without cramping his style. In public, Jay hid behind his accomplishments, turning his talent into a smokescreen to prevent outsiders from seeing the real man behind the machinery. He finally admitted to me that his extra fat probably served the same purpose.

Jay didn't consciously gain weight to keep the world at bay. But all the empty space in his life left room for him to fill out his cocoon with body fat, which in turn served as an excuse to avoid reaching out to others from within his safe, but lonely space.

In an increasingly confusing and hostile world, the urge to cocoon is perfectly normal. The danger is that too much sedentary time in the comfort of home and well-known company can cause you to grow a literal cocoon of fat.

The need to feel secure and protected is actually seriously threatened by the fat in which you might unconsciously wrap yourself. Extra body fat can prevent intimacy with those you love, make you feel unsure of yourself in public, and increase your risk of dietary disease. Though I would never ask you to rip yourself from the safe surroundings in which you function best, I do ask you, for the sake of your health and your self-esteem, to commit to a personal unwrapping. Your body longs to live free of its physical cocoon, in fitness and health.

Pat Yourself on the Back

Your Personal Prescription is specially designed to make you a *self-sufficient* healthy eater, to enable you to take those first steps from your cocoon on your own. But it's important to give yourself a pat on the back for your progress.

Plan some prizes to reward every move you make toward Eating By Design—small things that are easy to earn and enjoy, and enhance your daily life. Begin now to look forward to treating yourself to:

- Books
- Magazine subscriptions
- Compact discs
- Videotapes
- Cookware (see the Low-fat Gadget List in Part Four for ideas)
- Kitchen appliances
- A home shopping spree

Promise yourself one of these now just for finishing this book. Everybody deserves a round of applause for self-improvement.

✳

Soloists are so focused and self-aware that they rarely come to me before they're ready to make a change and a commitment. Chances are that if you've come this far, your moment of truth has arrived. But likewise, your sense of independence can make it hard to incorporate big changes into your life just because I tell you to.

Your Personal Prescription leaves the decisions in your hands, turning your independence and analytical ability into natural allies in a healthy eating effort, and enabling you to beat your own path to living well. The payoff is the genuine and permanent independence that comes from good health.

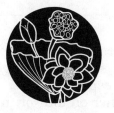

8

THE LOTUS EATER

"The best mind-altering drug is truth."
—LILY TOMLIN

✳

I think the world is still confused about why Elvis Presley got fat. An international sex symbol, a talented performer, and a *man*—none of these attributes jibed with the body ballooning outward right before the public eye. But we know the basic fact behind Elvis's fat: Elvis Presley was an addict.

✳

I met Jenni a year after she checked out, clean and sober, from a drug and alcohol rehabilitation center. Apparently, said Jenni, she was clean, sober, and *hungry*, because she had gained forty pounds over the course of the year. I already knew about Jenni's problem from the newspapers—she was a famous pop singer, and the press had been following her postrecovery weight gain with great interest. I was sad and angry when journalists joked about Jenni's insatiable appetite, because I could see what they cruelly overlooked or ignored. Jenni wasn't physically hungry. Jenni was a food addict.

Jenni's nemeses were no longer cocaine and Valium, but Green Room banquets, huge studio spreads, a house in the Hollywood Hills—and a serious hand-to-mouth habit born of a lifetime of stuffing away feelings and surrendering control with mood-altering substances. These days, that substance could be anything from filet mignon to Fritos. Jenni ate automatically, repetitively, and uncontrollably, trying to fill the emptiness she felt inside. Of course, Jenni's emptiness was emotional, not physical. But food is much easier to come by than self-esteem.

After a succession of publicly failed diet attempts, I was truly grateful that Jenni had come to me. More than a food plan, she needed an approach that treated her eating as addictive behavior, a legal but potentially life-threatening substitute for the drugs she had relinquished the year before.

67

Jenni had always wanted to be a singer. Like many other addictive performers, the only time she felt good about herself was when she was onstage in front of adoring fans who fed her sense of self. Offstage, especially alone, she felt incomplete and hollow. Her musician's lifestyle, whether on tour or in the studio, offered a plentiful supply of substances to dull her pain: first alcohol, then drugs, now food.

I immediately referred Jenni to a professional therapist for treatment of the core emotional causes of her compulsive eating. Then I put her on a special meal plan stripped of potentially addictive foods such as sugars, refined flours and grains, and caffeine, with the emphasis on simplicity and a careful balance of protein and carbohydrates to control cravings. As in a drug rehabilitation program, I emphasized to Jenni that our first task was to break the addictive cycle. But she wasn't condemned to this restrictive recovery diet forever; our ultimate goal was to get her eating a normal array of foods in a nonaddictive fashion. Unlike drugs and alcohol, food is a substance from which you can't abstain, and the wider the variety of foods you can safely eat, the healthier you are.

Initially, Jenni struggled through therapy and her food plan, revisiting the nightmare of drug rehabilitation in her mind, and feeling extremely anxious about having her last recourse—food—restricted. She dutifully ate her Diet Designs meals in public, and acknowledged that they filled her up and satisfied her physical hunger. But whenever she could sneak a moment to herself, her emotional hunger took over, and she binged on whatever food she could get her hands on. She would confess to me afterward, full of shame and a new sense of disgust as she discovered just how little control she had over her eating behavior. "I wasn't that surprised that drugs got the better of me," she said. "I've seen so many others crash and burn. But food??"

I forgave Jenni again and again, gently asking her to go back on her meal plan every time she fell off. I prayed that with my support and her work in therapy, Jenni would be able to forgive herself for her food dependency. That would be the key to breaking her addiction.

As the time between binges lengthened, Jenni told me that on the days she stuck to her diet, she felt healthy—a feeling so good it almost scared her. But she was constantly fearful of two things: an emotional crisis that might reactivate her hand-to-mouth motion, or a chance encounter with one of her "trigger-foods"—ice cream, macaroni and cheese, and peanut butter seemed to set her off on binges every time she touched them. We planned each week together, looking at her calendar, envisioning what foods she might come across in the course of her schedule, and strategizing around potential disasters by having Jenni avoid risky situations, write out rules, or enlist a buddy to help her through.

Jenni told me she had never expected to take her eating so seriously—but only when she did so did she realize how serious her addiction was. This admission made me breathe a big sigh of relief. Things were going well—Jenni had gone weeks without a binge and was making progress in therapy. She understood that she was addicted and was working on other ways to soothe and value herself more. We agreed together to lift the strictures against sugar and refined flour. Jenni thought she could handle it and was ready to return to the real world.

When I examined Jenni's next food diary, something seemed wrong. Though her meals were exactly as prescribed, she was consistently skipping her snacks—between-meal energizers that, initially, had made her feel "safe" on the eating plan. When I questioned her, she admitted to having drifted from her healthy snacks into a hard candy habit. All day, every day, she popped sugar-sweetened candies in her mouth the minute she started feeling low. "They're fat free!" Jenni defended herself, "And only ten calories apiece. I can eat ten of them for the same calories as a granola bar." Indeed, compared to her past bingeing, Jenni's candies seemed relatively harmless. But they were loaded with sugar, she was eating them without counting or recording them, and she was taking them for mood boosts just like a junkie.

I told her so, taking the blame on myself for giving her the green light on sugar. She stormed out, furious at being called a junkie. I thought I'd lost her forever, and I was saddened. Maybe Jenni was just doomed to transfer her compulsion from one behavior to another, all her life.

But Jenni had made so much progress, I refused to give up on her. Instead, I scoured the market for a hard candy sweetened with fructose, the natural sweetener in fruit that digests more slowly than other forms of sugar. I sent a boxful to Jenni and asked her to try them instead of her brand—and come see me if the switch was successful. A week later she showed up at my office, a bit suspicious of my intentions, but converted to the fructose candy. She said the rush they gave her (at last, she admitted to a rush!) was less immediate than the sugar-sweetened brand, but it lasted longer. I told her she could continue to pop her candies, but with just one rule: She had to log every candy she ate, just as she did all the other food that passed her lips. She groaned, but she got the message—no uncharted food allowed.

Soon, I asked Jenni to stay off the candies for a few hours a day and substitute a low-fat, high-carbohydrate snack bar. She reported fewer candy cravings, steadier energy, and an even longer-lasting "hit" from the snack bar. But she was still scared, most of all to report progress, as if just by saying that she was feeling better, someone might snatch it away. I assured her that the good feeling was hers to keep; all she was losing was body fat. Fifteen pounds lighter, Jenni was modeling new costumes for her upcoming tour with enthusiasm.

To prepare Jenni for the next twenty-five pounds and the big tour, we got her down to a two-candy limit each day and took a trip together to the frozen yogurt shop to see if she could snack on a sugar-free ice cream alternative without triggering a binge. She could, though with some trepidation. "Thank God for single-serving cups," she said.

As for macaroni and cheese, I gave Jenni a recipe for a fat-free version; she admitted she wasn't much of a cook, but it was nice to know that she could have it if she wanted it. And peanut butter? "What does an adult really want with peanut butter, anyway?" joked Jenni. When it came down to it, Jenni had learned that some things are better left untouched. Why jeopardize her newfound freedom from food's control with a spoonful of ground-up nuts?

✳

Addiction seems to be woven right into human nature. Throughout time and across social strata, people have leaned on substances to cope with feelings of powerlessness, usually ending up even more disempowered as they offer up careers, relationships, and health to their habit. One of these addictive substances is food, and one of these habits is compulsive or disordered eating.

Though most humans seem to have some sort of addictive tendencies, Lotus Eaters are particularly vulnerable to the power of substances. This is generally because they are acutely sensitive to the stress and trouble of life. As a Lotus Eater, you would probably rather do anything than suffer the pain of loneliness, failure, or fear. Repeated habits and actions give you relief from the uncertainties and disappointments of daily life. Whatever it is that you pick up when times get tough—a pill, a glass of wine, a cup of coffee, a doughnut—you know that you can rely on that relief. In an uncontrollable world, this seems to make things manageable.

The chemical properties of food as addictive substances have only recently been recognized by professionals in nutrition and psychology. The notion of

LOTUS EATER STYLE

BRIGHT LIGHTS	PERSONAL INFERNOS
+ You are blessed with brains and talent.	− You are a brilliant self-critic.
+ You have high imagination and energy levels.	− You have low reality tolerance.
+ You do the right thing in public.	− You self-destruct in private.
+ You feel deeply.	− You sublimate feelings with substances.

food addiction—or food using—has challenged both communities because unlike other addictive substances, such as drugs, alcohol, cigarettes, shopping, even sex, food isn't something you can give up.

Many Lotus Eaters are highly creative people, haunted into their habit by their own active imaginations. But don't romanticize the cliché of the creative addict. Habitual use of any substance saps your power, energy, and health, turning the creative addict into the comatose, alienated, fat, sick, or dead addict. Don't let a food habit eat away at your self-esteem.

※

Profile of a Food User

Feeding Instead of Feeling

Food users experience food not as fuel for the body, but as a mood-altering substance to weather the emotions and stresses of life. Stripped of their own self-esteem, usually by deep histories of unhappiness or abuse, they learn to distrust and devalue themselves. What should be life-affirming—the act of feeding yourself—becomes self-punishing and self-destructive. I don't deserve any better, the food user thinks. I don't have a right to feel good. For the user, food is a substitute for the expression of human feelings, and a relinquishment of the responsibility to face the painful issues at the source of those feelings.

Low self-esteem makes a food user loath to depend on other people. A private bingeing habit constructs walls to keep other people out. Conversely, a food user might abstain from food for the same effect—to gain control over uncontrollable feelings and attain a sense of autonomy.

Food users demonstrate three different responses to this same set of issues, all of which can be termed eating disorders: compulsive overeating, anorexia nervosa, and bulimia. Though I've worked with anorexics and bulimics, they require specialized care outside the scope of my practice. I work extensively with compulsive overeaters, the most common and misunderstood of the disorders.

I'll Have the Steak Stuffed with Feelings, Please

Compulsive eaters eat repetitively, automatically, and uncontrollably to feed an emotional hunger and alter their mood. They find relief in food's familiarity; the simple actions of moving hand to mouth, chewing, and swallowing; and the secure sense of feeling full. Eating is a course of action, something to do in the face of self-doubt or inexpressible emotions. With each bite swallowed, compulsive eaters are actually stuffing their feelings back inside.

An extended session of compulsive overeating—when you lose control of your consumption and eat without hunger, pleasure, or perhaps even conscious awareness—is a binge. A binge can act just like a drug in your system, soothing you, dulling your thoughts and feelings, helping you to forget or ignore the cries and screams in your heart. For the food user, there's a binge inside every diet. The diet symbolizes being "good," controlling the shameful desire for food. The binge symbolizes being "bad," providing a secret source of gratification too shameful to be shared with the outside world. This constant judgment of the self as "good" or "bad" takes over the food user's mental landscape. Dieting and bingeing come to express all possible moral behavior in a self-perpetuating cycle of shame.

Many psychologists describe habitual bingeing as binge eating disorder. Though not officially classified as a psychological disorder, repeated bingeing appears to be a behavior distinguishable from other eating disorders, requiring a different approach to treatment. Researchers are currently exploring the physiological and psychological roots of binge eating disorder and experimenting with treatment alternatives.

An even more extreme manifestation of using food to be "good" and "bad" is bulimia nervosa, characterized by recurrent episodes of binge eating; a feeling of lack of control over binges; self-induced vomiting; vigorous exercise; the use of diuretics, strict dieting, or fasting to prevent weight gain; and persistent overconcern with body shape and weight. People with this disorder make repeated attempts to control their weight by dieting, vomiting, or the use of cathartics or diuretics.

Anorexia nervosa is characterized by an extreme fear of being fat, manifested in a self-imposed inability to eat. Gross disturbances in eating behavior usually begin in early childhood or adolescence. The essential features of the disorder are refusal to maintain normal body weight for age and height; intense fear of gaining weight or becoming fat; a distorted body image; and amenorrhea (cessation of menstrual periods). People with this disorder are preoccupied and dissatisfied with their bodies, starving themselves to achieve a sense of control. Anorexics are fearful of food, thinking, "If I don't control food, food will control me."

Fear and Loathing in Adolescence

Teenage years are tough on everyone, and many people begin using food in this tumult of hormones, shifting social relationships, new responsibilities, and self-doubt. As puberty realigns fat cells to prepare the body for reproduction, many girls, taught by society to be thin at any cost, learn to hate their newly emerging shapes. Trying desperately to turn into self-controlled adults, teenagers see their changing bodies as a betrayal. Now, along with the pressure to score well on their SAT tests, attract the opposite sex, and handle the family car responsibly, they feel they must diet away what looks like bodily evidence of personal weakness. This response can turn into any of the three eating disorders.

I grew up with intense fear of fat. Watching my mother battle her weight throughout my adolescence, I saw her pain and sense of personal devaluation and wondered if this would happen to me. I would have done anything to make sure that it didn't. For many girls, this kind of experience is the beginning of an eating disorder. For me, it was the inspiration behind my decision to become a nutritionist. Instead of using food, I decided to explore its role in healthy living.

Most children are not as fortunate. Brought up in families in which food is used to communicate feelings or plays a part in family dysfunctions, many children develop a basic distrust of their bodies and their relationship with food that can explode during adolescence and haunt them for the rest of their lives.

Whenever it was that you went from an eater to a food user, the time to deal with it is now.

A Necessary Substance: From Cold Turkey to Turkey Sandwich

The transition from eating to using food involves the subversion of your basic pleasure cues. Anorexics convince themselves that the pain of starvation feels good; compulsive overeaters, that being stuffed with food is comfortable; bulimics, that vomiting is welcome relief. What happens as you live this kind of physiological lie is that you become increasingly alienated from the basic process of feeding your body. Then, food is no longer fuel. It becomes a substance.

Anorexia can seem like a somewhat logical response to food addiction. With other types of addiction, society and the medical profession recommend you just say no—avoid the addictive substance altogether! Like other users, anorexics reason that if they don't start, they won't have to worry about not being able to stop. Unlike kicking a drug habit, however, going cold turkey on a food addiction causes starvation and death.

✳

The Diet Yo-Yo

One of the greatest dangers of food using is a tendency to get caught in a repetitive cycle of dieting and weight regain as you skitter in and out of control. Yo-yo dieting is a widespread and debilitating behavior that threatens the health of many Lotus Eaters. Research shows that losing weight over and over again can slow metabolic rate and make weight easier and easier to gain, harder and harder to lose. Repeated weight loss also puts a tremendous strain on vital organs, including your heart. Here are the frightening details:

- Losing and regaining weight can increase your risk of death by heart attack by as much as 70% in comparison to maintaining a steady body mass.
- Studies suggest that yo-yo dieting increases the risk of breast cancer.
- Caloric restriction can lower resting metabolic rate by up to 45%.
- Each cycle of weight loss can lower resting metabolic rate even further, to the point where the decrease overcompensates for any calories you cut from your daily diet.
- Rapid weight regain is likely to be fat, not lean muscle mass.
- One animal study showed that in just the second cycle of weight loss and gain, subjects took twice as long to lose the weight and only one third the time to regain it.
- "Set point theory" suggests that dieting can't change your long-term body composition, because your hypothalamus reacts to conserve your "natural" level of body fat. Only exercise can lower your set point, by encouraging the breakdown of fat and raising the metabolic rate.

Your Personal Prescription in Part Three is designed to break the diet cycle and give you a permanent solution to your food using problem. *My healthy eating plan is always there for you*—even if you have a slipup. So use Eating By Design to yo-yo no more.

※

Get Help

You need help to kick the Lotus Eating habit. Most people can't give up an addiction alone. A food user needs more than just my food and nutrition advice; a user needs to work on the underlying emotional roots of addiction to develop the self-esteem that supports a healthy, trusting relationship with food. I recommend that you seek therapy—individual, family, or group—to explore and resolve the inner conflicts that underlie your habit.

Meanwhile, your Personal Prescription provides a simple recovery diet and lots of tips on how to let yourself eat while remaining in control. Many users are justifiably scared of the substance that controls them. As you work on basic inner issues in therapy, your Personal Prescription eliminates potential addictor foods from your diet and delivers maximum healthy, feel-good fuel with minimum hassle. The goal of both the therapy and the diet is to refocus your energies and attention from your *food* to your *self*.

Check In

Extreme cases of eating disorders can require hospitalization, when food abuse or starvation has caused a chemical imbalance in the body. Though this sounds extreme to some people, it is standard practice for drug addictions, providing medical support for your overtaxed body and a structured environment in which to break the habit. Most people fear the loss of autonomy inherent in hospitalization. But if you're using food as a substance, you've already relinquished control.

Check Out Your Options

There are many kinds of therapists, and I've found that different people click with different approaches. Finding the right relationship is crucial to your progress, and I encourage you to keep looking until you find one that makes you comfortable. Remember, this is something you're doing for you. It's not a punishment. It's a positive step toward making your life easier and easier.

Begin your search by identifying the philosophy that appeals to you, then seek out a therapist who agrees. Here are some of the most common approaches:

Cognitive therapy proposes that emotional problems result from the way you think and your attitude toward yourself and others. Correct the thinking process, and the problem disappears. Treatment takes a behavioral approach, focusing on skills such as relaxation training, anxiety management, and problem-solving to get you thinking on a positive, self-loving track.

Humanistic therapy contends that abnormal behavior begins when a part of the self is denied through too many "shoulds" and environmental strictures. It strives to create a setting in which the patient can self-cure by connecting with his or her true inner self. The emphasis is on enhancing self-esteem and making constructive changes.

Psychodynamic therapy explores your personal history, to uncover unconscious areas of conflict in the past and bring them to the forefront, where they can be resolved in the present. Sigmund Freud made this kind of therapy famous.

Whom to Invite?

Most therapy seeks first to help you accept yourself, and then enhance your ability to connect to other people. Some patients prefer to undertake this in a sociable atmosphere; others prefer privacy. Choose the therapeutic context that offers you the most comfort and support:

- **Individual therapy** allows you to confront issues in the safety of a one-on-one interaction.

- **Family therapy** offers a chance to resolve conflicts with family members—often a source of deep emotional pain—in an arbitrated environment, and creates family support for your undertaking.

- **Group therapy** helps you to connect and share with other people, teaching you to accept yourself as you reveal yourself to others. An example is the twelve-step approach practiced by Alcoholics Anonymous, which has several offshoots, including Adult Children of Alcoholics, CODA (for codependency), and Overeaters Anonymous.

✳

You're on the road to recovery when food becomes nutrition, not a substance in which you choose to indulge or from which you choose to abstain. Food is not moral, "good" or "bad." Your Personal Prescription for Eating By Design is the best way to give yourself the care you deserve, putting yourself in charge of very precious cargo: you.

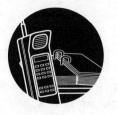

9

THE POWER PLAYER

"There is no such thing as a free lunch."
—MILTON FRIEDMAN

❋

There's a scene in the novel *The Player* where the hero, Griffin, a young studio executive, is at a power lunch with Levy, his archrival who has just been hired above him. Griffin has clearly already lost the battle for dominance at the studio, but takes this opportunity to pretend otherwise at the table. After Levy orders a salad, Griffin gleefully asks for a pizza, then butters up a roll, flouting his willingness to dig into the bread as a symbol of strength. During the meal, Griffin feels Levy "staring at his carbohydrates," but his offer of a slice of pizza is refused. High on the hubris of his culinary daring, Griffin even orders up a piece of chocolate cake for dessert. He finishes lunch feeling that he has won.

But there is, perhaps, a reason that Levy has catapulted above Griffin, landing a plum production position directly out of Business Affairs. While Griffin dines on sedatives, a load of carbohydrates releasing veritable opiates into his brain, Levy truly "power lunches" on the light food that gives Power Players the mental edge to close the deal and kill the competition. Who knows if it's a matter of nutritional savvy, but by the book's end, Levy is running the studio, and Griffin is out.

❋

Cynthia was the CEO of a large manufacturer of an exclusive cosmetics line. A chance complaint to a colleague about outgrowing her favorite suits as she tucked into yet another business dinner referred her to me. After many rounds between her assistant and mine trying to schedule a consultation into her busy calendar, we finally agreed that I would meet her while she was having her hair put up for a black-tie event. The struggle to schedule the appointment signaled to me right away: Here was a woman without any time for herself. Personal nutrition was probably at the bottom of her list of daily priorities.

I arrived to find Cynthia holding court, surrounded by her stylist, a manicurist, her assistant, Marcie, and a vice president trying to talk her into the merits of a new distribution deal. I wondered how we were going to have a consultation—an intimate, confessional occasion for most of my clients—amidst such a crowd. But Cynthia launched right into a briefing on her current diet dilemma, joking about the irony of accumulating cellulite while heading up one of the nation's top beauty companies. She had no trouble identifying and discussing the private details of her eating and body image; she just had trouble making the time to do it.

Cynthia's days were nonstop and hectic, and her eating followed suit. A typical morning began with a chocolate croissant and coffee. From there on, her meals varied wildly with her schedule and her stress levels. Lunch could be anything from a grilled cheese sandwich from the company cafeteria, to a three-course meal with bread and wine at one of L.A.'s better restaurants, to a burger and Coke from a coffee shop near the company's Orange County manufacturing plant, to nothing at all when the pace got really hectic. Dinner ran the same gamut. On the rare evenings when Cynthia and her husband both made it home for dinner, they loved to order up several dishes from their neighborhood Thai restaurant and spread their exhausted selves in front of the television.

"What about between meals?" I asked. "Do you snack at all?"

Cynthia looked at me like I was crazy. Marcie giggled. "What, are you kidding? I eat nonstop, constantly, all the time!" Marcie kept a bowlful of change on her desk, which she plugged into the vending machines every time her boss felt her blood pressure surge or her blood sugar plummet. This was partly self-preservation on Marcie's part, who was sure to hear some shrieks if she let Cynthia crash. Unfortunately, Marcie was no health expert. Cynthia was running a multinational company fueled mainly with M&M's and diet sodas.

Cynthia was concerned about her creeping weight, period. When I asked about her overall health and energy, she looked blank and replied, "Well, of course I'm always exhausted and stressed out, but I think that just comes with the territory." She rarely exercised, was subject to headaches, chest pains, and shortness of breath, and had a hard time getting out of bed in the morning. "But, when I get too dragged out"—she winked at Marcie—"there's always sugar!" She sighed. "Hence, the cellulite." Cynthia didn't even know the full picture—that along with the high calorie count of her candy, research has linked diet soda with the formation of cellulite. Her snack packed a double whammy.

I could see the pattern clearly: Here was a superachiever so absorbed in her work that she was ignoring her own discomfort and fatigue, presuming she could stay at the top of her game through sheer strength of will and chutzpah. This misconception can be especially tough on female executives, who worry that showing concern about issues of diet and health will seem soft. I prayed I could penetrate Cynthia's power shield in time to save her from her own determination.

Interested as she was in Diet Designs, Cynthia couldn't even begin to imagine how a complete meal plan could fit into her busy life, full of business lunches, social obligations, and travel. Taking my cue from Cynthia's style, I negotiated, extracting from her before I left a promise to start on the program for dinners only, to follow my restaurant guidelines at lunch, and to hand my list of healthy stress snacks over to Marcie to substitute for the vending machine ventures. "After all," I said. "You're head of the company. I think you deserve your own private stash of snacks."

By the time I finished with Cynthia, I had negotiated far beyond our original agreement, pulling my own power play on the state of her health. I helped her to choose and time her meals for energy and alertness all day long, to snack for stable blood sugar and stress control, and to control her fat and calories as closely as she did her marketing team and balance sheet. The newly energized chief executive officer announced that as part of the one-year plan for the company, she intended to pull the vending machines from the building, install healthy snack counters in their place, and revamp the menu in the cafeteria. "It's a hard-headed business decision," said Cynthia. "I see how much eating right enhances productivity—and this is the year I plan to edge out the competition."

✳

The nation's top companies and institutions seek out Power Players with "type A" personalities for good reason: They are self-starters, decision makers, motivated, committed, aggressive, and capable of getting the job done.

Unfortunately, Power Players are also singled out by stress, heart disease, hypertension, stroke, elevated cholesterol levels, and chronic fatigue. They are one of the most health-endangered personality types in our society.

I often see clients when the demands of highly pressured and tightly scheduled lives have aggravated these conditions to crisis point. A leading film director called me when his blood chemistry panel showed astronomical cholesterol levels; a trial lawyer arguing a headline-making case was referred to me by his doctor when his blood pressure shot through the roof; a publishing magnate came in complaining that the ten pounds she'd put on during a difficult acquisition made it impossible to complete her customary aerobic workout without chest pains and shortness of breath. All three came in emergency situations after the damage had been done, desperate to keep functioning in their overextended lives.

As a Power Player, you expect to feel tired and burned out most of the time; it's hard to convince you that it's possible to feel otherwise and still be a productive member of society. Likewise, you expect the medical profession to fix you when you're broken, administering emergency solutions like tranquilizers, medications for blood pressure, ulcers, and cholesterol, and, at the extreme, performing bypass surgery.

But often, the key to a Power Player's health lies not in major medication, but in simple self-care. The director cut back on fat by avoiding heavy sauces and dressings in his frequent restaurant meals; the lawyer gave up junk food and learned to love herbs and spices as much as salt; the publisher learned portion control. In addition to surmounting their immediate problems, each client reported increased productivity on the job. Eating more carefully not only corrects your pressing health problems, but also enhances your daily performance and energy levels. Your investment in healthy eating pays off not just in disease intervention, but in the invaluable currency of personal power as well.

As a Power Player, you are dedicated to your profession and to achieving high standards and goals. This drive to succeed, though it might provide you with plenty of psychic energy, can leave your physical body far behind. Morning impatience might be fueled by coffee and a greasy doughnut as you dash for your desk. Lunchtime could find you simultaneously talking on the phone, sending an E-mail, and scarfing down a greasy sandwich, chips and a Snickers bar, or tossing back a martini and a steak while cutting a deal with a client. At the end of the day, though you appear to be relaxing over dinner with your

POWER PLAYER STYLE

CREDIT	DEBIT
+ You are always on the "A" list.	− You neglect the ABCs of self-care.
+ You have the whole world in your hands, or at least in your Rolodex.	− The heavy weight of the world can contribute to stress, high blood pressure, and heart disease.
+ You are driven to get the job done.	− You can drive others to distraction and yourself to poor health with heavy demands.
+ You perform the deeds of gods and superheroes.	− You are trapped in a mortal body.

family, your mind is chewing through the deal you're trying to put together by tomorrow. Extended work hours, pressure-laden days, business lunches, frequent flying, hotel living, and your busy brain stand between you and healthy eating habits.

Workaholism is one of the few addictions not only allowed but actually encouraged by our society. Committed people like you contribute immeasurably to our economy and culture. But like any addiction, workaholism has its price. Fortunately, the costs of commitment to work can be negotiated downward with a healthy eating plan.

❊

The Work Ethic

In a world where work is everything, eating can get shoved aside like a frivolous activity. How can you stop for mere food when there's a memo to be written, a problem to be solved, a client to be wooed? Our cultural affiliation of food with relaxed and social times encourages us to make fueling up a leisure activity. But the harder you perform, the more important is a power nutrition plan. Eating is a crucial source of energy for performance, as important to your success as strategic planning.

Cynthia lived with her calendar in hand, juggling multiple obligations. Though she seemed committed to the program, Cynthia was having trouble taking the Diet Designs principles with her to restaurants, meetings, airplanes, and hotel rooms across the country. She was constantly canceling our consultations because she was too busy, so I had to improvise a solution. I asked myself what is the most direct route to a Power Player's stomach? I found the answer in front of my nose: I wrote Cynthia's meals right into her busy schedule.

You are well accustomed to scheduling meetings, committing to projects, and making deadlines. Your Personal Prescription in Part Three will help you to use that decision-making capability to decide in favor of health by scheduling healthful meals into your busy day, at times and intervals carefully calculated to optimally enhance your performance.

❊

The Neural Connection

As an achiever, you like to make the most of your native intelligence. Your driving ambition is to do things right and smart. You know that mental energy translates into accomplishment.

Now imagine that there was a simple, natural treatment to enhance your brain power on a daily basis. Imagine that it was part of something that you already do, in fact must do to live. Imagine that it could be enjoyable—and tasty.

This wonder drug is right here in Eating By Design. Your Personal Prescription contains a power nutrition plan that actually enhances your neurotransmitter activity for peak mental performance. Simply by following my meal plan, eating familiar foods according to principles only recently discovered by scientists, you will sharpen your thought processes as you attain a leaner and healthier body.

With your Personal Prescription, food is not just a necessary fact of life competing with other responsibilities for your precious time. Food is a tool for reaching your performance goals, full of healthy energy and with all your neurons firing.

※

The High Price of Pressure

When stress makes the nervous system run amok, adrenaline and other hormones are stimulated that prepare you to fight: They make your heart beat harder and faster, raise blood pressure and metabolism, tense your muscles, and disrupt digestion. All this internal action can deplete your blood sugar, tear away at cell walls, and depress your immune system. Other effects of a high-pressure lifestyle include:

- Increased risk of hypertension, heart disease, and stroke.
- Mindless eating, smoking, and drinking alcohol to alleviate tension.
- Use of sugary foods for a quick energy hit, resulting in low blood sugar and cyclical mood swings.
- Disrupted eating and exercise patterns.
- Stimulation of a hormone that promotes the storage of abdominal fat, which is in turn associated with increased risk of heart disease, hypertension, and diabetes.

An erratic eating schedule and poor-quality nutrition can both gravely compound the ill effects of stress. Eating well, on the other hand, goes a long way toward enabling you to embrace the urgent challenges you thrive on without creating a medical emergency in your body. Your Personal Prescription incorporates stress-busting strategies into your eating plan to keep all systems go no matter what pressures are at play in your working day.

✳

Bodies in Motion

Many Power Players are involuntarily members of the jet set, required by professional obligations to spend a lot of time in the air and away from home. Unfortunately, traveling often serves as an excuse to escape from the healthy eating plan you faithfully follow at home. Cynthia, for instance, comforted herself for the inconvenience and loneliness of business trips with elaborate room service meals. But remember that though you may leave your home, you take your body with you everywhere, and it will come back reflecting how well you treated it while you were away.

Furthermore, the physical demands of traveling require that you eat right for alertness and energy. Flying across time zones interrupts your internal rhythms and external food cues. Add stress, canned air, and high-fat, low-nutrient airplane food and you have a surefire formula for fatigue and weight gain.

Your Personal Prescription will feed your body's need with tips for healthy traveling, adding power nutrition to your business trips.

✳

Webster's Dictionary defines *power* as "1. ability to do or act. 2. vigor; force; strength. 3. authority; influence. 4. physical force or energy: as, electric *power.*" Use your ability to do or act to follow your Personal Prescription. Call upon your authority and influence to delegate any difficult details to your valued support system. Then prepare to enjoy the advantage of unparalleled vigor, force, and strength in body and mind. This will be the best investment you ever made. Ambition becomes electric.

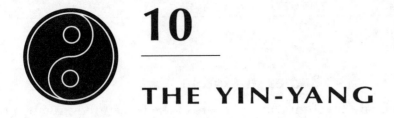

10

THE YIN-YANG

Ask the way
Straight to Nirvana
While you're healthy:
Before you set out on a journey
To the other world.

—JAPANESE FOLK SAYING*

※

Susanna came to me sick of being sick and ready for a new way of living. My initial intake with her—usually an hour-long conversation and a page of notes—required a two-hour interview, a week of follow-up with a battalion of doctors to piece together her medical history, and the compilation of reams of paperwork covering her treatments, prescriptions, hospitalizations, blood workups, and tests. There was no single theme to Susanna's checkered medical past. Her complaints ranged from colds and flu to viruses, respiratory illness, chronic yeast infections, fatigue, and foggy thinking.

Susanna remembered being sick with one thing or another all her life, dating back to her childhood in a high-rise apartment building in Manhattan. She had dealt with constant confinement by immersing herself in books, ideas, philosophies, and religions, finding power in her spirit that her body couldn't provide. Between the stressful environment of urban living—in Manhattan as a child and Los Angeles as an adult—and the frailties of her own immune system, Susanna literally didn't know what it felt like to be well. But her spirit knew what it felt like to soar free.

Susanna didn't suffer from imagined maladies. Each one was scrupulously documented and diagnosed by an acclaimed expert. She'd had to use many different doctors because, she said, everyone seemed to have a different specialty. It was impossible to envision herself as a healthy person when she was constantly undergoing different treatments to different body parts, as if each problem were isolated and separate from the whole. "I wish I could find a doctor who would just treat *me!*" she exclaimed.

---

*The Zen sayings in this chapter are from *A Zen Harvest*, compiled and translated by Soiku Shigematsu.

Hmm, I thought. I'm no doctor but it's definitely time Susanna was treated as a whole person. No matter what, I'm going to give her a good dose of mind-body nutrition.

Susanna was married to a prominent film director who led a high-energy life, working on the set and jetting around to distant locations. Susanna would have loved to spend more time with him, but she was usually housebound by one sickness or another, reluctant to leave the range of her doctors' beepers and the local pharmacy with all her prescriptions on file. This sense of restriction tortured Susanna; she felt as if she wasn't really *living*, or realizing the potential of her relationship with her husband.

Susanna heard about me from a friend who followed my diet and couldn't stop raving about her increased energy levels, an attractive prospect to a woman who had felt fatigued all her life. Susanna hoped that shaping up her eating habits would do something—anything—for her health. She would be happy with a marginal improvement in quality of life. But she had a loftier ambition: In six months, her husband was leaving to shoot on location in India, a country she had always dreamed of visiting, and she wanted desperately to go with him. Could I recommend an eating plan that could possibly help her get healthy enough to dare to leave the country for the first time in years?

I've always felt that the wonderful thing about nutrition is the way it treats everything at once, not attacking individual ailments, like an antibiotic, but strengthening the body's systems to enable every element to do its job. I had a visionary moment where I saw Susanna not as a shattered battleground for a war chest's worth of prescriptions and treatments, but as a strong, integrated, whole person working at top natural power to fight off intruding illnesses and acquire a new lease on life. I saw her exploring India, the dark circles beneath her eyes wiped away by good health and the excitement of her adventure. This picture was the gift I wanted to give Susanna.

Susanna's current diet was unremarkable but typically American: lots of things out of packages and cans, junk food, and eating on the run. She was a child of the big city with hurried urban eating habits, and she just didn't pay much attention. Likewise, she took little notice of her exercise or relaxation activities, doing only what she could "manage" between medical crises. She admitted that after so many years of betrayal by her body, she had started to feel alienated from it. But she was yearning to reunite with her physical self and feel at home in the earthly vessel she had been awarded at birth. After suffering for so long, she saw this as her destiny.

I started Susanna out with a bang: a month on an immune-boosting diet that cut out all yeast-producing foods, such as wheat, sweets, refined carbohydrates, yeasted breads, most fruits, and anything processed, focusing instead on whole grains, organic vegetables, and the purest poultry and seafood. I eased the transition by recommending a routine of yoga and meditation to make her increasingly mindful of her body's needs, and achieve the state of deep relaxation that creates the best space for healing. Mind and body would work together to go where medication couldn't reach: a holistic sense of wellness.

Susanna embraced her new meal plan enthusiastically and worked with the fervor of a zealot to get in touch with her thoughts and physical feelings. The result was like a miracle: a complete and dramatic turnaround in her health and energy. An immediate surge of strength inspired her to stop taking antibiotics (under her doctor's supervision, of course), which in turn energized her even more. She didn't succumb to sickness all month. Susanna's body was clearly buying this new line of treatment. But then came the inevitable moment of culinary truth.

"I really, truly want to do this," said Susanna. "I *believe* that this is the right way to eat. My mind knows it. My body knows it. But if I have to look at one more plate of grilled chicken, brown rice, and carrots, I swear I'm going to scream." Susanna had reached yeast-free burnout. I wasn't surprised—most people do.

Nor was I worried. Susanna's body was strong enough now to fight its own fights, without such a restricted diet. What it wanted was a variety of whole, unprocessed foods, including fruit, whole wheat, and all the superfoods that boost immunity and promote longevity with naturally occurring vitamins and phytochemicals. I sent her off to the organic markets and health food stores to buy the most wonderful natural foods. I gave her a superfoods shopping list literally dripping with vitamins and health-enhancing properties. We celebrated each time she erased a doctor's number from her telephone speed-dial and substituted that of a friend or family member. And before long I was seeing her off to India, where she explored yoga, Hinduism, and tabla drumming to her heart's content.

Susanna came back from her trip feeling healthy and wise. She signed off from the Diet Designs program with a statement worthy of a philosopher from the ancient world. "If yin is my extra sensitivity to the world—which made me sick for so long—and yang is my urge to explore it, then I think they're in balance at last."

✳

The Yin-Yang is on a constant quest for the perfect balance of mind and spirit, inner and outer, light and dark, looking for ways to understand the world and the force that quickens it. You are eager to explore alternate planes and possibilities, experiment with the interaction between self and environment, and embrace enlightened approaches to life, work, relationships, and health—

both personal and planetary. Life on the cutting edge of human possibility and potential keeps you keenly attuned to the music of the spheres.

A sojourning spirit like yours naturally roves the horizon like a free bird, seeing vistas that few others see. But sometimes these pilgrimages through the realms of the spirit, the inner reaches of the mind, and the outer limits of the universe can leave your body far behind.

The bird flies with an integrated effort of instinct and perception. Bring your body into your mind's eye with an eating plan that nourishes yin and yang in perfect balance and accord.

YIN-YANG STYLE

HARMONY	IMBALANCE
+ You are sensitive to the infinite possibility of things.	− You are swept along by sunbeams and subject to the winds of change.
+ You are spiritually attuned.	− You can live life as an out-of-body experience, letting the physical self fall out of tune with the whole.
+ You seek beauty in balance and hope in harmony.	− You live in a postindustrial world ruled by the forces of disequilibrium.
+ You are deeply intuitive and perceptive of energies invisible to others.	− You can be vulnerable and overly susceptible to the forces of the universe.
+ You are questing, questioning, dialectical.	− Your quest can obscure the venerable nutritional truths that have supported human life since ancient ages.

✳

The Mind-Body Connection

Wind is your breath;
The open sky, your mind;
The sun, your eye;
Sea and mountains,
Your whole body.

It's All in Your Mind and Your Body

Contemporary science is finally catching on to what many ancient philosophies have proposed for centuries: that physical, emotional, and spiritual health are intricately and inseparably linked. Happy minds make healthy bodies, and vice-versa. Though our initial fascination with modern medicine and technology caused a swing away from this time-honored understanding and toward a test-tube, cellular-level analysis of health, recent developments suggest that this isolationist approach to healing has been but a blip in the evolution of our self-understanding. Scientific evidence continues to mount in the medical community indicating that the mind has a big say in the body's state of sickness or wellness.

As a nutritionist taking a personal approach to my practice, I've always known about this connection. Much of my counseling work is directed toward helping clients work with their mental habits, thoughts, and feelings to get healthy in their head. Healthy instincts soon follow in their bodies, including natural desires to eat right, exercise, and relax. Such a mind-body approach to wellness, the basis of my Personal Prescription for the Yin-Yang, is known as holistic health.

Holistic health seeks to reassemble the human being, which has been dissected by the science lab into an unconnected conglomeration of organs, fluids, tissues, and bones. While conventional Western medicine treats individual ailments of these parts as isolated problems to be attacked with an arsenal of drugs and surgical invasion, holistic health practitioners address the health of the whole person with natural remedies such as nutrition, exercise, herbs and homeopathic preparations, acupressure and acupuncture, massage, chiropractic, biofeedback, and other stress reduction techniques. Americans are just beginning to tap the deep potential of holistic approaches to everything from basic health management to treatment of major diseases such as cancer.

THE BODY AS WAR ZONE

Have you ever noticed how much of our medical terminology is couched in the words of war? We speak of sickness "attacking" our immune system, of antibiotics "defending" against the invaders, of science "conquering" cancer. Countless children are counseled to rise victorious against tonsilitis with a preemptive strike. Is your appendix acting up? No problem—just remove it, like a pesky political agitator.

No wonder our bodies feel like battlegrounds for hostile forces. With this kind of combative attitude toward health, yin and yang are sworn enemies on opposite sides of the wellness line.

Holistic therapies are designed to help mind, body, and spirit work together to heal and keep you well. The central actor in this process is a sophisticated piece of human technology awarded everyone at birth: the immune system.

Enlightened Immunity

The immune system is a complex network of reactions, secretions, hormones, antibodies, and antigens that are the body's answer to the host of germs and stressful situations presented by the outside world. If you believe that a divine intelligence designed us without doctors in mind, a perfectly balanced immune system should in theory protect and heal us from all kinds of injuries and illnesses. In practice, certain diseases might just be stronger or smarter than the immune system. Even shamans get cancer. But evidence indicates that we might be missing out on much of our natural healing and preventive power. Most people's immune systems are moderately to severely depressed by poor eating habits, stress, and mind-body disjunction.

In prehistoric times, negative emotions usually stemmed from life-threatening situations, like a charging mastedon. In evolutionary accord, the immune system recognizes bad feelings such as fear as potential precursors of physical pain and injury, and responds by clicking into gear. But if these bad emotions stretch out over time, as they do in modern conditions of stress and postindustrial angst, the immune system gets worn down from being in a constant state of alert, and finally goes into recession. Severe and long-term unhappiness actually causes the body to secrete hormones that weaken the immune system, compromising its basic ability to fight off flu, colds, and infections—and, perhaps, killers such as cancer and heart disease.

The brain and the immune system are clearly talking to each other. To live a life of natural health as our original designer intended, we need to find a way to listen in.

Listen to Your Body Talk

> The serene mind
> Like the thread untied
> From the tangled lump:
> I see it in the moon.

There are many ways to eavesdrop on your mind-body conversation. The first step in Eating By Design is to tune in to this voice to find out what your body really needs and how well you're providing it. Remember, as you seek this line of communication, it's not how you get there but what you hear that matters. Here are some possibilities:

- **Meditation** is one of the most portable and ultimately powerful "listening" techniques. There are many approaches offered in books, classes, and meditation centers. Their shared goal is to quiet your mind and let your thoughts flow out by focusing on a sound, vision, or your breathing. Here, in this space of mental quiet, you can truly hear your body.

Many philosophies and religions use meditation to align thoughts, movements, mind, and energy with the force of the universe. For some people, meditation is a profound spiritual experience; for others, it's an effective but simple relaxation technique that promotes the peace of mind and body essential to health. A basic exercise is outlined in the sidebar to get you started.

A MEDITATION

Sit still in a quiet place with your eyes closed. Slowly, starting with your toes and working all the way up to your face and scalp, begin to relax your muscles one by one. As you focus on each part of your body, breathe in deeply; as you exhale, say a "prayer," phrase, or affirmation to yourself that makes you feel calm and positive. Focus on your breathing and your repeated phrase and let every other thought flow out of your mind. Let go of the inner voice chattering about "what ifs" and "did I?" and live only in this moment of peace and silence.

It should take ten minutes or so to complete this exercise. But don't worry about the time. Just be sure to attend to every part of yourself and stay still until your mind is clear.

- **Yoga** is a calming mind-body discipline you can pursue on your own or in a class. The most common and physical (as opposed to spiritual) practice, called hatha yoga, involves long, held stretches and deep breathing. The held positions help to focus the mind on the life force flowing into and out of the body through the breath. Both physically and mentally challenging, yoga is a gentle but deep exercise for mind and body.

Talk Back to Your Body

So, what if you're listening in on your body and you hear it say "Ow"? A fundamental Eating By Design principle is that you talk back, beginning with the basics: Eat well for fitness, immunity, and healing as outlined in your Personal Prescription in Part Three. Exercise. Sleep and relax. Then complement and complete your personal health management program with nonintrusive therapies that mobilize your own healing powers to realign your body and mind.

- **Massage, reflexology, acupuncture, and acupressure** use touch to nourish and destress the body, and treat conditions ranging from tension to organ dysfunction. Acupressure and acupuncture are particularly treatment oriented, as they work by manipulating the meridians that connect to various organs and important physical centers.

- **Biofeedback,** a technique administered with the guidance of a psychologist, physical therapist, or holistic practitioner, allows you to monitor and eventually control your nerve impulses. Electronic equipment makes visual the inner workings of your nervous system; as you watch your internal activities, you work to control them. Biofeedback helps you to get in touch with the physical manifestations of your emotions, and is especially useful for reducing stress and headaches.

- **Herbology** is based on the precepts of traditional Chinese medicine. Properly practiced, herbology draws on diagnostic techniques and herbal formulations dating back two thousand years to stimulate physical functions inhibited by your constitution or lifestyle. Traditional practitioners diagnose patients with the combination of a detailed questionnaire and a look at your tongue, the color and texture of which indicate the state of your energy, systems, and organs. Herbal treatments for both health maintenance and specific complaints are often administered in conjunction with acupuncture and acupressure.

  It's important to note that both the FDA and consumers are justifiably concerned with the unregulated sale of herbs, some of which are therapeutically ineffective, dangerous to your health, or even fatal. The best way to explore herbal treatments is under the care of a certified doctor of traditional Chinese medicine or other reputable health professional.

- **Homeopathy** treats conditions ranging from minor "constitutional" complaints, such as cold hands or insomnia, to a variety of major illnesses using low doses of natural substances that, like a vaccine, are known to create the symptoms of the condition. An ancient Greek and Indian medical practice that translates as "like illness," homeopathy contends that these low doses, obtained through a series of dilutions of substances derived from plants, animals, and minerals, stimulate the immune system to combat the condition and heal the body. Diagnosis and treatment involve a detailed assessment of the individual's health and emotional history, as well as basic traits such as height, weight, coloring, and personality. Properly practiced, homeopathy takes into account both the physical and mental state of the whole patient.

  Homeopathic medicine was resurrected from antiquity in Germany during the 1800s and remains a popular and perfectly legitimate form of health care in Europe today. It was commonly practiced in the United States until the early 1900s, when a surge of technological and pharmaceutical developments industrialized our concept of health care, and the natural and intuitive elements of homeopathy fell out of favor. Despite current enthusiasm for homeopathy as a health care option, training in the field remains unregulated, and it is difficult to assess the skill and experience of practitioners of this complex discipline. Confounding the case for homeopathy are a variety of over-the-counter remedies billed as "homeopathic" but which, lacking the specific, holistic interchange of individual diagnosis, tend to be ineffective, especially over time. Your best bet is to seek out an established homeopathic practice with satisfied patients.

※

The concept of yin and yang is based on balance, uniting opposed forces to form a harmonious whole. Western civilization has done its best to drive a stake between the body and mind, creating a dissipated and disease-ridden society rich in knowledge but poor in the potential of the physical self. As a Yin-Yang, you have the power to mobilize your awareness to reunite body and mind in a productive and integrated system ready to receive all the universe has to offer. You are constituted from everything you feed yourself, including food, thoughts, words, and your relationships with other people and the world. Use your Personal Prescription to create a healthy self and spirit.

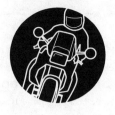

11

THE THRILL-SEEKER

"Between two evils, I always pick the one I never tried before."
—MAE WEST

✳

Skydivers always check their parachutes before jumping out of the plane. Rock climbers use a complex web of gear to keep them firmly anchored to the rock and out of gravity's way. And divers don't plumb the depths until they've learned how to safely return to the ocean's surface.

Shouldn't you be taking the same kind of elementary precautions when you introduce substances to your innermost organs?

✳

I met Bruce via a crackling intercontinental telephone line—a common route of communication for this thrill-seeking free spirit. He was calling from Paris, on one of his frequent forays out of the country as a photojournalist. He had met some of my vacationing clients there at a party; he was just dipping into a mound of steak tartare and mentioning how bored he was becoming with feeling weighed down with food, when his new acquaintances told him they had negotiated France with the help of Diet Designs guidelines.

Intrigued, Bruce called me right up and told me that he had recently quit smoking and seemed to be substituting an appetite for croissants and multiple-meat meals for his nicotine hunger. He couldn't afford to take any extra fat into the field—he'd been shot at on a recent assignment in Sarajevo and couldn't risk moving too slowly—and his current heavy French eating habits were making him feel stodgy and sedated. He needed a quick trim. "But convince me it's not boring. If it's boring, I would just as soon fast, which I'm perfectly capable of doing."

"Fasting is one of the most dangerous things you can do to your body!" I said. Then I rose to Bruce's challenge with a report on the latest research linking a low-fat diet with high energy and enhanced mood, on the many low-fat foods naturally found in cuisines around the world, and on the exciting new low-fat food products now available in the U.S. I faxed Bruce my European game plan, which is adapted to eating customs there. In a return fax, he told me he loved it.

Bruce finished his assignment and returned to L.A., telling me he was bored out of his skull between assignments and that he planned to spend his month of downtime exploring L.A.'s best restaurants. I knew it would be a *healthy* exploration only if I could keep his taste buds continually stimulated and his mind convinced that health and peak physical performance were goals worth pursuing. I gave Bruce the most innovative, flexible meal plan I could dream up and cheered him on through his healthy eating adventures. He ordered a special fish-blackening stove all the way from Louisiana and had the fire department at his door three times as he searched for the perfect charred catfish; he took a camera crew into a Chinese restaurant to investigate the headlines condemning the fat content of Chinese restaurant food in America; he conducted a comparative tasting of octopus in fifteen different sushi restaurants and, after locating an obscure, hotter-than-hot chile pepper in the South American Andes, he took a brief jaunt to Peru to pick up a case.

"Okay," said Bruce as a trip to Korea neared, "what are we going to do about my menus in the land of beef a billion ways and pickled everything?"

I racked my brain for nutritional advice on a cuisine about which I knew virtually nothing. "Go get yourself a book on Korean cooking, take a look at the recipes, and make yourself a list of what to look for—the names of low-fat dishes with vegetables, rice or noodles, poultry, seafood—and what to avoid—oil or fried things, heavy beef, high salt. I think you're ready to figure it out for yourself."

Bruce jumped to the task like a runner to the starting line and came back a few days later carrying a detailed list with both English and Korean food names. "Excellent!" I said. "Now you have a mission—to search far and wide for the best versions of these dishes in all of Korea."

I emphasized to Bruce the importance of packing snacks for his extended days in the field and had him buy a second camera bag for the purpose. The padded, zippered compartments were perfect for protecting fresh fruit and crushable crunchy things. In Korea, I knew Bruce would be able to get fruit and items like toasted soybeans to fill his snack stash.

My work with Bruce was an international education. By the time we were done, I had reviewed menus and selected best bets from the top restaurants in Singapore, Tokyo, Moscow, Paris, Florence, and London. I had helped compile hit lists for the cuisines of Finland, Argentina, and Ethiopia. Perhaps most challenging, I had helped Bruce devise a strategy for nourishing himself while he shot a photographic essay on the roadside diners of America.

Fortunately, I had an easy client. Bruce would eat anything anywhere. With a truly adventuresome and inquisitive palate, he had a whole wide world of food to choose from. He returned from Australia boasting about an outback walkabout on which he nourished himself on nothing but low-fat bugs and slugs; I told him I didn't really want to know. Though he was initially apprehensive about hemming himself in with a healthy eating plan, Bruce turned his willingness to try new things into an exciting exploration in eating well. A little knowledge and a few reminders of the energy benefits of good food spurred Bruce toward the achievement and maintenance of his peak personal potential.

✳

Thrill-Seekers love the excitement of adventure, challenge, and risk. Whether trekking through a faraway jungle, bungee jumping, or speculating on the stock market, they seek thrills and intense sensations. As a Thrill-Seeker, you are an individualist who believes in yourself; you're willing to commit to goals out of a certainty that you can achieve them.

As you explore the unknown, your health and safety are probably last on your mind. Thrill-Seekers don't worry about collisions when they drive one hundred miles per hour, or about frostbite on an Arctic expedition, or heart disease and cancer when they eat. Yet you require enormous energy to propel you through your interesting and active life, and the same healthy eating plan that will provide maximum and long-term energy will also protect you against disease and help prevent some manifestations of the aging process. As you take big chances and thrill to their challenges, why gamble with your ability to embark on further adventures?

THRILL-SEEKER STYLE

THRILLS	CHILLS
+ You are constantly on the go, burning calories by cliff-hanging and other exhilarating activities.	− You live and eat experimentally, without nutritional traffic laws.
+ You are a resourceful risk taker, expert at outwitting the elements.	− You are reluctant to follow rules, consult maps, or read the label.
+ You are exciting, adventuresome, and independent—the last action hero.	− At this rate, each of your actions could be the last.

※

Survival of the Fittest

Darwin's evolutionary maxim is currently in full evidence in America as millions die from not being fit. It seems that in the face of fatty foods and sedentary lifestyles, a good portion of society has lost its survival instinct. Though Bruce could dodge bullets in Sarajevo, he hadn't learned to elude the lipids in steak frites. As the evolutionary law states, only those who continually adapt to their surroundings meet the ultimate challenge: survival.

To be fit is:

- To eat little fat and to carry little on your body.
- To eat plenty of whole grains, fruits, and vegetables for essential energy and the antioxidants, phytochemicals, and fiber that ward off cancer and heart disease.
- To round out your diet with moderate amounts of lean protein for cell construction and repair.
- To exercise regularly for strong muscles, bones, and cardiovascular condition.
- To release or manage stress.
- To have access to medical care and resources to battle injuries and illnesses to the extent of human knowledge and technology.

Many Thrill-Seekers pride themselves on their survival instinct in dangerous situations, without stopping to consider the greatest challenges presented by daily habits and practices. History and the news media tell us the odds are against us. Use Eating By Design to rise to that challenge and turn them to your advantage.

※

Eat to Feel Alive

We have to eat to live—but why settle for that when you can eat to feel really, truly alive? A healthy, high-energy eating plan can heighten the very sensation of being human by sharpening your physical and mental powers, and stimulating your taste buds with the wide variety of fresh and naturally intense foods necessary for nutritional balance.

Consider the following arguments for following your Personal Prescription in Part Three:

- Adopting new dietary guidelines is a great excuse to explore new flavors, textures, and techniques.

- The complex carbohydrates at the base of your Personal Prescription provide the best energy there is for sports, outdoor activity, and other Thrill-Seeking requirements. They fill the glycogen stores that fuel your muscles, so you can sow your wild oats (and rice, and wheat, etc.) every day.
- Dietary fat slows you down by diverting blood from other organs to your stomach as it digests at a sluggish pace.
- Are you carrying extra body fat? Imagine climbing the mountain with an extra twenty-pound pack on your back. Is this your peak performance?
- Most unhealthy processed and packaged foods have been made bland for the average unadventuresome consumer, with flavor and seasonings replaced by sugar and salt. By returning to the fresh, real foods of a healthy diet you can reclaim the intense flavors and textures of fresh produce, poultry, seafood, herbs, spices, and grains. The soft juiciness of ripe mango, sharp tang of fresh yogurt, velvety brine of ahi tuna tartare, and piney bite of fresh rosemary all await you.
- Increasing awareness of the low-fat, low-additive imperative in the food industry has produced a vast assortment of restyled foods that make every trip to the supermarket an adventure.
- Much of today's most innovative restaurant cooking emphasizes healthful, low-fat preparations and ingredients. Only the stick-in-the-muds continue their public assault on America's health.
- Nobody, no matter how strong, smart, or resourceful, outwits or outwrestles heart disease, stroke, or cancer.
- Much of what we consider the "natural" aging process—loss of energy, muscle mass, and skin resiliency; increased body fat; and the onset of disease—is preventable with proper diet and exercise.
- A fit and well-fed body is powerful and ready for anything.

The only time to begin a healthy eating plan is the present. Take this challenge and run with it, and the future will take care of itself.

✳

Eating for health and energy is the great experiment of the coming century, as we deepen our understanding of how food creates mental and physical power. Don't let your freewheeling lifestyle leave you with food lag! Use your Personal Prescription as a map to guide your exploration of the vast Casbah of culinary treasures. Take the plunge into peak performance by using good food to fuel the fire for all your Thrill-Seeking adventures.

12

THE DREAMER

"Dream a little dream of me."

—MAMA CASS

✳

Luella grew up in Georgia, one of six children in a family of genteel lineage but no money to speak of. A beautiful woman, Luella realized in her early twenties that the world was bigger than the state of Georgia, and she set off for Los Angeles in pursuit of her dreams.

L.A. is certainly a land where dreams are encouraged, if not always realized. Luella's first job was as part of the Southern California dream-making machinery, playing Snow White at Disneyland. Though she had never aspired to be an actress, she pulled an ebony wig over her blond hair, posed for pictures with the kids, and patiently awaited her prince.

With her Southern accent and state of mind, Luella fit the role of the debutante perfectly. She was swamped with social engagements, out nearly every night at trendy restaurants with baffling menus. Crostini, sashimi, and chèvre were all Greek to Luella's Georgia-educated palate, so she quickly adopted the habit of letting her date order for her. She ate with curiosity, wonder, and joy. But, like a true Southern lady, she also ate like a bird. She knew that to be rescued from her current straits of being single and poor, she had to be fit and attractive.

Luella's candor and sincerity won her many admirers in L.A.'s social scene. She had plenty of offers for more serious relationships, but nobody stood out as Mr. Right. Nobody had the larger-than-life aura that she had come to Los Angeles to find. Through many witty screenwriters and handsome actors, Luella awaited her destiny.

Luella knew when her prince had come. A globe-trotting businessman, he took her to Paris on their second date. Don was loving, generous, and full of hope for a life with Luella in the unnamed future. There was just one hitch. Don had a wife and family.

When Luella became pregnant, her helpless surprise and happiness inspired

Don to offer his support despite the difficult circumstances. Luella had her lover's illegitimate baby, whereupon he installed her in a mansion with a house-keeper, a nanny, and an annuity. But the demands of his own family and his business made Don's personal appearances less and less frequent. Luella's prince had come and gone, leaving a castle but no masculine presence upon which to lean for the rest of her days.

When I met Luella she was listless and unhappy, rattling around the house with no one but her one-year-old daughter to talk to, and reverting to the culinary comforts of childhood—fried chicken, casseroles, gravy, sweet potato pie. With no admirers at hand, gone were the Southern belle habits of delicate eating; Luella's hearty helpings had added fifteen pounds to her tiny figure. Her upbringing hadn't prepared her for this curious situation, and without a clear understanding of her role or her future, she surrendered to her appetites. "Help me," she implored. "Save me from myself and my stretch marks!"

I immediately put Luella on the full Diet Designs program. At her request, I gave her a daily schedule of meal and snack times, and extra meals for the weekends, when I usually let everybody fend for themselves. Luella was an amazingly gracious and grateful client, sending constant flowers and thank-you notes, referring her friends, and foreseeing a great future for my company. It soon became apparent that Luella would happily eat my prepared meals for the rest of her days if I allowed it, never once reverting to fried chicken as long as she had Diet Designs food in the fridge.

Because I believe that everyone ultimately needs to take some responsibility for feeding themselves, I recommended to Luella that we do a cooking instruction session in which I would give her recipes and teach her the basics of low-fat cooking. As always, she was agreeable. During the lessons, she was warm and receptive, attending to my every word. At the end of three sessions, she thanked me effusively, saying how happy she was to have the recipes, the cooking techniques, and the freshly stocked healthy kitchen. "But, Carrie," she added, "you know I can't do this without you. I can't stand the thought of not seeing you. Can we continue with our weekly consultations, even if I'm cooking for myself?"

Much as I wanted to help Luella through the transition to taking care of herself, I also wanted her to start turning some of the energy she'd been putting into our relationship in a different direction. I suggested that I could continue to see her if she would also join some other weekly activity to expand her social outlets and self-esteem. As we started to review possible groups and classes, Luella told me she'd always been secretly fascinated with martial arts. She hadn't had the opportunity to explore them in Georgia, but L.A. was full of studios. It was perfect. She would meet people and tone her body at the same time.

Six months later, she reported progress in her tae kwon do class, and agreed to move from weekly to monthly consultations. I gave her housekeeper a rotating menu with recipes and explicit instructions for feeding her employer, and now I only hear from Luella two or three times a year.

✳

Snow White, Cinderella, and Sleeping Beauty were all rescued by their princes. But have you ever wondered if, after the wedding, the honeymoon, and the first flush of love, these fairy-tale princesses got fat?

Dreamers have an optimistic outlook on life, expecting the best for themselves and others. As a Dreamer, you are probably upbeat, trusting in your loved ones, and hopeful for a better world. You like to think great thoughts and build castles in the air. However, your castles rarely have a blueprint, and usually require the support of someone else to keep them from tumbling down. And when it comes time to fight off demons, you cry for help. You would rather depend than defend.

Your rich fantasy life might keep you out of touch with the realities of here and now, including the importance of a healthy self to a happy future. Though you may be in love with beauty, you would rather wait for it than make it happen. Blind Dreamer faith—you dream with your eyes closed, don't you?—that you will be rescued from all evil leaves you susceptible to the nutritional goblins of unconscious eating, procrastination, and diet myths. Without a recipe for success, you can float through life without making your dreams come true.

DREAMER STYLE

DREAMS	DEMONS
+ You think lily-white thoughts about the world and other people.	− You fall easy prey to frogs in princes' clothing.
+ You dream of a beautiful and happy future.	− You are slow to wake up and smell the coffee in the present—is it burning?
+ You love to love and be loved.	− You hate to make hard choices.
+ Hope springs eternal in your wait for the knight in shining armor.	− You could be waiting for Godot.

✳

Dream a Little Dream of Perfect Health

The Allegory of the Diet Deluder

Once upon a time, there was an innocent young maiden who had an unfortunate encounter with a burger, shake, and fries while on a date with her boyfriend. Bursting out of her ball gown the week before the big event, she packed
her saddlebags with all the wealth of her father's kingdom and set out in search
of a solution.

Following the clues in magazine ads, the maiden visited many meccas of diet
magic, begging each guru for the secret to quickie weight loss so that she could
go to the ball in her fabulous gown. Many pills, powders, drinks, and enzymatic
concoctions later, she returned home five pounds lighter with her father's fortune spent. She had a lovely time at the ball until she confronted the banquet
table. Deprived of solid food for a week, she fell to the wild boar and mead with
enthusiasm, devouring nonstop until she split a seam and fled the scene in
shame and disgrace. Thus abruptly ended the maiden's social season.

Dreamers love the stuff of myth and legend, including tall tales of diet witch-
craft. I've met many diet deluders in my practice who are drawn to the romantic
possibilities of special solutions to unhealthy eating and body fat—especially
ones that promise to shape you up in time for next week's ball. Plans that work
outside the regular routines of daily life are particularly alluring, promising an
exotic escape from your own imperfections.

Unfortunately, you always have to return to being you. No pill, short-term
plan, or even valiant prince can ward off the invasion of the hot fudge sundae.
Only an understanding of your own hungers and a knowledge of how to fulfill
them healthily will keep you fit now and into the future.

Envision Inner Beauty

So what kind of you do you dream of being? Luella had a vivid and positive
imagination that she could apply to all aspects of life except her physical self.
Though she could imagine a better world on a grand scale, the details of her
own personal picture were fuzzy. She was accustomed to thinking of herself in
the context of other people and circumstances, not as an autonomous, physical
individual. I asked Luella to apply her creative optimism to her own body, to
help internalize her new way of life. The most positive and effective change
begins with a dream.

Here's an exercise to help you dream for health, to start you down the road to Eating By Design:

Picture your most energetic, vital, dynamic, and vigorous self. See yourself as beautiful, healthy, and fit, as attractive as the most attractive person you know, with one major difference: This person is you. See how your unique shape, features, and coloring work together to make one harmonious whole.

Keep this picture for yourself alone. Though others might be looking and admiring, no one is in the picture with you. Your radiance fills the entire frame.

Now let the perfect person in the picture move. Watch yourself breathe, talk, eat, and drink. Witness a healthy you moving through time, changing, learning, and growing. There's no ending to this picture, no freeze frame, but a limitless, happy future.

Gaze into Your Crystal Ball

To complete her dream picture, I asked Luella to tell me her vision of life at age sixty. "Well, there will be a husband, of course, dozens of beautiful grandchildren, and a big house and grounds to hold everybody." And Luella herself? "Oh, I'll age gracefully, with just the occasional nip and tuck. Happiness will make me glow." No wheelchairs, walkers, or gaunt look of disease in the picture? "Gosh no," said Luella, looking slightly shocked.

"Then, Luella, I suggest you lay off the fried chicken and gravy, to make sure your dream lasts a lifetime."

Hope for a happy future is essential to a Dreamer's sense of well-being. When you tell your own fortune, does it include cancer, stroke, or heart disease? If you have a history of any of these diseases in your family or are yourself overweight, any crystal ball that doesn't predict the possibility of suffering from them is cracked or warped. And even if you're fortunate enough to be free of obvious risk factors, statistics show what soothsayers cannot: Hundreds of thousand of Americans die from one of these diet-related illnesses each year.

Fortunately, you can alter destiny. Electing to eat well and maintain a fit body now can contribute to a bright future and help you fulfill your personal promise—all the way through grandchildren and the golden years. Your Personal Prescription in Part Three holds the key to a happy and healthy future.

✳

Make Your Healthy Dreams Come True

Have a Will for Every Wish

Though a dream is a great way to initiate change, it requires waking action to make your dream come true. If imagining is your strong point, then taking action is your Achilles heel. Why? Because in your dreams, action comes in the form of an arriving prince, an outside agent carrying a complete package of solutions to whatever ails you.

In reality, other people may help you toward your goals and dreams, but profoundly personal issues, including how you feed your body, remain yours alone. Once you know how you want to feel, look, and be, you need to formulate a plan to make your dream reality. For every wish, you must have a will. Idealize, then realize.

Take a moment now to make a list of things you truly wish for your body and health. Then fill in the steps you're going to take to get there.

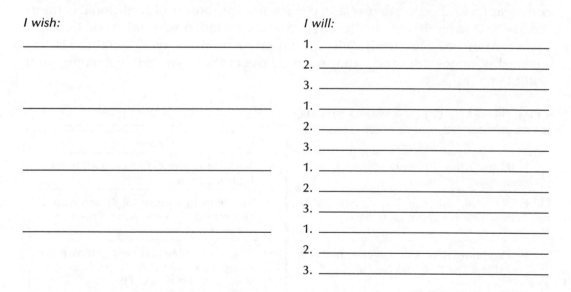

I wish:

_____

_____

_____

_____

I will:

1. _____
2. _____
3. _____
1. _____
2. _____
3. _____
1. _____
2. _____
3. _____
1. _____
2. _____
3. _____

Your Personal Prescription will give you more ideas for turning your wishes into actions and making them come true.

Feeding Your Inner Child

Your childhood and family background shape the way you feed yourself for life. First, childhood relations with your family directly impact your personality, which in turn dictates how you eat. Second, family life is closely intertwined with food. As you grow up, family meals function as a microcosm of the social structure, power relations, and caretaking functions of the household. With every morsel of food, your parents indoctrinate you with their morals, values, expectations—and eating habits. They feed you because they love and care for you, and this message is never lost.

The association of certain childhood foods with comfort and security can be lifelong, especially for the Dreamer. When your happy dreams for the future seem far away, your inner child might want to crawl back into the safety of simpler times. Luella returned to the heavy Southern foods of her childhood when her lover deserted her, roaming the halls of her mansion in a silk bathrobe with a slice of pecan pie. If a bad day has you reaching for a Three Musketeers bar or a mound of mashed potatoes, you are feeding that inner child—not your adult body.

But don't worry. The Eating By Design philosophy on comfort eating is: No problem! Food should nurture and cheer you. The danger of traditional comfort food is that it tends to come in large quantities, laden with fat. Your Personal Prescription provides healthfully grown-up versions of traditional foods like mashed potatoes and gravy that comfort the child in you while keeping your adult body fit.

COMFORT EATING PLUSES AND PITFALLS

DREAMS	DEMONS
+ Familiar foods provide comfort.	− Traditional comfort foods tend to have high fat content.
+ You feel joy and spontaneity when reaching for childlike foods.	− You tend to choose foods and quantities outside of your normal plan when eating for comfort.
+ Psychologically, eating like a child provides a return to simpler times.	− Physically, things are only getting more complicated—you can't get away with what you did as a child.
+ Eating is a safe place to express feelings of vulnerability.	− Eating without good, adult judgment makes you even more vulnerable by lowering your energy, damaging your self-esteem, and aging your body.

COMFORT YOURSELF

Sometimes a slice of meatloaf isn't really what you need. Here are some other ways to comfort yourself when you crave a little TLC:

- A facial
- A manicure
- A deep hair conditioning
- A hot bath
- A massage
- A romance novel
- Gardening

✳

A Happy Ending Is a Healthy Beginning

I've had many clients think they had finished my program when they hit some major marker in their lives—they met their body fat goal, landed the movie role, received the promotion, got married, ended the marriage, or whatever event seemed sure to fix life and make it perfect. As the moment of victory faded and life went on, they often came back, realizing that the apparent ending was just a transition point presenting a whole new set of challenges. The maintenance client has to learn to eat normally without reverting to old high-fat habits; the actor who becomes unnaturally thin for a role has to regain muscle mass instead of body fat to keep him healthy and attractive for the next role; the newlywed has to adapt to the eating habits of a partner; the divorcée has to confront the new challenges of dining alone.

There are no happy endings. There are only healthy beginnings.

PART

2

THE EATING BY DESIGN PROGRAM

Though I work with a melting-potful of different food personality types, a basic nutritional blueprint guides all the diets I design. This section introduces you to the Eating By Design program, my low-fat, high-nutrient, portion-controlled formula for fitness that works for everyone from the most demanding Perfectionist to the most volatile Shooting Star.

You'll begin by taking a quiz to assess your basic nutrition knowledge. Then you'll take another to check your body composition and pinpoint your Eating Quotient—a personalized calorie count to match your body type to your fitness goals. Then you'll learn the Eating By Design Proportions for your Eating Quotient—how much to eat of which foods, and what they do for you. Armed with this unique insight into your body, you'll have all the elements at hand to follow the Personal Prescription for your food personality type.

✳

How Healthy Are Your Eating Habits?

The following quiz completes the picture of your eating style by assessing your current daily eating habits and nutritional know-how. How big a challenge do you face in moving toward health and fitness? Circle the appropriate answer for each question. Choose only one answer unless otherwise indicated.

1. On average, how many servings of vegetables do you eat per day? (1 serving = ½ cup; don't count iceburg lettuce or anything deep-fried.)
   a) 0–2
   b) 3
   c) 4
   d) 5 or more

2. How big is your average serving of pasta?
   a) 1–2 cups
   b) 3 cups
   c) 4 cups
   d) 5 cups or more, or don't have any idea

3. How often do you eat breakfast?
   a) Every day
   b) Usually
   c) Sometimes
   d) Never

4. Which of the following contains the most fat?
   a) 1 tablespoon cheese spread
   b) 1 tablespoon olive oil
   c) 3 ounces turkey breast
   d) 4 Oreos

5. On average, how many servings of fruit do you eat per day? (1 serving = 1 piece, ¾ cup diced, or 1 glass juice.)
   a) 0–1
   b) 2
   c) 3
   d) 4 or more

6. How big is your average serving of meat? About the size of a:
   a) Deck of cards
   b) 3-by-5-inch index card
   c) Pocket rack-sized paperback book
   d) Bigger than a paperback

7. How often do you skip a meal (breakfast, lunch, or dinner)?
   a) Rarely or never
   b) 1–3 times a week

    c) 4–6 times a week
    d) 7 or more times a week

8. Which of the following sugars is metabolized most slowly, resulting in the mildest "sugar rush"?
    a) Table sugar (sucrose)
    b) Brown sugar
    c) Fructose
    d) Honey

9. How often do you choose pasta, grains, legumes or a baked potato as a *main dish?*
    a) 0 times a week
    b) 1–2 times a week
    c) 3–4 times a week
    d) 5 or more times a week

10. How many snacks do you eat per day?
    a) 0–2
    b) 2–4
    c) 4–6
    d) 7 or more

11. When do you usually eat?
    a) Scheduled meal and snack times
    b) When I'm hungry
    c) When I have time
    d) Whenever I feel like it

12. Which of the following fatty foods is most implicated in an increased risk of heart disease?
    a) Pecans
    b) Chocolate
    c) Palm Oil
    d) Olive Oil

13. What do you usually dress your salad with?
    a) Regular dressing
    b) Light dressing
    c) Fat-free bottled dressing (not low-sodium)
    d) Fat-free dressing (bottled low-sodium or homemade), plain vinegar or lemon juice, or nothing

14. What do you usually order at a fast food restaurant? (Circle *everything* you would include in *one single* meal. Imagine what you would order even if you don't generally eat fast food.)
    a) Large burger, sandwich, or salad
    b) Small burger, sandwich, or salad
    c) Baked potato
    d) Baked potato topping
    e) Large order fries
    f) Small order fries
    g) Nondiet soda or juice
    h) Shake or dessert

15. Do you snack?
    a) Yes, regularly
    b) Yes, sporadically
    c) No
    d) Yes, when something irresistible is presented to me between meals

16. Which of the following is *not* a low-fat source of protein, carbohydrates, and fiber?
    a) Soybeans
    b) Black-eyed peas
    c) Kidney beans
    d) Sesame seeds

17. On average, how much red meat (beef, lamb, pork chops) do you eat each week? (4 ounces is a quarter-pound burger, or a piece about the size of the palm of a woman's hand.)
    a) None or less than 4 ounces per week
    b) 4 ounces
    c) 8 ounces
    d) 12 ounces or more

18. In a restaurant, do you usually
    a) Eat the full portions served?
    b) Split portions with a companion or take half home?

19. How often do you eat dinner less than three hours before going to bed?
    a) Every day
    b) 3–6 times a week
    c) 1–2 times a week
    d) Never or on special occasions only

20. Which group of vitamins are called "antioxidants"?
    a) A, B, E
    b) A, C, E
    c) B, K, E
    d) A, D, K

21. How many times a week do you eat a meal out of a package or can? (I.e., frozen dinners, pasta mixes, canned soups and stews, vending machine burritos. Don't count whole, healthy foods like chicken breast wrapped in plastic or fat-free granola in a box.)
    a) Less than once a week
    b) 1–2
    c) 3–4
    d) 5 or more

22. How do you usually negotiate a buffet?
    a) Take small servings of your very favorite foods
    b) Fill your plate once, eating only as much as you want
    c) Fill your plate once and clean it
    d) Make two or more trips to the buffet

23. How do you usually feel when you sit down to meals?
    a) Ravenous
    b) Still full from your last meal
    c) Hearty appetite
    d) Moderately hungry

24. Which of the following foods contains the most sodium?
    a) Stouffer's Lean Cuisine Lunch Express
    b) 3 ounces baked salmon
    c) 1 cup Campbell's tomato soup
    d) 1 ounce Kellogg's Corn Flakes

25. Which do you most often choose as an entree?
    a) Cheeseburger with all the trimmings
    b) Beef, lamb, or pork chops, or a cheese- or egg-based dish
    c) Poultry with the skin
    d) Skinless poultry, seafood, or pork loin, or pasta or grains

26. How do you usually serve meals at home?
    a) Family style, with dishes passed at the table for everyone to help themselves to as much as they want

    b) Served onto plates with second helpings

    c) Served onto plates with no second helpings

27. When you know you'll be out of your normal eating environment at meal or snack time, do you:
    a) Put off eating until you return?
    b) Eat whatever you can find wherever you are?
    c) Search out a restaurant, deli, or store with healthy food?
    d) Pack your own meal or snack, or make definite plans for a stop at a restaurant that you know has healthy options?

28. Which of the following contains the most calcium?
    a) 1 cup yogurt
    b) 1 cup soy beverage
    c) 1 cup broccoli
    d) 1 ounce cheddar cheese

29. What do you snack on most often?
    a) Burgers, tacos, meat or cheese sandwiches
    b) Chips, nuts, cookies, cakes, doughnuts, french fries, muffins
    c) Fat-free products: chips, cookies, bagels, granola bars, pretzels, etc.
    d) Fruit or vegetables

30. What do you usually eat for breakfast? (Circle *everything* you normally eat in *one single* meal.)
    a) Juice or fruit
    b) Muffin
    c) Toast or bagel
    d) Cereal
    e) Milk, yogurt, or cottage cheese
    f) Pancakes or waffles
    g) Eggs
    h) Potatoes
    i) Bacon or sausage

31. How do you usually feel at the end of a meal?
    a) Satisfied
    b) Full
    c) A touch stuffed
    d) Can't even imagine eating again

32. From which of the following foods is iron most easily absorbed?
    a) Vegetables
    b) Fruits
    c) Meats
    d) Seafood

33. What do you usually put on bread or toast?
    a) Butter, margarine, or olive oil
    b) Cream cheese, peanut butter
    c) Fat-free or light cream cheese or ricotta, fruit preserves
    d) Nothing

34. What do you usually eat for lunch? (Circle *everything* you normally eat in
    one single meal.)
    a) Whole sandwich, entree, or entree salad
    b) Half sandwich, entree, or entree salad
    c) Soup or green salad
    d) Deli salad
    e) Roll
    f) Fries or potato chips
    g) Dessert or fruit
    h) Nondiet soda, fruit juice, or alcoholic beverage

35. How many times a day do you eat? (On purpose, and in the context of your
    regular meal plan. Don't count binges or unusual impulse eating.)
    a) 2 or less
    b) 3
    c) 4
    d) 5 or more

36. Which of the following contains the most fiber?
    a) 1 cup brown rice
    b) 1 slice whole wheat bread
    c) 1 cup canned vegetable juice
    d) 1 apple

37. How many glasses of water do you drink per day?
    a) 0–1
    b) 2–4
    c) 5–7
    d) 8 or more

38. What do you usually eat for dinner? (Circle *everything* you normally eat in *one single* meal.)
   a) Salad
   b) Soup
   c) Appetizer
   d) Full entree
   e) Half entree
   f) Bread or roll
   g) Dessert or fruit
   h) Nondiet soda, fruit juice, or alcoholic beverage

39. By what time of the day have you eaten the majority (more than half) of your daily calories? (Adjust times if you live by an unusual schedule.)
   a) 2:00 p.m.
   b) 6:00 p.m.
   c) 8:00 p.m.
   d) After 8:00 p.m.

40. Which of the following supplies the most protein?
   a) 4 ounces chicken breast
   b) ½ cup soybeans
   c) 1 slice whole wheat bread with 1 tablespoon peanut butter
   d) ½ cup cottage cheese

Score Sheet: How Healthy Are Your Eating Habits?

Fill in the number of points corresponding to your answer in the box for each question, then add each column to get your score for the four healthy eating areas. See pages 116 and 117.

Interpreting Your Eating Habits Scores

Food Choices

34–40: Excellent
Congratulations! You're making good choices in your daily diet. Keep it up, and focus on tips for timing and portion control to perfect your design for eating well.

27–33: Good
You're choosing healthy foods most of the time; now it's time to aim for "always."

20–26: Not Great
You could be choosing better foods for health and fitness. Be prepared to make some changes in your daily menus.

10–19: Needs Work!
Prepare to revamp your pantry from the bottom up; you're about to discover a whole new world!

Portion Sizes

9–20: Delicate Eater
You eat like a bird; be sure your food choices and timing are on target.

21–34: Moderate Eater
You seem to have reasonable control over your portions and meal size, but might need to fine-tune your intake to your body's needs.

35–44: Hearty Eater
Your caloric intake is on the high side; are you a field hand or ski instructor?

45–60: Portion Overload
Whoa! The day of groaning boards is over. You need to take a firm hold of how much food goes in your mouth each day.

   For further information on targeting your portions to your body's needs, take the Eating Quotient Quiz in Part Two.

Food Timing

34–40: Excellent
You're fueling your body regularly and frequently, just as it requires for maximum energy and metabolic burn. Just beware of portion overload!

27–33: Good
You're pretty good about fueling your personal machine, but might be mismatching your calorie intake to energy expenditure from time to time.

20–26: Not Great
You're probably going hungry when you need fuel the most, and feeding when you need it the least.

10–19: Fueling Fiasco!
You seem to have forgotten that food fuels your body! Pay close attention to the tips for timing your meals in the following chapters.

Question # **1.** a-1 b-2 c-3 d-4	4	**2.** a-1 b-2 c-3 d-4	1
5. a-1 b-2 c-3 d-4	2	**6.** a-1 b-2 c-3 d-4	1
9. a-1 b-2 c-3 d-4	1	**10.** a-1 b-2 c-3 d-4	2
13. a-1 b-2 c-3 d-4	3	**14.** (Add your total: 2 points for a and e, 1 point for every other item.)	1
17. a-4 b-3 c-2 d-1	3	**18.** a-4 b-2	2
21. a-4 b-3 c-2 d-1	4	**22.** a-1 b-2 c-3 d-4	1
25. a-1 b-2 c-3 d-4	4	**26.** a-4 b-3 c-2	4
29. a-1 b-2 c-3 d-4	3	**30.** (Add your total, 1 point for each item circled.)	1
33. a-1 b-2 c-3 d-4	3	**34.** (Add your total: 2 points for a, 1 point for every other item circled.)	1
37. a-1 b-2 c-3 d-4	3	**38.** (Add your total: 2 points for d, 1 point for every other item circled.)	3
TOTAL	30	TOTAL	17
Your Food Choices Score (10–40)		**Your Portion Sizes Score (9–60)**	

Nutrition Savvy (The correct answers are 4:b, 8:c, 12:c, 16:d, 20:b, 24:c, 28:a, 32:c, 36:d, 40:a.)

34–40: Excellent
You know your nutritional facts! Now just be sure to apply your knowledge.

27–33: Good
You're hip to the healthy eating scene, but could bone up on a few fine points.

20–26: Not Great
A little more knowledge could go a long way toward helping you make healthy food choices. Polish up your glasses and read those labels!

3. a-4 b-3 c-2 d1	4	4. a-2 b-4 c-1 d-3	4
7. a-4 b-3 c-2 d-1	4	8. a-1 b-1 c-4 d-2	4
11. a-4 b-3 c-2 d-1	4	12. a-2 b-3 c-4 d-1	4
15. a-4 b-3 c-2 d-1	4	16. a-1 b-1 c-1 d-2	2
19. a-1 b-2 c-3 d-4	3	20. a-2 b-4 c-1 d-1	4
23. a-1 b-2 c-3 d-4	4	24. a-3 b-1 c-4 d-2	3
27. a-1 b-2 c-3 d-4	3	28. a-4 b-1 c-2 d-3	4
31. a-4 b-3 c-2 d-1	4	32. a-2 b-1 c-4 d-3	2
35. a-1 b-2 c-3 d-4	3	36. a-2 b-3 c-1 d-4	4
39. a-4 b-3 c-2 d-1	3	40. a-4 b-2 c-1 d-3	2
TOTAL	36	TOTAL	33
Your Food Timing Score (10–40)		**Your Nutrition Savvy Score (10–40)**	

10–19: Nutritionally Naïve
Danger—you are eating in the dark! Read Part Two from start to finish, and begin to get friendly with your food and its nutritional content.

✳

How do you score? Don't worry if your results indicate that you're in need of major nutritional first aid—your Personal Prescription will cure you with savvy eating strategies specially tailored to help *you* eat according to Eating By Design principles in a contemporary and metabolically calibrated fat-burning system offering:

- Low-fat foods packed with fiber, vitamins, and minerals.
- Properly proportioned proteins and carbohydrates.
- Personalized portions to key calories to your metabolic needs.
- Fueling intervals for optimal satisfaction and metabolism.
- The right flavors at the right time for maximum gratification, zero deprivation.
- REAL FOOD!

What are the results you can expect to see from following your Personal Prescription for Eating By Design?

- Weight management; fat loss and lifelong maintenance of a lean physique.
- Protection against diet-related illness, including heart disease, stroke, cancer, and diabetes.
- Enhanced energy and stamina.
- Improved inner and outer functions, from digestion, to sleeping patterns, to the appearance of skin and hair.
- Sharper mental performance.
- Increased self-esteem.
- The healthful enjoyment of the natural pleasures of Eating By Design.

13

YOUR EATING QUOTIENT: A Personalized Calorie Count for Your Body's Unique Nutritional Needs

✳

What's Your EQ?

You don't have to be a brain surgeon or even a nutritionist to know that different people require different amounts of food. But it can be much more difficult to know exactly how much food you need to be satisfied while still losing weight or maintaining the body you want. The Eating By Design solution is a personalized calorie count—based on your body composition, background, and lifestyle—that I call your Eating Quotient.

Your Eating Quotient, or EQ, is the amount of food energy you need to take in for *your body.* This no-guesswork equation eliminates the frustration of diets that don't burn fat because your metabolism is slower than the norm, or leave you starving because your body frame is bigger than the national average. Your EQ is the key to matching your diet to your body type and fitness goals.

Compose Your Body

Forget about the numbers on your scale. Your enemy in the fight for fitness and health is not weight, but body fat. Your Eating Quotient zeroes in on the elements of a healthy, attractive body by measuring not just pounds but body composition, or the relationship between lean body mass (bones, muscles, organs, tissues, water) and body fat. By assessing your Body Mass Index, or weight-to-height ratio, and your body frame size, along with age, gender, family background, and activity level, you'll arrive at an Eating Quotient that takes

119

your whole physical structure into account. The Eating By Design goal is to optimize your body composition. (You do need some essential body fat to insulate you from the cold, cushion your internal organs, and regulate hormonal function.)

We accomplish this by using your EQ to key your calories to the needs of your metabolism, the process by which your body burns calories by converting food into energy. A basic Eating By Design principle is to keep your metabolism revved up through interval eating and exercise, because the faster you burn calories, the easier it is to lose weight. As extra incentive, keep in mind that the more you progress toward your goal, the faster your metabolism burns, because lean body mass requires about 25% more energy (or calories) for basic maintenance than body fat. So generally, the higher your lean-to-fat ratio, the higher your metabolic rate, and the more calories you burn simply by being alive.

However, if you try to diet too hard by skipping meals or following a very low-calorie regime, your metabolism immediately acts to prevent starvation by slowing down and burning fewer calories. **Shooting Stars, Nurturers,** and **Lotus Eaters** are particularly prone to the bad habit of starving themselves and dragging down their metabolic rate; **Power Players,** too, can become so goal-oriented that their "power dieting" becomes counterproductive. Following your EQ helps prevent this. See the upcoming chapter on interval eating for more information on eating for metabolic burn.

The metabolic equation states that if you balance energy input and output, your body will maintain status quo. If the balance tips in either direction, you will gain or burn body fat. The Eating Quotient Quiz that follows on page 124 assesses your own unique nutritional needs to find that point of balance, then shows you how to run a deficit for healthy fat burning. Your personalized calorie count is the first step toward Eating By Design.

❋

Calculate Your Eating Quotient

Your age, sex, body composition, frame, family background, and activity level all affect how many calories your metabolism burns. The Eating Quotient quiz will take you step-by-step through each of these metabolic variables. After calculating your EQ, a quick glance at the Eating By Design Mosaic will always show you how much of what foods you should eat each day.

Your Eating Quotient will only be as good as your assessments are honest. You'll begin by measuring your Body Mass Index, body frame size, and activity level. Perform each of these exercises carefully, then plug your results into the quiz to arrive at your EQ.

Better than the Scale: The Body Mass Index

The Body Mass Index (BMI) is a snapshot of your body composition that relates your weight to your height. Though only a rough substitute for a good body fat test, the BMI gives you a way to judge your body composition at home. On the following chart, mark your weight without clothes on the left-hand scale, and your height without shoes on the right. Draw a straight line between the two points, and read your BMI where the line crosses the center scale.

Your Body Mass Index _____

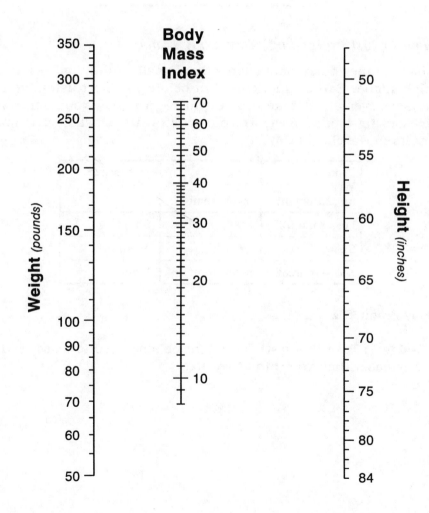

Use the chart below to translate your BMI into your body composition.

The goal of the Eating By Design program is to hit the Fit or Lean zone.

If your BMI is:	Then your body composition is:
Under 20	Lean
20–25	Fit
26–30	Overweight
Over 30	Obese

Big-Boned or Just Pretending? Your Body Frame

Bigger body frames burn more energy than smaller ones, and result in correspondingly higher Eating Quotients. But before you start using big bones as an excuse for overeating, take this test to see just how your frame sizes up: Use a measuring tape to measure your wrist at the smallest part and check your results in the chart below.

Women Wrist measurement	Men Wrist measurement	Frame size
Less than 5½"	Less than 6½"	Small
5½"–6½"	6½"–7½"	Medium
More than 6½"	More than 7½"	Large

Your Body Frame Size ___*Medium*___

Artful Dodgers: Take this test! You might be surprised to discover that your bones are smaller than you think they are.

Moving and Shaking: Your Physical Activity Level

Your exercise habits are a very important factor in your Eating Quotient. In each column, circle the score in the category that applies to your *regular* activity level. Write your score for each column in the blank at the bottom. Add the three numbers and divide by 3 to reach your activity rating.

EXERCISE RATING

Frequency	Intensity	Duration
4 6–7 times per week	**4** High-impact aerobic activity (including running and intense swimming or biking; can be mixed with strength training)	**4** 60 minutes or more
3 3–5 times per week	**3** Intermittent high-impact aerobics (including tennis, racquet ball, squash; can be mixed with strength training)	**3** 30–60 minutes
2 1–2 times per week	**2** Moderate aerobic activity (biking, jogging, low-impact aerobics; can be mixed with strength training)	**2** 10–20 minutes
1 Less than once a week	**1** Light aerobic activity (walking, golfing)	**1** Less than 10 minutes
_____ Frequency Score	_____ Intensity Score	_____ Duration Score

Total Score (Frequency + Intensity + Duration) _____ divided by 3 = Your Exercise Rating: _____ (round fractions downward)

Artful Dodgers and **Shooting Stars:** Don't pad the numbers. **Nurturers:** Your workout schedule might seem too erratic to judge; just use your best efforts. **Perfectionists:** Don't sell yourself short: 59 minutes is close enough to an hour. **Dreamers:** Thinking about exercise is not the same as doing it. But don't forget to count your long walks by the lake. **Power Players:** Can't remember? Check your calendar for all your tennis or golf dates in the past month. **Lotus Eaters:** Don't count excessive, "purge" type exercise sessions.

The Eating Quotient Quiz

Now, with all your metabolic variables measured, you're ready to take the EQ Quiz to arrive at your personalized calorie count for weight loss or maintenance. Simply write the appropriate point value in the blank next to each question.

1. **Age**
   12–18 (4 points)
   18–30 (3 points)
   30–50 (2 points)
   50 or older (1 point)

   1

2. **Sex**
   Male (2 points)
   Female (1 point)

   1

3. **Body Mass Index**
   Below 20 (1 point)
   20–25 (2 points)
   26–30 (3 points)
   30 or above (4 points)

   4

4. **Body frame size**
   Small (1 point)
   Medium (2 points)
   Large (3 points)

   2

5. **Family background**
   Two overweight parents (1 point)
   One overweight parent (2 points)
   Normal weight parents (3 points)

   2

6. **Dieting history**
   I have lost ten pounds or more:
   Never or once (4 points)
   Twice (3 points)
   Three times (2 points)
   Four times or more (1 point)

   3

7. **Activity level** (1–4)

   1

   TOTAL SCORE *14*

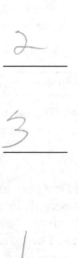

SCORING YOUR EATING QUOTIENT

If your score is:	Your Eating Quotient for Weight Loss is:	Your Eating Quotient for Maintenance is:
7–12	1 Low	1 Low
13–16	1 Low	2 Low–Medium
17–20	2 Low–Medium	3 Medium–High
21–24	3 Medium–High	4 High

DAILY EATING QUOTIENT COUNTS

	EQ 1 Low	EQ 2 Low–Medium	EQ 3 Medium–High	EQ 4 High
Calories	1,200	1,600	2,000	2,400
Carbohydrates (65–70%)	195–210 g	260–280 g	325–350 g	390–420 g
Protein (15–20%)	45–60 g	60–80 g	75–100 g	90–120 g
Fat (15–20%)	20–27 g	27–36 g	33–44 g	40–53 g

How to Use Your Eating Quotient

The only thing you need to do to put your EQ to work for you is make a decision: Do you want to lose fat, or maintain your current body composition? Look back at your BMI at the beginning of this section. Are you in the "Fit" or "Lean" zone? Great! You get to choose whether to follow your weight loss EQ (1–3) to shave off those last few pounds of fat, or, if you're happy with your body, to use your maintenance EQ (1–4) to keep it in its current good shape.

If you're in the "Overweight" or "Obese" zone, use your weight loss EQ to progress toward "Fit." When you reach your goal, take the EQ test again to reassess yourself for maintenance. It's that simple.

The Eating By Design Mosaic and the meal plans in the Personal Prescriptions are keyed to your EQ, with portions appropriate to your daily needs. There's no need to count calories or make unscientific guesses about how much to eat. Your EQ makes for smart nutrition.

Please remember, any written quiz can only provide an estimate of your actual needs. If you follow your EQ for weight loss for a week and find that you're uncomfortably hungry and have lost more than five pounds, try adjusting your EQ up by one level. On the other hand, if your EQ seems to provide more food than you really need and you're losing less than two pounds a week, try adjusting downward by one level. Reassess at the end of a month; you should be comfortable and satisfied, losing about 1–3 pounds a week for weight loss and remaining at a stable weight for maintenance.

How to Assess Your Progress

You can assess your progress on the Eating By Design program any time simply by retaking the BMI test and logging your progress toward the "Fit" or the "Lean" zone. If you move from one zone to another, you should recalculate your EQ—your calorie needs may have changed.

An even more accurate assessment of body composition is a body fat test, which actually measures the ratio of fat to lean body mass. Perfectionists will certainly want to have this done, for the most precise self-profile science can offer. You can have your body fat tested at many health clubs and fitness centers, usually for a fee. The best method is water displacement, in which you immerse yourself in water and compare the volume you displace with your weight. Other ways to test body fat include electrical impedance, infrared beam, and skinfold caliper measurement (less accurate unless used in conjunction with another method).

Your body fat is expressed as a percentage of your total weight. The "fit" range is 18–25% body fat for women, 12–19% for men. If you are a woman with less than 18% body fat, you are lean; 25–30% is generally overweight, and over 30% is considered clinically obese. Lean men have less than 12% body fat; 20–25% is overweight, and over 25% is obese.

✳

Now that you know what your Eating Quotient is, let's find out how to put it into action by talking about my favorite topic: Food, glorious food!

14

THE EATING BY DESIGN MOSAIC: Food Proportions

Every design contains proportions, the relationships between its parts that make it graceful and give it form. This chapter describes the Eating By Design Mosaic, the food proportions that underlie my fat-burning program.

In 1992, the United States Department of Agriculture replaced its Basic Four Food Groups with a Food Guide Pyramid that *introduced* the idea of proportions to the old pie-shaped portrayal of a balanced diet. Based on findings that our high-fat, high-protein diet is linked to numerous diseases, the Pyramid put the complex carbohydrates contained in bread, cereal, rice, and pasta at its base, followed by high-fiber and vitamin-rich fruits and vegetables. The next layer consisted of moderate amounts of lean protein, with fats, oils, and sweets occupying the very tip.

Though the USDA's new design was a big improvement on the proportion-neutral Basic Four, the Food Guide Pyramid was still an oversimplified depiction that failed to distinguish between the fat content, preparation, and processing of different foods in the same category. What, for instance, is the nutritive difference between a hot dog, skinless chicken breast, and a lentil salad? Which should you choose for optimum health and weight management? And how do you know where you stand in the range of recommended servings? If you eat at the upper end, you could rack up 2,800 calories a day even without buttering your bread or sautéing your vegetables in oil. This regime would turn most of us into the Goodyear blimp! My feeling about the Food Guide Pyramid is that its architects got hot in the midday sun and went off to take a premature siesta. The work is unfinished.

The Eating By Design Mosaic goes far beyond the Food Guide Pyramid to tell you which foods work for fat-burning, and how to put them together to meet your EQ. Here are some of the Mosaic principles:

- I group legumes with complex carbohydrates rather than with high-protein foods such as meat, poultry, and fish. Rich in carbohydrates and fiber, legumes definitely deserve a space at the base of a healthy diet.
- I break vegetables and fruits into two separate groups. Both contain valuable vitamins, minerals, fiber, and antiaging compounds. But since vegetables deliver these benefits with fewer calories and less sugar than fruit, I give them extra emphasis, and allow them in unlimited quantities.
- I also break poultry and seafood apart from the daily group, to depict my belief that you should eat from the first category primarily for protein, from the second primarily for calcium.
- To account for the little "add-ons" that make food fun without being nutritionally necessary, I have a special group for extras that lets you indulge in sweeteners and garnishes in a controlled manner. Fun is fine, as long as you account for it!

EATING BY DESIGN MOSAIC

Complex Carbohydrate Group	
EQ:	Servings:
1 (Low)	5
2 (Low–Medium)	7
3 (Medium–High)	8
4 (High)	10

1 serving (about 100 calories each) =
✓ ½ cup cooked grains, pasta, or legumes (white, brown, or wild rice; bulghur; couscous; quinoa; pasta; black, navy, pinto, or cannellini beans, lentils, etc.)
✓ ½ baked potato (sweet or regular), 1 small white potato, or 4 new potatoes
✓ 1 slice white, wheat, rye, pumpernickel, or sourdough bread; 1 English muffin; 1 small roll; ½ pita, bagel, bun, or large roll; 1 low-fat waffle; 1 small or ½ large fat-free muffin; ½–1 fat-free toaster pastry; 2 corn tortillas; 1 flour tortilla
✓ 1 ounce fat-free or low-fat breakfast cereal, oatmeal (uncooked measure), or granola
✓ 1 cup fat-free or low-fat soup
✓ ½ low-fat grain, legume, or pasta cup-of-soup
✓ 1 complex carbohydrate snack (see Master Snack List)

Vegetable Group	
EQ:	Daily Servings:
1 (Low)	4
2 (Low–Medium)	6
3 (Medium–High)	7
4 (High)	8

1 serving (about 30 calories each) =
- ✓ ½ c. carrots, peas, lima beans, broccoli, cabbage, brussels sprouts, cauliflower, summer or winter squash, peppers, tomatoes, mushrooms, corn, turnips, rutabagas, beets, asparagus, string beans, okra, sprouts, etc.
- ✓ 1 c. leafy greens: lettuce, spinach, chard, kale, mustard greens, escarole, endive, radicchio, etc.
- ✓ ½ c. vegetable sauce (tomato, marinara, primavera, etc.)

Fruit Group	
EQ:	Daily Servings:
1 (Low)	2
2 (Low–Medium)	2
3 (Medium–High)	2
4 (High)	3

1 serving (about 75 calories each) =
- ✓ 1 small apple, pear, orange, kiwi, or summer fruit
- ✓ ½ banana, ½ grapefuit, 15 grapes or cherries
- ✓ ¾ c. diced fruit or mixed berries
- ✓ ½ c. juice
- ✓ 1 fruit snack (see Master Snack List)

Protein Group		
EQ:	**Daily Servings:**	
1 (Low)	1	
2 (Low–Medium)	2	
3 (Medium–High)	3	
4 (High)	3	

1 serving (about 150 calories each) =
✔ 3 oz. cooked chicken or turkey breast, seafood, leanest beef, pork tenderloin
✔ 6 egg whites
✔ See vegetarian proportions for protein guidelines

Dairy Group		
EQ:	**Daily Servings:**	
1 (Low)	2	
2 (Low–Medium)	2	
3 (Medium–High)	3	
4 (High)	3	

1 serving (about 100 calories each) =
✔ 1 c. nonfat milk or plain yogurt
✔ ½ c. nonfat cottage cheese or sweetened nonfat yogurt
✔ 1 oz. low-fat cheese (part-skim or reduced-fat)
✔ 1½ oz. nonfat cheese
✔ 1 dairy snack (see Master Snack List)

Extras Group	
EQ:	**Daily Servings:**
1 (Low)	5
2 (Low–Medium)	6
3 (Medium–High)	7
4 (High)	8

1 serving (about 16 calories each) =
✓ 1 teaspoon sugar, fructose, honey, fruit-sweetened preserves, fruit or maple syrup, fat-free fudge sauce, dried fruit, or Parmesan cheese
✓ 1 tablespoon fat-free cream cheese or ricotta, fat-free mayonnaise, sweet fat-free salad dressing, barbeque sauce, fat-free granola as garnish

Water
2–3 quarts a day

Let's summarize how the Eating By Design Mosaic breaks down for each EQ:

DAILY SERVINGS

EQ	Complex Carbohydrates	Vegetables (minimum)	Fruits	Protein	Dairy	Extras (maximum)
1 (Low)	5	4	2	1	2	5
2 (Low–Medium)	7	6	2	2	2	6
3 (Medium–High)	8	7	2	3	3	7
4 (High)	10	8	3	3	3	8

MOSAIC POINTERS

A few reminders on keeping your food low-fat and flavorful:

- No butter, oil, cream, mayonnaise, or fried foods.
- Perk up flavors with mustard, salsa, Tabasco, Worcestershire, low-sodium soy sauce, balsamic vinegar, lemon or lime juice, fresh herbs, lettuce, tomato, and onion.
- Use sweet fat-free salad dressings and fat-free mayonnaise in accordance with the servings in the Extras Group. Unsweetened fat-free dressings (vinaigrettes, etc.) are "free."

The Personal Prescriptions in Part Three will provide you with a meal plan utilizing the Eating By Design Mosaic and specially tailored to your food personality type and EQ. So you don't need to memorize these proportions. Use them to acquaint yourself with the program's basic principles, and, if you wish, to make substitutions in your meal plan. You can't go wrong if you use your EQ!

✳

I know, you're burning with curiosity: What do all these foods actually *do* in my body? Why can't I go on a diet of nothing but baked potatoes or nonfat yogurt? Is protein a dirty word? Why do you favor seafood over beef? And what is all the flap about antioxidants and other multisyllabic words? Reading the constant barrage of magazine articles on these topics can feel like taking one of those superauthentic, go-native trips abroad, only to suddenly realize you don't speak the language.

Here, then, is a brief nutritional tour of the Eating By Design Mosaic, the tourist-friendly type of trip where you don't even have to get off the bus. Just look out the window and see the sights.

✳

Water, the Staff of Life

The majority of your body is composed of water—60–65% for men, 50–60% for women. Water carries nutrients to cells and flushes them of waste, and provides your basic internal biochemical environment. It stabilizes blood pressure, regulates body temperature, and provides an internal cushion for organs and joints. And though you might think that your brain is all intelligence apparatus, it's actually three quarters water.

Furthermore, water makes a great snack. Research shows that many people confuse hunger and thirst, reaching for food when water would satisfy better.

You should drink a minimum of two quarts of water a day. Here are some hints on getting your daily drench:

- **Nurturer** and **Soloist:** Keep a two-quart bottle in the refrigerator. Fill it every morning and make sure it's empty by the time you go to bed.
- **Artful Dodger, Blue Rose, Lotus Eater,** and **Dreamer:** Keep a glass at your side at all times. Finish off a tall one every time you think you're hungry.
- **Passionflower:** Explore the wide variety of bottled mineral waters, identifying the differences in flavor by source and mineral mix. Enjoy sparklers flavored with fruit essences (not juice) floating a slice of fresh lemon or lime.
- **Shooting Star** and **Thrill-Seeker:** Carry a bottle of designer water with you in one of those nifty bottle holders. The Thrill-Seeker might prefer an all-in-one bottle with a built-in straw.
- **Perfectionist:** Designate a water glass. Measure its capacity and be sure to drink at least eight ounces every hour during the working day.
- **Power Player:** Take a carafe to all your meetings. Choose mineral water instead of cocktails at social functions—hydration with a mental advantage!
- **Yin-Yang:** Think of water as the liquid analogue to breath. It should be constantly flowing through you, cleansing and purifying.

More than Bread Alone: Complex Carbohydrates

Once considered the dieter's nemesis (remember diets of all cottage cheese and tuna fish but no bread?), carbohydrates are now proven to be 100% nutritionally correct. In fact, these long, branched chains of glucose that form starch or fiber provide the best energy and are reluctant to convert into body fat. Most of the Eating By Design meal plans derive 65–70% of their calories from complex carbohydrates, prepared without added fats. But each food personality type has a slightly different carb profile.

Complex carbohydrates are a **Blue Rose's** best friend, full of soothing serotonin power. **Power Players,** however, have to watch the timing of your carb intake so you don't snooze through a deal-making moment. **The Dreamer** might discover that many of your favorite comfort foods, like mashed potatoes, are based on healthy complex carbohydrates, once you siphon off the fat. **Yin-Yangs** will find lots of carbohydrate superfoods in your meal plans, like lentils, quinoa, and yams. **Lotus Eaters** must beware the carbohydrate craving cycle, but your Personal Prescription will walk you through having your bread and eating it too. **Thrill-Seekers** should remember that carbohydrates provide the most energy for action. Bring on the granola bars; this stuff is *pure fuel.*

COMPLEX CARBOHYDRATE MERITS AND PERILS

Merits:

- Very low-fat and accessible source of energy.
- Gradual release of energy into the bloodstream.
- Whole grains contain fiber, vitamins, and minerals.

Perils:

- Easy to underestimate portion size.
- Can lead to craving cycle in sensitive individuals.

Vitamins by the Pound: Fruits and Vegetables

First the good news: I hereby declare vegetables free foods! Packed with vitamins and minerals, phytochemicals, fiber, and fat-free flavor, veggies are the food of the gods. I never met anyone who got fat eating vegetables—so add them with abandon to any of the Eating By Design meal plans.

Fruits are fabulous too, but nature's way of sweetening them makes them more caloric than their vegetable cousins, so stick to your EQ in this group.

Next, more good news: Vegetables and fruits are enhancing their reputation every day as study after study shows them to have virtually medicinal properties. Scientists have long known that the vitamins and minerals found in vegetables and fruits are required for a huge range of essential life functions, ranging from blood clotting to nervous system control. But exciting new evidence also suggests that natural compounds in these foods have powerful anti-aging properties with major medical benefits.

Focus on Phytochemicals and Fiber

Broadly, these food compounds are known as phytochemicals. Naturally occurring in vegetables and fruits ranging from broccoli to garlic to grapefruit, phytochemicals act to prevent disease, particularly heart disease and cancer. Among the phytochemicals are the antioxidant vitamins C, E, and beta-carotene, which have been shown to neutralize free radicals that can damage cell walls.

HOW DOES A PHYTOCHEMICAL SPEND ITS DAY?

- Helping along in the production of anticancer and detoxifying enzymes.
- Inhibiting tumor growth and lipid oxidation.
- Binding cholesterol and bile acids.
- Lowering cholesterol.

The only good deed phytochemicals don't do is help little old ladies across the street!

WHERE DO PHYTOCHEMICALS LIVE?

Phytochemicals seem to take up residence in just about all the fruits and vegetables, but the highest population densities are in the following:

- Broccoli, cabbage, cauliflower, brussels sprouts.
- Onions, garlic, scallions.
- Yellow and orange fruits and vegetables.
- Dark greens.
- Citrus fruits.
- Soybeans.
- Whole grain cereals.

Fruits and vegetables are also diamonds in the rough, full of fiber (or "roughage," as our mothers used to say), which fills you up while fending off troubles ranging from digestive disorders to colon cancer.

FIBER FACTS

Fiber is a noncaloric substance of two types:

- Insoluble fiber passes essentially intact through the digestive system, cleaning it out like a Brillo pad. It also absorbs water and expands in the stomach, making you feel full. Whole grains, wheat bran, celery, beets, and lentils are good sources of insoluble fiber.
- Soluble fiber, so named because it dissolves in water, flushes cholesterol and carcinogens from the blood. It also slows the release of glucose into the bloodstream, leaving you satisfied longer after eating. Soluble fiber is found in oat bran, citrus fruits, and legumes.

The government recommends 25 grams of dietary fiber per day. As a benchmark, note that ⅓ cup of dry oatmeal or one medium apple contains 3 grams of fiber. Food labels are now required to disclose fiber content.

FRUIT AND VEGETABLE MERITS AND PERILS

Merits:
- Intense fat-free flavors.
- Vitamins and minerals, including antioxidants and phytochemicals.
- Fiber and great filling power.
- Low in calories.

Perils:
- Some people have trouble digesting certain fruits or vegetables. Cooking often solves this problem.
- The calories in fruits, juices, and smoothies can mount up if consumed indiscriminately.

Yin-Yangs love the "superfood" properties of fruits and vegetables, and your Personal Prescription gives you free rein for exploration. **Shooting Stars** and **Dreamers** will discover the joys of the perfect salad, while **Thrill-Seekers** and **Soloists** will focus on quick and efficient ways to get your daily dose. The **Blue Rose** and **Power Player** will be happy to learn that vegetables don't interfere with the neurotransmitter activation built into your diets, and you can always add them to any meal you like. The **Artful Dodger** uses vegetables as the first line of defense against diet sabotage, and the **Nurturer** can match the kids snack for snack—as long as you choose carrots!

The Building Blocks of the Body: Protein

Many people are puzzled by protein. The meat-heavy diet of the American majority has caused justifiable concern about the overload of fat and calories that goes along with it. But proteins, the building blocks of cells and body tissues, are an indispensible element of the human diet. Absolutely everybody needs them.

Proteins make up your organs, tissues, blood, hormonal and immune systems, skin, and other parts of the body. They are composed of amino acids, many of which are produced by your body, but eight of which, called the "essential" amino acids, must come from your diet. Complete protein foods, including meat, poultry, seafood, dairy, and eggs, contain all eight essential amino acids. Plant proteins are incomplete, and their amino acids can only be used in the presence of the missing ones, as provided by another "complementary" food.

PROTEIN POINTERS

- The protein requirement for a 2,000-calorie diet (EQ 3, Medium-High) is about 75 grams per day.
- 3 ounces of skinless turkey breast provides 26 grams of protein, or about one third of the above requirement, for just 115 calories and 0.6 grams of fat.
- Excluding water, 50% of the body's weight consists of protein, in the form of muscle, bone, cartilage, skin, blood, enzymes, and hormones.

All forms of animal protein except skimmed dairy products contain saturated fat and cholesterol. But in its leanest forms, including skinless breast of chicken and turkey, seafood, and lean beef or pork, animal protein can be the most calorie-efficient way to meet your daily protein requirement. Whole grains, legumes, nuts, and seeds in complementary combinations provide protein too, but for more calories per gram. See the Vegetarian Proportions section [pp. 144] for further pointers on getting your protein from plants.

PROTEIN PICKS

Leanest sources of protein:

- Skinless breast of chicken or turkey
- Fish
- Game meats and birds: venison, beefalo, pheasant, quail, etc.
- Whole grains and legumes in complementary combinations
- Fat-free dairy and soy products

Occasional sources of protein (these have slightly higher fat and/or cholesterol contents):

- Salmon
- Shellfish
- Lean beef
- Lean pork
- Regular tofu, soy beverage, soybeans

PROTEIN MERITS AND PERILS

Merits:

- Builds and repairs the basic cells and tissues that constitute the body.
- Produces antibodies for the immune system.
- Regulates the balance of water, acids, and bases in the body.
- Transports nutrients in and out of cells.
- Digests slowly, providing a steady stream of energy and long-term satisfaction.

Perils:

- Saturated fat and cholesterol content.
- Can "crowd out" the other essential components of a healthy diet.
- Can strain the kidneys, which must process the nitrogen contained in protein into urea to be excreted.

Who needs to pay special attention to getting enough protein? Most women, especially **Shooting Stars, Dreamers,** and **Perfectionists,** who are likely to try to live on salad alone. **Nurturers** should try to space protein throughout the day for steady energy during the stress of caring for others. The **Blue Rose,** though concentrating on carbohydrate minimeals, should try to get in the protein servings recommended for your EQ at dinnertime. **Power Players** who use protein for brainpower during the working day should be careful not to overdo.

Got Milk? Dairy Products

Nonfat and low-fat dairy products are the very best dietary source of calcium, a mineral in which many adults, especially women, are deficient. Calcium is a busy mineral, responsible for blood clotting, muscle contraction, nerve function, and strong teeth and bones. Evidence suggests that it also helps to control hypertension (hello, **Power Players!**). Two to three cups of milk or yogurt supplies the daily recommendation of 800–1,000 milligrams of calcium per day, warding off the threat of the osteoporosis that cripples 20 million older Americans each year.

The wide variety of fat-free dairy products now available can substitute for hidden fats, like butter on your bread or sour cream on your potato, that may sabotage an otherwise healthy diet. And as we go to press, soy products are starting to follow suit, with fat-free tofu making its supermarket debut.

FAT-FREE FINISHES

We're skimming the fat off a lot more than milk and yogurt these days. Top a potato or spread a bagel with nonfat versions of:

- Sour cream
- Ricotta cheese
- Cream cheese
- Cheddar, jack, swiss, mozzarella, and Parmesan cheese

SUPPLEMENT YOURSELF

Because many people are not in the habit of eating enough dairy to supply the Recommended Daily Allowances, or RDA, for calcium, I suggest a daily supplement of 500 milligrams. Supplementation is definitely required if you choose to avoid dairy products. I also strongly urge you to take a calcium supplement if your EQ is 1 or 2 (Low or Low-Medium), as servings of dairy in your daily diet only supply about 60% of your calcium requirement.

DAIRY MERITS AND PERILS

Merits:

- The best source of calcium, an essential nutrient in which many people, especially women, are deficient.
- The only complete protein that can be completely skimmed of fat.
- Nonfat dairy products make good substitutes for fatty toppings and spreads.

Perils:

- Unskimmed dairy products are high in saturated fats.
- Dairy is difficult to digest for those who are lactose intolerant.
- Cows treated with antibiotics can pass residues into their milk. Human consumers of such residues might experience reduced response to antibiotic treatment.
- The FDA has recently approved the manufacture and sale of a bovine growth hormone that boosts cows' milk production. Though naturally occuring and deemed safe for humans, the long-term impact of synthetic BGH is still not known.

Fat: Villain, Scapegoat, or Fact of Life?

From fat love to fat phobia, Americans tend to have highly charged opinions of the lipids in their lives. Dietary fats provide the most concentrated source of energy in the diet and transport vitamins, hormones, and fatty acids. You do indeed need them to live—but unless you are a growing infant or have an eating disorder, chances are you aren't deficient. In fact, fat makes up 34% of the average American diet, well above the 10–30% range recommended by most health experts.

THE FAT FLAP: HOW MUCH IS TOO MUCH?

Though everybody agrees that Americans need to lower their fat intake, there is no clear consensus on how much. Here's a synopsis of the recommendations:

Maximum % of daily calories:	Recommended by:	For:
30%	USDA American Heart Association	General health
15–20%	Eating By Design Various diet plans	Health and weight management
10%	Pritikin Longevity Center Dr. Dean Ornish	Reversal of heart disease

Fat in your diet is likely to become fat on your body, both because of its high calorie count—9 calories per gram, versus 4 calories per gram in protein and carbohydrates—and the small amount of energy required to digest it. This "eat fat-store fat" connection exists in every body, but research indicates that some people might be even more genetically disposed toward immediate fat storage than others.

The long-term dangers of an overfat diet include obesity and high serum cholesterol levels, which drastically increase your risk of heart disease, stroke, and cancer. High fat intake is the single most life-threatening dietary practice you can participate in—and one that can catch you by surprise. Fat seems to be invisible and everywhere. But don't panic. High-fat eating is a highly preventable problem.

Lower-Fat Eating: Evolution, not Revolution

High-fat eating habits have been built into human culture by an evolutionary desire to eat for as much energy as possible. But to survive as sedentary animals, we need to adapt to lower energy needs. Just as man learned to use tools and cultivate crops, we are currently learning to tame our taste for fat.

It is a proven physiological fact that you can reduce your desire for dietary fat. Recent clinical tests confirm what my clients have reported for years: The less fat you eat, the less fat you crave. The evolution away from fat is further fueled by the talented chefs, food manufacturers, food writers, and home cooks who are developing a diverse lower-fat American cuisine.

The Eating By Design meal plans derive 15–20% of their calories from fat. My practice has proven this to be the magic balance that keeps you satisfied and nourished, physically and psychologically, while weeding the overgrowth of fat taste buds from your palate. Once you clean up your diet, you'll lose the instinct to regress to higher-fat ways. Evolution is just too enjoyable!

THE FAT-TO-CALORIE EQUATION

Look at how quickly fat grams translate into calories:

	Fat (g)	Calories
✓ 2 tablespoons oil (easy to drizzle on your dinner salad)	28	240
✓ ½ cup peanuts (a mere handful while watching the game)	36	428
✓ Jack in the Box Colossus Burger (your fat allotment for 2–3 days)	75	1,095

Compare these counts to the 200 calories in a large baked potato or cup of pasta. Ah, the bountiful virtues of fat-free foods. . . .

Three Degrees of Fat

There are three types of fat in food, each with different effects on serum cholesterol. All are equally high in calories and potentially implicated in cancer risk, so don't make the mistake of adding any of them to your diet with healthy intentions. But the worst fat for your health is the saturated fat found in animal products and tropical oils.

First, a word about cholesterol, a complicated substance misunderstood by many people for its good-bad, Dr. Jekyll-Mr. Hyde function in the body. Cholesterol is a lipid produced internally by animals, including humans. Low-density lipoprotein (LDL) cholesterols in the bloodstream can build up as plaque deposits on artery walls, leading to risk of heart attack and stroke. High-density lipoprotein (HDL) cholesterols counteract this ill effect by flushing LDLs from the bloodstream. It's not certain what impact eating cholesterol has on the cholesterol levels in your blood, but evidence indicates that saturated and polyunsaturated fat might be at least as much to blame as dietary cholesterol for raising artery-clogging LDLs. The upshot? Worry more about the fat than the cholesterol in your diet, in the following order:

■ First-Degree Offender

Saturated fat, found in meat, poultry, whole dairy products, and tropical oils, raises the level of bad LDL cholesterol without boosting beneficial HDLs. Studies show that the "trans" fatty acids created by hydrogenating vegetable oil so they are solid at room temperature act like saturated fat in the body by raising LDLs—so margarine is as bad for you as butter.

■ Second-Degree Offender

Polyunsaturated fat, in vegetable oils such as corn and peanut, raises both bad LDL and good HDL cholesterol.

■ Third-Degree Offender

Monounsaturated fat, found in olive and canola oil, raises HDLs *without* raising LDLs. Suggestions that this quality might have preventive benefit against heart disease have yet to be supported with clinical research, and I believe the other health risks and calorie cost of dietary fat to be too great to recommend it as prevention.

If there is a good fat, it is the Omega-3 oil found in fish such as tuna, salmon, and mackerel. Omega-3 has been shown to protect against heart disease by reducing blood cholesterol and triglyceride levels, as well as inhibiting blood clots—all making fish your very best protein pick.

FAT IN FOOD LABELING

Food labels are now required to use standardized terminology to provide an instant read of fat content. Here's how these terms translate:

Fat-free	Less than 0.5 g fat per serving
Low-fat	3 g or less fat per serving
Fat- or calorie-reduced	25% less fat or fewer calories than the original
Light	⅓ fewer calories or ½ the fat of the original
Lean	Less than 10 g fat (!) per serving
Extra lean	Less than 5 g fat per serving

Note the importance of knowing the serving size, and the original fat and calorie counts for "light" or "reduced" foods. A light version of Häagen Dazs ice cream, for instance, could contain eight grams of fat in a half cup serving.

Don't be fooled by the "percent daily value" column on the label, especially when it comes to fat. These numbers are based on a 2,000-calorie diet deriving 30% of its calories from fat—too many calories for many people, and far more fat than the Eating By Design program!

FAT MERITS AND PERILS

Merits:

- Transports fat-soluble vitamins, hormones, and fatty acids.
- Controls the passage of substances into and out of cells.
- Promotes a feeling of satiety.
- HDL cholesterols in monounsaturated fats flush LDL cholesterols from the bloodstream, lowering serum cholesterol.

Perils:

- High calorie count and stimulation of LDL cholesterol production deeply implicates fat in heart disease, America's number one killer.
- Conclusively linked to obesity, stroke, and cancer.
- Takes up dietary "space" that should be filled with other nutrient-rich foods.
- Is often invisible, added with abandon to processed foods and restaurant meals.
- Coats the palate, preventing you from appreciating the full flavors of food.

Personality Fat Traps

Watch for these fat dangers in your food personality type:

- **Nurturer:** A lot of favorite family recipes and snacks are padded with fat. Keep them out of your kitchen altogether for the sake of your own health and your family's.
- **Artful Dodger:** Yes, fats are invisible, so it's easy to pretend they aren't there. But check out the tangible evidence of their presence: nutrition labels; the way they feel in your mouth and your stomach; the shape of your body.
- **Passionflower:** All those exquisite preparations you live for are likely to be landmines of fat—*until* you assert your own personal aesthetic upon them and recreate them in the image of contemporary cuisine.
- **Blue Rose:** Fat is your false friend—it pretends to satisfy you, but secretly inhibits the release of serotonin that will actually convey fullness and well-being to your brain. Keep it out of the loop.
- **Shooting Star:** You know those elegant little bacon-wrapped hors d'oeuvres at the fabulous parties you love so well? The rich desserts that you nibble at in tiny little bites? The beautiful glistening salads served at your favorite glamorous restaurants? Potential fat traps all. Remember: Fat on your lips is fat on your hips.
- **Perfectionist:** Scrutinize your favorite foods for fat content—but don't overdo it! Remember that *some* fat in your diet, up to the grams specified in your EQ, is okay.
- **Soloist:** Many prepared and convenience foods are laden with fat. Check those labels!

- **Lotus Eater:** Once you get the junk and the repetitive eating out of your diet, the fat will naturally follow. So don't worry—your Personal Prescription keeps your fat intake under control.
- **Power Player:** Your stressful lifestyle increases the urgency of keeping the fat out of your arteries, so be ruthless in your restaurant orders!
- **Yin-Yang:** Beware the fats in many so-called health foods—canola and soy oil, nuts and seeds, and full-fat tofu are all on your hit list.
- **Thrill-Seeker:** There's no telling *what* you'll run across in your travels, fat-wise—so always educate yourself in advance.
- **Dreamer:** In food talk, romantic and old-fashioned usually mean high-fat. Look for the romance in lighter, more contemporary preparations.

✳

Vegetarian Proportions

Since prehistoric times, humans have turned to animal foods for their generous supply of protein and certain minerals. The basic Eating By Design program updates this practice by singling out the leanest animal sources for your protein requirements. However, the program is fully adaptable to a plant-based diet for those who choose to eat low on the food chain for spiritual, environmental, or personal reasons.

A vegetarian diet, like any other, can set fat and calorie traps if you eat excess food to insure adequate protein intake, rely on high-fat dairy and soy products, or use abundant fats and oils in cooking. Careful planning is require to create a vegetarian diet with adequate protein and controlled caloric content.

THE PROTEIN-FAT TRADE-OFF

3 ounces of:	Calories	Fat	Protein
Firm tofu	126	8 g	14 g
Fat-reduced tofu*	90	4 g	8 g
Fat-free tofu	120	0 g	24 g
Cheddar cheese	342	29 g	21 g

The fat-free tofu clearly delivers the most protein for the least fat and calories. But notice how badly the fat-reduced tofu compares—the 9 ounces required to deliver a comparable amount of protein packs 270 calories and 12 grams of fat (an argument for reading the label). You need 5 ounces of regular firm tofu to get the protein in 3 ounces of fat-free, which weighs in at 216 calories and 14 grams of fat. And the cheddar cheese contains your fat allotment for a day while supplying only a third of your protein. Red alert!

*Nutrition numbers may vary.

An additional nutritional challenge of a meatless lifestyle is that all vegetable proteins are incomplete, lacking one or more of the essential amino acids necessary to make the protein available to the body. To provide complete protein, vegetable foods must be eaten in combinations that provide the full complement of amino acids.

COMPLEMENTARY FOOD COMBOS

The following combinations provide complete protein with low to moderate fat:

✓ Pasta with cannellini beans.
✓ Rice and lentils.
✓ Corn tortillas with black beans.
✓ Peanut butter (drain the oil off the old-fashioned style) on whole grain bread.
✓ Chickpea salad with pita bread.
✓ Tofu with sesame seeds or rice.
✓ Hummus (chickpeas pureed with sesame paste).
✓ Eggplant parmesan.
✓ Vegetable egg-white omelette with whole grain toast.
✓ Nonfat yogurt with fat-free granola.

Eating By Design Vegetarian-Style

Use these guidelines in conjunction with the Eating By Design Mosaic to get your portion of protein:

Vegetarian Proportions

Food:		=	Eating By Design Mosaic:

- 3 c. nonfat milk or yogurt *or*   = 1 Protein Group + 2 Dairy Group
- 3 oz. low-fat cheese *or*
- 4½ oz. nonfat cheese
- 6 egg whites   1 Protein Group
- 6 oz. fat-free or firm tofu *or*   1 Protein Group + 1 Dairy Group
- 2 c. soy beverage
- 3 c. complementary vegetable   1 Protein Group + 5 Complex
  combinations (see below)   Carbohydrate Group
- 3 T. Naturade protein powder   1 Protein Group
- 1 vegetarian burger   1 Protein Group + 1 Complex
                                   Carbohydrate Group

- Eat all vegetable proteins in complementary combinations, or at least within the same day:
  - ✓ Nonfat dairy or egg whites with grains, legumes (including soy), nuts, or seeds.
  - ✓ Grains with legumes.
  - ✓ Nuts or seeds with grains or legumes.
- Nuts and seeds are high in fat; limit their use to ¼ cup a day.
- Look for low-fat and fat-free soy products; eat other forms in moderation. In their natural state, soybeans have a relatively high fat content, but are important sources of protein and calcium for vegetarians, and may be anticarcinogenic. Strict vegans who don't eat dairy products must eat soy for protein and calcium; milk-drinking vegetarians should limit their full-fat soy intake to 1 serving per day.
- Take a B12 vitamin supplement; this nutrient is provided only by meat. Vegans should also consider taking a calcium supplement.
- Insure adequate iron intake by emphasizing dried beans and fruits. Get plenty of vitamin C, which enhances iron absorption; avoid drinking coffee and tea, which inhibit it, with food.

THE POWER OF POWDER

Though I generally advocate eating food in its natural state, protein powder can be a great help for vegetarians hungry for more of this cell-building nutrient. The trick is finding one that has everything you want and nothing you don't. Naturade brand wins on both counts. What it doesn't have: sugar, yeast, soy, wheat, or dairy. What it does have: corn and rice bran, apple and pea fiber, rice, potato, barley, spirulina, B12, amino acids, and 100 calories, 22 g protein, 0 g fat, 3 g carbohydrate, and 290 mg sodium per 2-tablespoon serving.

VEGETARIAN MERITS AND PERILS

Merits:

- Little saturated fat.
- Emphasis on complex carbohydrates, fruits, and vegetables provides plenty of fiber and antiaging compounds for health, prevention, and longevity.
- Minimized risk of food contaminants and hormones.
- Morally, personally, and physically preferable for some people.

Perils

- Typical vegetarian food in restaurants, stores, and cookbooks can be full of fats (including saturated fat in whole dairy products).
- Difficult to get adequate complete protein, essential to cells, tissues, life itself.
- Deficiency of vitamin B12, iron, and for vegans, calcium and vitamin D.
- High volume of food required for proper nutritional balance bears high-calorie price tag—and associated risk of obesity—unless you eat very carefully.

✳

Nonnutritional Extras: Sugars, Sodium, Caffeine, and Alcohol

Sugars, Simple and Sweet

Sugars, the sweetest link of the food chain, are also the simplest members of the carbohydrate family. As you might suspect, sweetness and simplicity translate into nutritional emptiness. Like a vacant pretty face, sugar serves only a decorative value to the diet, while increasing your risk of tooth decay and providing a hard sugar "hit" that can lead to fatigue and craving cycles. This is true for any sweetener, including maple sugar, grain-based syrups, molasses, and honey. Nutrition, nil; calories, mucho.

Average per capita sugar consumption in this country is nearly *one cup* per day, representing 20% of our daily caloric intake. I join other experts in recommending that you limit sugars to no more than 5–10% of your daily calories. You'll notice that the foods in your meal plans contain little to no added sweeteners, but I do allow them in many snacks and desserts. Real food shouldn't be loaded with flavor-masking, calorie-adding sugars, but sweet indulgence can have its place. Enjoy sugar in small amounts where it really counts. Your Personal Prescription will tell you more.

There is one sweetener slower to attack your insulin levels than the rest: fructose. Naturally occurring in fruits and currently used in powdered and juice concentrate forms to sweeten a wide variety of foods, fructose must travel to the liver before entering the bloodstream, so its release is much more gradual. Many diabetics can safely digest the naturally occuring fructose in whole fruits. I use powdered fructose at Diet Designs to keep my clients out of the sugar craving cycle.

Sodium, the Salt of the Earth

We come from the sea, and our systems are naturally full of salt, which regulates the body's fluid and chemical balance. But since we've started loading our supermarket foods with salt—75% of the sodium in the American diet comes from processed foods—people are dying of hypertension and related conditions. We are eating much more of this essential mineral than we need.

You perceive saltiness in your food in relation to the amount of salt in your saliva, which is in turn directly related to how much salt you eat. So the more salt you consume, the more salt needed to register on your taste buds. That's right, your craving spirals upward just like an addiction. **Lotus Eaters,** listen up!

Though the relationship between sodium intake and high blood pressure is still not completely understood, reducing dietary sodium has proven effective in treating existing cases of hypertension. Even if your blood pressure is normal, your total sodium intake should be no more than 2,000–3,000 milligrams per day—somewhere around a teaspoon of salt. **Power Players** should be especially vigilant on this front.

The Eating By Design program allows salt and salty foods in moderation; if you have high blood pressure, you should consult your doctor regarding your sodium intake.

SODIUM STATISTICS

Some sodium suppliers are more obvious than others.

	Sodium	% Daily Value
1 t. salt	2,132 mg	71–106%
1 c. vegetable juice cocktail	883	29–44%
2 T. Italian salad dressing	324	11–16%
2 T. barbeque sauce	260	9–13%

Stimulants and Soothers in a Cup: Alcohol and Caffeine

Hey, that beverage you're sipping for a break that refreshes? If it contains alcohol or caffeine, it's actually a mood-altering and habit-forming substance. Do not confuse it with water, the liquid staff of life!

Most health experts agree that one to two cups of coffee per day pose no significant health risk for most people (unless you are pregnant or on certain medications). Though past studies have suggested links between coffee and various cancers, heart disease, osteoporosis, and birth defects, all have been called into question by studies with conflicting, if not contradictory results. I feel that caffeine is a matter of personal choice, but advocate moderation. **Lotus Eaters** should definitely cut it out to liberate yourselves from addition. **Power Players** should keep tabs on your intake, to make sure you're not powering your high-performance work style with caffeine instead of healthier energy sources.

Alcohol is also the subject of recent nutritional controversy, as some evidence suggests possible health benefits from one to two alcoholic drinks per day. However, alcohol damages your brain cells and liver, alters your mood, impairs your judgment, and adds empty calories to your diet. If you choose to drink alcohol, I recommend limiting your choices to beer or wine, drinking in moderation, and counting each one as a snack in your Eating Quotient. **Lotus Eaters,** again, shouldn't even go close; **Blue Rose** should beware; and premenstrual women might want to reconsider that glass of white wine—it might plunge you further into hormonal despair. Pregnant women should not drink alcohol at all.

✳

As form follows function, the Eating By Design Mosaic follows proven nutritional principles to provide the right foods to burn off extra fat, energize your body, and pump you full of natural preventive medicine against life-threatening disease. Stay tuned to see how the Mosaic works for your own food personality type.

15

PORTION CONTROL:
A Personal Imperative

"Enough is enough is enough."
—DONNA SUMMER

✳

Calories Do Count

My Diet Designs clients in Los Angeles have a tremendous advantage in their weight loss efforts: I portion all the food they eat into individual containers in serving sizes targeted to their personal needs. They are never served more food than they should have. By controlling their portions, I control their nutritional balance and their total caloric intake.

Your Eating Quotient is formulated to serve the same purpose, controlling the nutritional mix and calorie count of your daily diet as closely as I do those of my clients. But your EQ, no matter how personalized, is only as good as your portions are precise. If your serving sizes don't correspond exactly to those in the Eating By Design Proportions, your equation will never balance. So the secret to making your EQ work for you as well as it works for Diet Designs clients is portion control.

Portion control is one of the most controversial topics of contemporary weight management. Everybody is rightfully burned out on an outmoded concept of dieting that essentially translates to eating less than everybody else. The deprivation strategy of eating little and infrequently is neither gratifying, sustainable, nor healthful. Tiny bites of food and the rumbling of hunger have made "diet" a four-letter word.

So when we discovered that *what* you eat is as important to the equation as *how much*—that is, that fatty foods make you fat, and fat-free foods *help* to keep you thin—there was a national fat-free frenzy. Would-be dieters downed

PORTION POWER IN THE CALORIE COUNT

Take a look at the way the calories count during a day of fat-free and low-fat foods. In the first column are the portions you might unthinkingly eat, while praising yourself for a virtually fat-free day. But compare those unthinking calories to those of EQ 1, weight loss portions for most women:

	Typical portion	EQ 1 (Low)
Breakfast		
Bran flakes cereal	2 c.	1 c.
Nonfat milk	1 c.	½ c.
Sliced banana	1	—
Orange juice	1 c.	¾ c.
	576 calories	263 calories
Snack		
Fat-free potato chips	4 oz. bag	1 oz.
	400 calories	100 calories
Lunch		
Pasta	3 c.	1 c.
Fat-free marinara sauce	1½ c.	½ c.
Salad	2 c. mixed greens with 2 T. fat-free dressing	
Sourdough bread	2 1-oz. slices	—
	990 calories	290 calories
Snack		
Nonfat fruit yogurt	8 oz.	4 oz.
	190 calories	95 calories
Dinner		
Swordfish	12 oz.	6 oz.
Baked potato	Large (10 oz.) with 4 oz. nonfat sour cream	½ medium (3.6 oz.) with 1 oz. nonfat sour cream
Steamed broccoli	2 c.	1 c.
Entenmann's fat-free cake	4-oz. slice	1-oz. slice
	1,318 calories	489 calories
DAILY TOTALS	*3,474 calories*	*1,237 calories*

The difference between typical and portion-controlled menus adds up to 2,237 calories per day. On your body, that translates into four pounds of fat per week—even with almost no fat in the food!

mounds of pasta and pounds of fat-free cookies and cakes in an orgy of celebrating this new, no-holds-barred religion. Unfortunately, in the furor of the forged license to eat, everybody forgot about the tried and true metabolic equation, which makes its math quite clear: *Calories do count.*

As a result, even though the proportion of fat in our diet has gone down (mostly because the total number of calories consumed has gone up, for all you math whizzes out there), Americans are fatter than ever. Our metabolisms have no choice—they convert those extra calories, even the fat-free ones, into body fat. Observe the following statistics:

- 33.4% of American adults are 20% or more heavier than they should be—up 8% from ten years ago.
- The average adult weighs eight pounds more than he or she did ten years ago.
- Despite all our fat-free foods, 58 million Americans are currently overweight. In a fit of misfired fat consciousness, innocent people are being encouraged to eat limitless quantities of low-fat foods, without regard for the essential fact that any unburned calorie is stored as body fat, whether it comes from an extra rice cake or a bite of steak.

It's true that for many people, simply switching to a lower-fat diet higher in fiber and complex carbohydrates will automatically shave off calories and provide the preventive benefits of a healthier diet. But two in three Americans continue to pay the daily emotional toll and run the serious health risks of being overweight. The Eating By Design program is based on the premise that this is largely due to a lack of portion control.

Portion Savvy: Ignorance Is the Kiss of Death

Humans are the only animal to regularly and systematically overeat. Why? Most of us simply don't know how much we're eating. Who can tell, offhand, what a cup of pasta looks like? Four ounces of chicken breast? How many people realize that a small slice of sourdough contains 100 calories even without a pat of butter, and that if you break a hunk off the loaf you might end up with a piece four times that size?

After years in the weight management business, my conclusion is clear: Most people have no idea what the right-sized portions look like or feel like in their stomachs. Ignorance of the caloric value of the food you eat is the kiss of death to your metabolic balance.

THE HAND-TO-MOUTH MISCOUNT

Studies show that people tend to underestimate what they've eaten by up to 1,000 calories a day. Exceeding your daily energy requirement by this amount adds up to a pound of body fat in just three and a half days! The problem stems less from "forgetting" about that chocolate eclair than it does from misjudging portion size. Being just half a cup off on your serving of rice will add 100 calories to your meal, and chances are you wouldn't know half a cup of rice by sight.

Here are four easy ways to add 100 calories to your diet. Do that every day for about a month and say hello to a new pound of flesh:

- 1 c. dry cereal
- ½ c. pasta or rice
- ½ bagel
- ½ c. sweetened yogurt

But in a busy world full of work and fun, most people don't like to count calories. ("Yes!" I hear the **Shooting Stars, Power Players,** and **Thrill-Seekers** exclaiming.) I've designed the Eating By Design program so that you don't have to count calories. But you *do* have to measure your portions.

Use Your Portion Sense

Personally, I'm quite comfortable going through life with a measuring cup in my hand. Many **Perfectionists** may feel the same way. But if you're not one to break out the scale and the tablespoons in a restaurant or at your mother-in-law's table, then you need to sharpen your serving skills until you can eyeball a plate and pronounce authoritatively, "That's *just my size!*"

How do you do this? Spend one week measuring your servings at each meal and studying them, hard. Visualize what that mound of rice, that fish filet, that bowl of cereal would look like on another plate, in another light, at a different time of day. Note how you feel after eating your proper portion. Concentrate and focus on portions until you carry the information around, encoded in your eyes, your brain, and your stomach. Soon, you'll have a sixth sense for serving size.

Refresh your memory every once in a while with another measuring session. It's amazing how that cup of pasta can grow in your mind's eye while you're not looking. Just like that spare tire that appeared out of thin air!

Portions by Personality

I have yet to encounter a food personality type that didn't benefit from a lesson in portion control. But of course, not everyone has the same portion-related issues. That would be too easy. Here's a brief summary of some of the most burning personality-driven concerns:

- **Nurturer:** If food is love, then it sure seems as if more should be better—but actually it's just potential body fat. DON'T feed yourself every time you feed someone else, pile your plate as high as your growing son's, or have seconds with the rest of the group. You deserve your very own portion size, as reward for all your hard work.

- **Artful Dodger:** Your portion perception tends to be made of smoke and mirrors. Of course this pile of pasta is okay to eat, you say to yourself. That man over there is scarfing down one the same size. And besides, they gave it to me. And I really didn't have much for lunch. . . . Cut short the internal dialogue with an external act: Check your portion against your EQ, and remember that numbers don't lie.

- **Passionflower:** "What?! Cut short a pleasurable experience?" you protest. Yes, you should because there are many exquisite flavors in the world. Stop now for increased enjoyment in the future.

- **Blue Rose:** Constant cravings can result in constant eating, especially if you've cancelled your social plans to stay home and nurse your sadness. Keep *all* your meals small to control your cravings, and stick strictly to your snacking schedule.

- **The Shooting Star:** An instinct toward impetuous gobbling can turn that *taste* of cake into an empty plate of crumbs in a nanosecond, especially if life's little distractions have made you starve yourself by mistake. Master your serving size sixth sense, especially the way your stomach feels when it's flat and just comfortably fed, since your patience with measuring cups won't last long.

- **Perfectionist:** You've probably bought the same size fish filet or frozen yogurt for years, and it might rankle a bit if your EQ asks you to do something differently, or waste food by throwing away the dark meat or sending extra back to the kitchen. But if you want results you can count on, break out the measuring cups—there's no greater peace of mind than portion security.

- **Soloist:** Solo meals come without built-in social limits on your consumption—no watching eyes, no distracting conversation. But that's no problem, because you're strong enough to set healthy boundaries for yourself, with the help of an impartial measuring device to prevent any solitary self-deception.

- **Lotus Eater:** Portion control probably looks like a big enemy, the archnemesis that defeats you every time. Don't worry—ease gradually into your EQ. You'll soon find that it's your friendly guide in satisfying your needs without deprivation or excess.

- **Power Player:** Yes, waiters persist in presenting plates laden with protein and pasta, and you've got more important things to think about than how many ounces you're going to eat. So keep your serving sizes written down in your Filofax or wallet and let someone else—a waiter or assistant—worry about it for you. Meanwhile, remember how oversized meals can slow your synapses and make you less productive.

- **Yin-Yang:** Have you ever downed a huge plate of brown rice and vegetables while discussing matters of the heart and spirit with a dear friend, only to realize that your body feels as full and dull as your mind feels clear and bright? Therein lies the case for portion control—to keep your body as clear as your mind.

- **Thrill-Seeker:** The wide world has a way of offering you more, and more, and more. . . . But while faster is more fun and higher is more thrilling, bigger plates of food will only weigh you down. Carry your visual portion memory with you everywhere—it doesn't take up any extra space and always clears customs!

- **Dreamer:** Happy memories of childhood abundance can make you lose yourself in mountains of mashed potatoes and buckets of warm, creamy gravy. . . . Wake up and dig yourself out with a measuring spoon!

No matter what your food personality type, portion control is an imperative for fitness. Part of Eating By Design is choosing a quantity that works for you. This simple equation of metabolic math will keep you fit for a lifetime.

16

EAT EARLY AND OFTEN

Traditionally, many dieters have made a great show of "saving up" calories for as long as possible through the day, looking forward to the delayed gratification of food as if it were a reward for good behavior instead of fuel for the body.

If you were about to embark on a long automotive trip, would you drive right by the gas pump, telling your car to look forward to a fill-up at the end of the journey?

✳

My meal scheduling philosophy is analogous to the old joke about voting: Eat early and often. Your body's energy needs start with the beginning of your day and taper off as you approach your bed.

Your metabolism's monitoring system is vigilant and pays attention all day long. Just like Santa Claus, it knows whether you're naughty or nice *and when you skip a meal*, and it slows down if it perceives an energy need beyond available calories. The best way to maintain a brisk metabolism is to feed it energy the same way you expend it—in small increments throughout the day, trailing off as you slow down to sleep. Decades of strange diets have distanced many people from the simple good sense of this schedule.

Frequent feedings keep your stomach feeling full and cared for, unlike that grumbling black hole you might have encountered on other diets. This makes the **Artful Dodger** happy, for whom grumbling stomachs can cause grumpy behavior. Another happy recipient of frequent meals is your brain. Small amounts of food eaten at intervals digest more easily than larger, more concentrated loads, drawing less blood away from the brain and other vital organs. **Power Players** know that spreading food intake out over the day keeps your mind alert and ready for action.

Interval eating has other benefits too. It stabilizes your blood sugar to give you maximum, steady energy all day long. For the **Thrill-Seeker,** this means plenty of energy for daredevil activities. For the **Blue Rose,** steady blood sugar spells fewer cravings. For the **Lotus Eater,** it means control over food choices and quantities when you sit down to eat. Interval eating gives the **Soloist** plenty of good breaks to look forward to when time seems to be stretching out into eternity. **Nurturers** are happy for increased energy during crazy days. **Perfectionists** like the reassurance of knowing that they will eat again soon.

Finally, spreading food intake out over the day has been shown to lower cholesterol levels. This is important for everyone, but especially for at-risk and high-pressure people like **Power Players.**

So eat early and often. Don't skip meals, especially not breakfast, and schedule healthy snacks into your day according to your Eating Quotient. Use interval eating to cast your vote for health and energy.

✳

Now you know the principles of the Eating By Design program, including all the nutritional details that inform the Personal Prescription for your food personality type. Read on to find out how to mobilize the Eating By Design concepts in a daily nutritional plan that works for *you.*

PART 3

PERSONAL PRESCRIPTION FOR YOUR FOOD PERSONALITY TYPE

Now that you've determined your food personality type (and subtypes), calculated your Eating Quotient, and discovered the fat-burning principles of the Eating By Design nutrition plan, you're ready to put them all to work for *you*. This section contains a Personal Prescription just for you, specially designed to work with your own quirks, habits, and foibles to make you a naturally healthy eater for life.

You have one dominant food personality type. You have two or three subtypes that color your eating style. Follow the Personal Prescription for your dominant food personality type. As you get to know your food personality better, customize your prescription by mixing and matching with recipes and tips from your subtypes.

You're about to embark upon a personal nutrition consultation that delves into your deepest eating issues and presents easy, sustainable solutions—a way of eating that feels, well, *just right.*

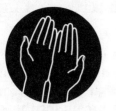

17

THE NURTURER'S PERSONAL PRESCRIPTION

Caretaking requires a cross between the administrative skills of a CEO and the hard labor of a construction worker. In a long career of caring for others, I've learned firsthand the importance of interval eating for optimal energy, portion control, and a well-organized healthy kitchen to keep me going from one crisis to the next. Healthy people give the best help.

Your Personal Prescription is about planning, scheduling, and preparing healthy food on a daily basis for your whole family—*and for you.* It provides a framework for the repetitive task of feeding a crowd of which you are a very important member, and stocking an Eating By Design kitchen that will serve as the center of a family-based healthy lifestyle. As you follow your Personal Prescription, not only will your energy level improve, but you'll find your concerns for your family effortlessly alleviated as you provide them with healthy food alternatives. There will be no more need to worry when your daughter raids the snack cabinet or your husband starts to rustle around in the refrigerator. You know that anything they find will nourish and nurture their bodies, while educating them in one of the important lessons of a lifetime: protecting your health.

An Eating By Design household provides total care for you and those you love.

✳

The Cross-Culinary, Nutritionally Sensitive Dietary Diplomat

Nurturers tend to be dietary diplomats, accommodating tastes, needs, and schedules as diverse as the United Nations. You can use these negotiating skills to move toward a healthy accord for the whole family with a few simple tactics.

161

Care Enough to Share

As you feed your flock, you might find that you shop and cook for a real or imaginary audience of bottomless and unhealthy hungers. If you've ever gone to the store with good intentions and come back with ice cream for the kids, steak for your husband, ribs for the neighborhood cookout, and Brie, crackers, chips, and cookies for drop-in guests, you are a victim of self-sacrificing shopping syndrome. Ironically, this fat-laden basket of goods does more to sabotage than to nourish your loved ones. And though you bought it all for them, you need to eat too, and you will end up with steak and ice cream when you meant to have fresh seafood and vegetables.

The first step toward caring for everybody, including yourself, is to develop a repertoire of healthy foods with mass appeal. If you think of *sharing* rather than *providing* food, you put your own needs on the same plane (and plate) as everybody else's, and avoid the risk of buying unhealthy foods for others and then eating them yourself. Better to find yourself idly nibbling on a fat-free pudding than a Ding Dong.

WHY SHOP SMART FOR YOUR FAMILY?

A recent study of second and fifth graders by Cornell University found the following:

- They all eat too much fat in the form of pizza, macaroni and cheese, cookies, and ice cream.
- Over half are deficient in their fruit and vegetable intake.
- 7% of second graders and 16% of fifth graders skip breakfast—a bad habit for health and hard on the learning curve.

Here's a shopping list specifically targeted toward feeding a family or noshing with the neighbors, including the makings for healthy sandwiches, snacks, and family meals. (For a more complete shopping list designed to thoroughly stock a healthy kitchen, see the Master Market List.) You'll find yourself doubly nourished by nurturing others with healthy foods.

Nurturer Staples (see Master Market List for brand names)
_____ Low-fat breakfast cereals
_____ Nonfat milk
_____ Fat-free whole wheat bread
_____ Pure fruit jams and syrups
_____ Frozen fruit juice concentrates
_____ Nonfat egg substitute
_____ Low-fat frozen waffles
_____ Fat-free or low-fat soup

_____ Low-fat dried soups
_____ Egg- and oil-free pasta, noodles, macaroni
_____ Albacore water-packed tuna
_____ Fat-free salad dressings
_____ Fat-free mayonnaise
_____ Low-sodium barbeque sauce
_____ Whole and ground turkey breast

Family-Friendly Non-Junk Junk Foods
_____ Lite popcorn
_____ Fat-free potato chips
_____ Low-fat cheese puffs
_____ Fat-free pretzels
_____ Baked tortilla chips and fat-free dips
_____ Salsa
_____ Apple chips
_____ Fat-free or low-fat cookies, brownies, and crackers
_____ Frozen fruit bars
_____ Nonfat frozen yogurt
_____ Fat-free fudge sauce
_____ Fat-free toaster pastries
_____ Fat-free pudding
_____ Nonfat and low-fat cheese
_____ Sparkling mineral water

Once you've stocked up, remember to store staples and canned goods in cool, dry cupboards (not over the stove) to prevent nutrient loss.

∗

Take Care of the Caretaker

Feed Yourself First

Nurturers need to feed themselves first to effectively care for others. The trick to eating for your heavy energy requirements is to do so at regular intervals. Three portion-controlled meals and two to five snacks a day (depending on your Eating Quotient), starting first thing in the morning and following a planned schedule, are key to your performance as a provider. Note that while it's important to share a healthy pantry with your household (more on this later), you don't always have to share eating times with them.

To help Sophie remember that her mealtimes and portions might not always coincide with her family's, we wrote them down. You should do the same. Find the meal plan for your EQ in the pages that follow, then practice writing out your schedule in advance, including times and portions, so that no matter what's going on and who else is or isn't eating, you are clear on your own agenda. Then, when you serve food from communal dishes, you'll be conscious of sizing everyone's servings—*including your own*—to individual needs.

✳

The Nurturer Meal Plan*

EQ 1 (Low)

BREAKFAST   TIME_____

½ c. orange or apple juice
1 c. skim milk
Choose from:
✓ ½ or mini Orange Bran Muffin 🗒
✓ 1 oz. cereal
✓ 1 fat-free toaster pastry

LUNCH   TIME_____

Choose from:
✓ 1 Turkey Roll-Up 🗒
✓ 1 Barbequed Chicken Pizza 🗒
✓ Meatloaf sandwich (1 slice Meatloaf 🗒 , 1 slice bread, lettuce, tomato, onion, and mustard)
✓ Tuna sandwich (¾ c. Tuna Salad 🗒 , 1 slice bread, lettuce, tomato)

SNACK   TIME_____

1 piece fruit

DINNER   TIME_____

Raw vegetables
Mixed green salad with fat-free dressing
Choose from:
✓ 1 serving Cheese Lasagna 🗒
✓ 1 serving Southwest Casserole 🗒
✓ 1 c. pasta with ¾ c. oil-free marinara sauce and 1 oz. grated Parmesan cheese

Choose from:
✓ 2 Chocolate Chip Cookies 🗒 or store-bought fat-free cookies
✓ 1 fat-free brownie
✓ Frozen yogurt sundae (4 oz. frozen yogurt and up to 4 t. toppings)

---

* 🗒 = See recipe in Chapter 33.

EQ 2 (Low-Medium)

BREAKFAST   TIME_____

½ c. orange or apple juice
1 c. skim milk
Choose from:
✓ 1 Orange Bran Muffin 📄
✓ 2 oz. cereal
✓ 1 fat-free toaster pastry

LUNCH   TIME_____

Choose from:
✓ 1 Turkey Roll-Up 📄
✓ 1 Barbequed Chicken Pizza 📄
✓ Meatloaf sandwich (1 slice Meatloaf 📄 , 1 slice bread, lettuce, tomato, onion, and mustard)
✓ Tuna sandwich (¾ c. Tuna Salad 📄 , 1 slice bread, lettuce, tomato)

1 piece fresh fruit

SNACK   TIME_____

Choose from:
✓ 1 oz. fat-free potato chips
✓ 4 c. air-popped popcorn
✓ 2 T. Spinach Dip 📄 , Crab Dip 📄 , or 5-layer dip with ½ oz. fat-free crackers or chips
✓ The Master Snack List (Chapter 30)

DINNER   TIME_____

Raw vegetables
Mixed green salad with fat-free dressing
Choose from:
✓ 1 serving Cheese Lasagna 📄
✓ 1 serving Southwest Casserole 📄
✓ 1 serving Apricot Chicken 📄 with ½ c. rice or ½ baked potato and steamed vegetables
✓ 1 c. pasta with ¾ c. oil-free marinara sauce, topped with 3 oz. chicken or seafood and 1 oz.
   grated Parmesan cheese

Choose from:
✓ 2 Chocolate Chip Cookies 📄 or store-bought fat-free cookies
✓ 1 fat-free brownie
✓ Frozen yogurt sundae (4 oz. frozen yogurt and up to 4 t. toppings)

EQ 3 (Medium-High)

BREAKFAST   TIME_____

½ c. orange or apple juice
1 c. skim milk
Choose from:
✓ 1 Orange Bran Muffin 📄
✓ 2 oz. cereal
✓ 1 fat-free toaster pastry

SNACK   TIME_____

½ c. fruit-sweetened nonfat yogurt

LUNCH   TIME_____

Choose from:
✓ 1 Turkey Roll-Up 📄
✓ 1 Barbequed Chicken Pizza 📄
✓ Meatloaf sandwich (2 slices Meatloaf 📄 , 2 slices bread, lettuce, tomato, onion, and mustard)
✓ Tuna sandwich (1 c. Tuna Salad 📄 , 2 slices bread, lettuce, tomato)

1 piece fresh fruit

SNACK   TIME_____

Choose from:
✓ 1 oz. fat-free potato chips
✓ 4 c. air-popped popcorn
✓ 2 T. Spinach Dip 📄 , Crab Dip 📄 , or 5-layer dip with ½ oz. fat-free crackers or chips
✓ The Master Snack List (Chapter 30)

DINNER   TIME_____

Raw vegetables
Mixed green salad with fat-free dressing
Choose from:
✓ 1 serving Cheese Lasagna 📄
✓ 1 serving Southwest Casserole 📄
✓ 1 serving Apricot Chicken 📄 with ½ c. rice or ½ baked potato and steamed vegetables
✓ 1½ c. pasta with ¾ c. oil-free marinara sauce, topped with 3 oz. chicken or seafood with 1 oz. grated Parmesan cheese

Choose from:
✓ 2 Chocolate Chip Cookies 📄 or store-bought fat-free cookies
✓ 1 fat-free brownie
✓ Frozen yogurt sundae (4 oz. frozen yogurt and up to 4 t. toppings)

EQ 4 (High)

BREAKFAST   TIME_____

½ c. orange or apple juice
1 c. skim milk
Choose from:
✓ 1 Orange Bran Muffin 🗒
✓ 2 oz. cereal
✓ 1 fat-free toaster pastry

SNACK   TIME_____

½ c. fruit-sweetened nonfat yogurt

LUNCH   TIME_____

1 c. Cream of Tomato Soup 🗒 , or canned or dried low-fat soup
Choose from:
✓ 1 Turkey Roll-Up 🗒
✓ 1 Barbequed Chicken Pizza 🗒
✓ Meatloaf sandwich (2 slices Meatloaf 🗒 , 2 slices bread, lettuce, tomato, onion, and mustard)
✓ Tuna sandwich (1½ c. Tuna Salad 🗒 , 2 slices bread, lettuce, tomato)

1 piece fresh fruit

SNACK 1   TIME_____

1 piece fresh fruit

SNACK 2   TIME_____

Choose from:
✓ 1 oz. fat-free potato chips
✓ 4 c. air-popped popcorn
✓ 2 T. Spinach Dip 🗒 , Crab Dip 🗒 , or 5-layer dip with ½ oz. fat-free crackers or chips
✓ The Master Snack List (Chapter 30)

DINNER   TIME_____

Raw vegetables
Mixed green salad with fat-free dressing
Choose from:
✓ 1 serving Cheese Lasagna 🗒 with 1 slice French bread
✓ 1 serving Southwest Casserole 🗒
✓ 1 serving Apricot Chicken 🗒 with 1 c. rice or 1 baked potato and steamed vegetables
✓ 1½ c. pasta with ¾ c. oil-free marinara sauce, topped with 3 oz. chicken or seafood and 1 oz. grated Parmesan cheese

Choose from:
✓ 2 Chocolate Chip Cookies 🗒 or store-bought fat-free cookies
✓ 1 fat-free brownie
✓ Frozen yogurt sundae (4 oz. frozen yogurt and up to 4 t. toppings)

Simple Self-Nourishing Guidelines

Breakfast

- Try not to eat breakfast on the run—you're probably up for hours before you leave the house. Keep it simple and have it first thing in the morning.
- Choose a high-carbohydrate breakfast for instant energy. Share fat-free toaster pastries or frozen waffles with the kids.

Snacks

- Interval-eat for maximum helping energy by spacing your snacks evenly throughout the day.
- Every time you open a package of snacks for the kids, pack yourself two portions and put them away for later; don't touch the open bag again.
- Remember that you don't need to snack every time someone in the family does. You might pass the potato chips midmorning without eating any yourself.

Lunch

- While you pack the kids' lunch, make one for yourself if you won't be home.

Dinner

- Keep a bowl of vegetables at hand throughout dinner preparation.
- Split your meal into courses if you need to sit down with more than one set of family members.
- Be very careful with your dinnertime portions. End-of-the-day fatigue and the chaos of feeding others can easily end up in evening calorie overload.
- Measure and weigh everything onto your plate, differentiating your portions from everybody else's.
- Steer family conflicts away from the table to protect everyone's digestion.
- If your clan likes dessert, choose fat-free sweets that you can indulge in too. Remember to count dessert in your daily meal plan.
- Make dinner your last bite of the day. Resist the temptation to fill evening quiet time with snacking. Wind down with a cup of herbal tea and make this moment of relaxation your reward.

WORK YOURSELF OUT

- Take advantage of your rare downtime to join a daytime class—aerobics, stretching, toning, or all three—with a friend.
- Look for a facility with childcare to eliminate a common excuse for skipping your exercise!!

SUPPLEMENT YOURSELF

- Round out your meal plan with a well-balanced daily vitamin and mineral supplement that the whole family can use.

Road Warrior

Now that you know how to plan your eating day, you face the classic nurturing challenge: How do I do this in the context of my nonstop schedule? Sophie practically lived at the wheel of her Bronco, out and about for hours at a time on endless errands and child-moving missions. When she finally returned to her kitchen, she was ravenous and weak, subject to superfluous snacking.

When providing nonstop road service, make sure your meals are as mobile as you are:

- Pack portioned snacks in the car, to make sure neither you nor the kids have a carpool meltdown.
- Keep a bottle of water with you in the car to sip on all day long. Freeze overnight ahead of time to keep it cold.
- Take big bags of air-popped popcorn, fat-free pretzels, rice cakes, or fat-free cookies to the movies and sporting events. Preportion your own snack and let everybody share the rest.
- Take advantage of the healthy alternatives offered at fast food restaurants. If you order carefully, this can be a quick, efficient, and economical refueling stop for you or the whole family. See the Fast Food Guidelines in Chapter 30, and don't be shy—it might not measure up to your home-cooked fare, but it beats skipping a meal!

✳

Power Providing

As a Nurturer, you generally have one advantage when it comes to the kitchen: *You are in control.* Through the subtle power of providing, you can unobtrusively guide your group to healthy eating. There's no need to make a federal case out of your resolve to bring health to the household table. Chances are no one will notice.

- Look for low-fat versions of family favorites. I've included my favorite classics in the recipe section of this book 📄 . Many low-fat cookbooks and magazines on the market also focus on family-style dishes and easy entertaining menus. Look for those with fat and calories listed per serving, with recipes that appeal to your audience.

- Use the Low-Fat Cooking Techniques in Part Four to adapt your recipes to your new healthy lifestyle. Almost any dish can be lightened up to deliver favorite flavors without the fat. Read on for an example of recipe adaptation in action.
- Take small steps. Cut back the butter in the mashed potatoes gradually; serve steak once every two weeks instead of once a week.
- Once you know your healthy repertoire is approved, reveal your trump card and ask for a standing ovation. You deserve appreciation for your feat, and they deserve to know that they're eating well.
- The next time you think, "The way to a man's (or child's) heart is through his stomach," ask yourself: But what is this food *doing* to his *heart*? And how did it end up in *my stomach*?
- If your family insists upon keeping certain forbidden foods on hand, move them to a separate shelf, and do not, under any circumstance, invade that space yourself.

As you feed and care for your children, you are establishing their lifelong patterns of body composition and eating habits. The main predictor of your child's fat future is *you*. If excess body fat doesn't fit into your vision of your children's brilliant careers, now is the time to get them eating right.

In general, healthy babies should double their birth weight by five months, and triple it by age one. Faster weight gain could be a warning sign that you are overfeeding your baby, and should be discussed with your doctor. After age two, keep your children lean and healthy with a wide variety of low-fat food, an education on the role of good eating habits in fueling strong young bodies, and positive adult role models. You have a chance to condition your children's developing taste buds to love pure, honest foods without excess salt, sugar, and fat. Make your family table a forum for learning healthy eating habits.

You also have a chance to teach your children the difference between food and love. This is an important lesson to learn for lifelong physical *and* emotional health.

Recipe Redux

Cutting the fat from your family's food is a great way to lavish a little extra care on them. Here's an example of applying Eating By Design low-fat cooking techniques to rescue one of Sophie's treasured recipes from high-fat purgatory.

Cream of Tomato Soup

3 medium shallots, chopped
2 cloves garlic, chopped
¾ cup minced onion
5 tablespoons oil
4 cups chicken broth
1 cup white wine
1 35-ounce can tomatoes
2 cups heavy cream
1 teaspoon sugar
2 tablespoons lemon juice
1 teaspoon salt
3 fresh tomatoes, peeled and cubed

Portion 1 cup

Calories 350 (81% from fat)

Fat 31.6 g

Protein 4.8 g

Carb. 14.2 g

Chol. 81 mg

Sodium 391 mg

1. Sauté the shallots, garlic, and onion in 4 tablespoons oil until softened, about 8 minutes. Add the broth, wine, and canned tomatoes to the pot. Simmer uncovered for 30 minutes, and transfer to a blender or food processor. Puree the mixture and add the cream, sugar, lemon juice, and salt. Return the soup to the pot.

2. Sauté the fresh tomato in the 1 remaining tablespoon of oil for 2 minutes. Mix slowly with the soup. Warm, and serve.

Yields 8 one-cup servings.

You can redesign this recipe by substituting fat-free chicken broth for the olive oil, nonfat evaporated milk and yogurt for the heavy cream, low-sodium Pomi tomatoes for the standard canned brand, apple juice concentrate for the sugar, and dried herbs for the salt. By busting the fat and salt villains, you'll bring the calories per cup down from 350 to 142, the fat from 31.6 grams (!) to 1.0, and the sodium from 391 to 174 milligrams. Serve this for lunch with fat-free cheese toasts, or ladle up a bowl to warm the bones of anyone home with a cold.

Cream of Tomato Soup (Eating By Design version)

4 cups + ¼ cup fat-free chicken broth
⅓ cup chopped shallots
2 cups chopped onions
3 tablespoons minced garlic
1 cup dry white wine
2 bay leaves
¼ teaspoon dried thyme
¼ teaspoon dried tarragon
½ teaspoon celery seed
1 35-ounce box Pomi tomatoes
¼ cup apple juice concentrate
2 tablespoons fresh lemon juice
1 cup evaporated skim milk
1 cup plain nonfat yogurt
Black pepper
1½ cups seeded and chopped ripe tomatoes

Portion 1 cup

Calories 142 (6% from fat)

Fat 1.0 g

Protein 8.6 g

Carb. 26.3 g

Chol. 2 mg

Sodium 174 mg

1. In a large stockpot, heat 2 tablespoons of the chicken broth over medium-high heat and sauté the shallots, onions and garlic for 10 minutes. Add 4 cups broth, the wine, bay leaves, herbs, and Pomi tomatoes with their juices to the pan. Simmer uncovered for 45 minutes, remove bay leaves, and puree. Stir in the apple juice concentrate, lemon juice, evaporated milk, yogurt, and pepper to taste. Return the puree to the pan.

2. Sauté the fresh tomato in the remaining 2 tablespoons chicken broth for 2 minutes. Add to the soup. Gently warm over medium heat and serve immediately.

Yields 8 cups.

1 serving from the Vegetable Group
1 serving from the Complex Carbohydrate Group

Whether it's cream of tomato soup, taco salad, or vinaigrette dressing, use fat-reducing techniques to negotiate new life for any favorite recipe. Get a head start by studying my low-fat versions of traditional favorites in Part Four, such as Meatloaf in three varieties, or Cheese Lasagna.

Cool Cooking Begins at Home

Sophie told me that she subscribed to Murphy's Law Number 101: If she came home late and too tired to cook, the kids had always conspired to request patty melts and fries from the local burger joint. How could she refuse when she had nothing else to offer?

When the caretaker gets harried, cooking decisions get hasty. You can avoid emergency excursions to McDonald's by planning and cooking in advance, incorporating some mass production into your weekly cooking routine to form the backbone of easy menus:

- Bake one or more whole turkey breasts to serve for supper, then use the leftovers for sandwiches.
- Cook up a big vat of oil-free Marinara Sauce 📄 . Freeze some for later, then use the rest throughout the week:
  —Serve over pasta, either plain or with fresh vegetables, shrimp or clams, or ground turkey breast.
  —Sauce simple grilled chicken or fish.
  —Use a dab to dress up steamed vegetables or sandwiches.
  —Make a low-fat Cheese Lasagna 📄 with fat-free ricotta and part-skim mozzarella.
- Marinate chicken in the morning for easy prep in the evening.
- Make a home-style meal of Country Meatloaf 📄 , doubling the recipe to have leftovers for sandwiches—try it on sourdough with tomato and an extra brush of barbeque sauce.
- Make healthy soups, stews, and casseroles (such as Southwest Casserole 📄 , popular with Tex-Mex fans) in large quantities. Leave most of it in the refrigerator for the gang, then pack the rest in individual servings and freeze for quick meals for yourself.
- Make a pot of pasta for quick and healthy meals. Cook extra while you have the water boiling and store it in the refrigerator for even faster prep. Always keep low-fat sauces on hand, along with add-ins like ground turkey breast, shredded part-skim or nonfat cheese, sun-dried tomatoes, and fresh vegetables.

Rally 'Round the Kitchen

Though you may live to serve, long hours alone in the kitchen can start to feel like exile in Siberia when the rest of the household is happily interacting somewhere else. You might just keep yourself company with extra tastes—and extra calories—while you toil. The best way to promote eating well to your family and prevent excess solitary snacking for yourself is to invite the people you're cooking for into the kitchen. Encouraging others to share in making good food together helps them to gain an appreciation of the planning and effort that go into feeding a family.

Here are some projects to get you started:

- Bake a batch of low-fat Chocolate Chip Cookies 📄 . These are the best bait I know to snag kitchen helpers.
- Single out easy tasks for novices: forming the meatloaf, portioning the marinara sauce into freezer containers.
- Make a bunch of Barbecued Chicken Pizzas 📄 , with each of your helpers taking a turn at kneading the dough. Let everybody get creative with the toppings for a true designer experience.
- Call on a resident "taster" for preparation of each meal. Having the kids taste your work in progress saves you calories, insures that they'll like the dish when it gets to the table, and teaches them to appreciate the flavors of healthy food.
- Make a big weekend breakfast together of homemade Orange-Bran Muffins 📄 , waffles served with nonfat yogurt and pure fruit syrup, or assemble-your-own egg white omelettes with vegetables, herbs, fat-free cheeses, and nonfat sour cream.
- Have a make-your-own sundae party with frozen yogurt, fresh fruit, fat-free fudge sauce, fruit syrups, marshmallow topping, fat-free granola, and light whipped cream. Just be sure to watch your own portions while the gang goes wild!

Extend a Healthy Welcome

Nurturers make great hosts, holding out welcoming hands and platters of food—a tangible symbol of your hospitality. While you wouldn't dream of making brownies to satisfy your personal craving, news of your sister-in-law's impending visit has you melting chocolate and brewing coffee in a flash, unconsciously grateful for the excuse for a treat.

But though buttery brownies might be your old habit when guests drop by, the best welcome you can offer is an assortment of easy, healthy foods that allow you to relax, enjoy the company, and share without sacrificing your own plans. Most guests appreciate a healthy welcome, and will go home blessed with both your good advice and the brand name of the low-fat snacks they loved so much.

- Keep your favorite healthy entertaining foods on hand for unexpected drop-in guests.

- Make a classic five-layer dip with fat-free bean dip, salsa mixed with diced avocado (no more than one avocado per six people served), shredded nonfat cheddar cheese, and nonfat sour cream. Serve with baked tortilla chips.
- Whip up a Spinach Dip or Crab Dip 📄 to serve with pita wedges or fat-free crackers.
- Round out your party platter with fat-free cheese and crackers, fresh fruit and vegetables, and fat-free cookies, along with a selection of mineral waters.
- Air-pop popcorn with spices and seasonings for slumber parties or watching the game.
- Accompany your tea and sympathy with fat-free coffee cake or cookies.

Holiday Time

Holidays can be grand occasions for Nurturers, a chance to cherish your family with the preparation of special dishes. But add up all the holidays—religious, historical, and national—on the calendar, and you'll see several pounds of potential body fat staring you and your family in the face. Frequent festivities can derail the most determined healthy eaters.

Sophie, even after her Diet Designs education, was fully prepared to gain five or ten pounds in the course of the winter holidays. "How can I possibly prepare Thanksgiving, Christmas, and New Year's dinner for my family, host and attend several neighborhood parties, and participate in special church celebrations without adding some holiday heft?" I suggested that Sophie experiment with low-fat versions of holiday dishes, many of which are based on naturally healthy ingredients packed with nutrition and antiaging compounds. This would spare both the cook and her loved ones the agony of New Year's weight loss resolutions.

HOLIDAY PLUSES AND PITFALLS

PLUSES	PITFALLS
+ Festive, sharing occasions.	− Unusual emotional stress.
+ Traditional holiday foods often based on healthy ingredients.	− High-fat holiday preparations and the pressure to overeat.
+ Opportunity to share low-fat lifestyle with loved ones.	− Difficult to alter time-honored traditions.
+ Well-deserved celebration.	− Ill-deserved sabotage of your personal well-being.

No matter how joyful, holidays present special eating challenges exaggerated by the weight of tradition. The first step to functional festive eating is to recognize that you are constantly creating your own living tradition, and the happiest holiday celebrates a healthy life. Here are some hints for putting that idea into action:

- *Don't* try to lose weight during holiday times; you will only add to your stress and temptations. *Do* be determined to maintain your present weight and commitment to low-fat cuisine.
- Scour the holiday issues of low-fat cooking magazines such as *Eating Well* and *Cooking Light*—they're packed with recipes, menus, and techniques for lower-fat holiday fare.
- At Thanksgiving and Christmas, emphasize the naturally healthy staples of the holiday table: potatoes, yams, vegetables, fruits, breast meat turkey, cranberry relish, breads without butter.
- Serve fat-free cakes or cookies. Substitute egg whites for yolks and evaporated skim milk for cream in pumpkin pie and eggnog.
- Experiment with alcohol-free drinks made with exotic fruit juices, concentrates, and sparkling water.
- Use the tablespoon theory: One tablespoon of every dish—no matter what—makes a festive holiday plate.
- Or choose the one indulgent dish you love—gravy, pie, stuffing—and treat yourself to a small portion. Make sure everything else is "legal."

Realize that the bounty of holiday tables is *symbolic* of well-being and togetherness. In reality, you and your family will find greater happiness in moderation than in overindulgence, today and every day.

✳

Empty Nest

Nurturers are so devoted to feathering their nests that they are often at a loss when they find them empty. Watching your children grow up and move out, or losing a spouse or lover, can radically change the details of daily life, including the foods you prepare and when and how you eat them. Loneliness, boredom, and empty time can all interfere with your healthy eating habits. Food might seem like the only comfort or companion in an empty, echoing house. Or eating alone can become too much of a chore, causing you to skip meals or undereat.

If you find the population of your nest diminishing, the best way to get through the transition in good health is to establish new routines that reinstill a sense of predictability and self-nurturing to your mealtimes.

- Establish a new eating schedule that reflects your situation.
- Downsize your shopping! Buy food in small or individual packages: boneless, skinless chicken breasts (wrap and freeze separately), sliced deli meats, cans of soup, pasta-in-a-cup, granola and breakfast bars, eight-ounce cartons of milk and yogurt. Store sliced bread in the freezer and thaw only what you need.
- Use Tupperware and Ziploc bags to freeze foods in individual portions, anything from homemade soups and casseroles to store-bought fat-free cookies or cheese.
- Invite your friends over for special low-fat meals.
- Identify and enjoy your new freedoms. Pick yourself up from the TV tray and go out to a fabulous dinner (see the Restaurant Guidelines in Chapter 30). Reassess your cupboards, refrigerator, and freezer and make sure they're stocked with *your* favorite healthy foods.
- Join a social group.
- Volunteer your services to charitable, community, educational, or arts organizations.

✳

Whether your nest is empty or full to the chaos point, eating well is an affirmation of life, an act of caring for yourself that doesn't require anyone else's approval to be worthwhile and important. Healthy foods for your body will help your generous heart to do what it was meant to do: share and care.

Notes to Myself

Nurturers always have a lot to keep track of and remember, often a little more than humanly possible. You wouldn't go to the grocery story without a shopping list, right? Then don't go into your kitchen without these little reminders posted in strategic spots, like refrigerator and cupboard doors:

- Portion control!
- I shall not push provisions.
- The greatest gift I can share with my loved ones is HEALTH.
- I eat for *me*.
- I am the only one who can take care of the caretaker.

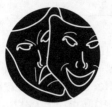

18

THE ARTFUL DODGER'S PERSONAL PRESCRIPTION

The first step of your Personal Prescription is to put the past behind you. No matter how your relationship with food and your personal body image has permutated in the past, there is always the possibility for new and lasting ways of thinking, being, and taking care of yourself that will enhance your daily life and happiness. You have opened one route to that possibility by opening this book. Your Personal Prescription is designed to help you develop your own easygoing approach to eating well that focuses on the process of feeling well, rather than the prohibitions of a dictatorial diet plan.

To prepare for Eating By Design, try using the form below to make a list of your motivating factors. Then ask yourself: Am I ready to make this decision for myself? If not, what stands in my way?

Reasons I want to embark on a healthy eating plan:

For myself:
_____
_____
_____
_____
_____
_____
_____

For others:
_____
_____
_____
_____
_____
_____
_____

Because I "should" (why?):
_____
_____
_____
_____
_____
_____
_____

If you've decided in favor of Eating By Design, it's time to get on with it. To help melt your suspicions away and give you a jumpstart on your Personal

Prescription, I've listed some common fears about healthy eating below, along with my suggested solutions. If you have additional fears, write them down too, along with a possible solution.

Common fears about healthy eating:	Suggested solution:
I won't like the food.	Try some of the foods that sound appealing from the Master Market List in Chapter 30, the Artful Dodger Meal Plan in this chapter, and/or the recipes in Part Four. Read healthy cookbooks or magazines such as *Cooking Light* or *Eating Well*. Are any of these foods or dishes pleasing?
I'll be hungry.	Calculate your Eating Quotient in Chapter 13 and try eating according to the Eating By Design Mosaic for one day, evenly spacing your meals and snacks.
Are you hungry?	Add a snack or serving of complex carbohydrates.
Too full?	Take a snack away.
It will be a lot of work.	Scan your meal plan and the Restaurant and Fast Food Guidelines in Chapter 30 to see how convenient it can be to eat healthfully. Remember that the calorie counts and exact proportions are initially less important than the process of eating healthy foods.
I won't lose weight.	Look at the fit people around you and imagine them twenty pounds heavier. Maybe some of them once looked this way. Everyone can lose weight, even people who never have before.
I won't have energy.	Spend a day eating low-fat, high-carbohydrate foods of your choice. Eat at least four times during the day. This is the kind of energy and well-being you have to look forward to with a healthy eating plan.

I'll go back to my old favorites when I get bored or something goes wrong.

Look at the list of "Legal Cheats" later in the chapter. Trust yourself to continually put the past behind you and move into a healthy present.

_____

_____

_____

_____

_____

_____

_____

_____

_____

_____

_____

_____

✳

Have It Your Way

It may be ironic to adopt the slogan of a fast-food hamburger restaurant for a book on healthy eating, but that company was on to something: You won't eat anything that's not right for you—at least not for long. And I want your long-term commitment just as much as the marketing managers who coined that phrase.

The Artful Dodger Meal Plan below suggests some of the possibilities from which you can choose for an easy approach to healthy eating, complete with the caloric control you need to enhance your health, weight, and fitness level.

But the Meal Plan is just a suggestion. You decide what you like and when. Do you hate turkey? Don't ever have it; chicken and seafood can provide all the protein you need. Love chocolate? Check out the Master Snack List in Chapter 30 for all the luscious low-fat chocolate options. Hate snacking? Skip your snacks and save them for dessert. Love snacking? Break breakfast, lunch, and dinner into mini-meals and eat them throughout the day. Do you prefer to eat a vegetarian diet? See the Vegetarian Proportions section (on page 144) in Chapter 14 for instructions on how to incorporate vegetable protein into the meal plan. You are in control of your eating plan, and no book can ever wrestle that control away from you.

Supermarket shelves and restaurants are now virtually packed with healthy, low-fat food choices. The food industry has done this for you, to empower your healthy self and make it easy to be fit. Forget "deprivation." Go with the low-fat flow. Revel in the abundance of good food and enjoy the feeling of being good.

The Dodger Diet

Here's a step-by-step framework for incorporating easy healthy menus into your lifestyle, nibbling away at your plan by working with a few simple ingredients.

Again, this is just a suggestion. You don't have to do it this way to succeed. But it's an easy approach that you can begin today.

Focus: Breakfast

Jump-start your entry into the world of healthy eating with breakfast, which, just like the cereal advertisements say, is the most important meal of the day. A light and low-fat breakfast wakes up your metabolism, stimulates a sense of well-being, and provides energy for your morning tasks after a long night's fast.

Right Now:

- Serve yourself some fresh fruit or juice.
- Go to your cupboard and scan the cereal boxes. Which one has the lowest fat content? If there's a tie, choose the one with the least added sugar. Add the lowest-fat milk in your refrigerator. Enjoy.

Whether this is your usual routine or a new experience, it's undeniably easy. And the epitome of healthy eating!

Follow-up:

Continue with this breakfast in the days to come. Start to measure your portions: 1 ounce of cereal, ½–1 cup skim milk. By the time this box of cereal is gone, have one or more new alternatives on hand.

Focus: Lunch and Dinner

A quick shopping trip will stock you up for eight easy quick-prep meals that you can choose from interchangeably for four days' worth of healthy lunches and dinners. The mini market list that follows contains everything you need to have on hand. The Dodger Diet does not require the dedication of a martyr!

Mini Market List (see Master Market List for brand names)

- _____ Ground chicken breast (ask butcher to grind skinless chicken breasts)
- _____ Smoked turkey breast
- _____ Fresh or frozen fruit juice
- _____ Eggs
- _____ Lettuce
- _____ Tomato
- _____ Onions
- _____ Assorted fresh vegetables
- _____ Salsa
- _____ Fat-free marinara sauce
- _____ Corn tortillas
- _____ Bread (sourdough or wheat)
- _____ Egg- and oil-free pasta
- _____ Canned fat-free black beans

_____ Tuna packed in water
_____ Canned bean or turkey chili
_____ Canned fat-free vegetable soup
_____ Fat-free mayonnaise
_____ Fat-free salad dressing
_____ Breakfast cereals of your choice without added fats
_____ Frozen entree (no more than 400 calories, 10 grams of fat, 15 g of sugar, and 550 milligrams of sodium)
_____ Frozen spinach
_____ Snacks of your choice (see Master Snack List in Chapter 30 [p. 341])

Congratulations! You've got a great start on the process of eating well. Now nothing can stand in your way. Choose from the wide array of possibilities in your meal plan, personalizing your program until you feel truly content and satisfied. Just don't bite off more than you can chew!

✳

Artful Dodger Meal Plan*

EQ 1 (Low)

BREAKFAST

½ c. fruit juice or ¾ c. mixed berries
Choose from:
✓ 1 Banana Chocolate Chip Muffin 🗒
✓ 1 oz. cereal

1 c. skim milk

LUNCH

1 c. Vegetable Soup 🗒 or canned fat-free vegetable soup
Choose from:
✓ Tuna salad (3 oz. water-packed tuna mixed with fat-free mayonnaise, chopped celery and onion, and any other vegetables and seasonings you like) on mixed greens
✓ Smoked turkey breast sandwich (3 oz. turkey, 1 slice bread, lettuce, tomato, onion, mustard, fat-free mayonnaise)
✓ 1 c. low-fat turkey or bean chili
✓ Joe's scramble (sauté 2 oz. ground chicken with chopped onions and spinach; scramble in 3 egg whites)

---

* 🗒 = See recipe in Chapter 33.

SNACK

Choose from:
✓ 2 fat-free cookies
✓ Master Snack List (Chapter 30)

DINNER

Mixed green salad with Poppyseed Dressing 📄 or bottled fat-free dressing
Choose from:
✓ Black bean burritos (2 corn tortillas, ½ c. canned black beans, and salsa, onions, and tomatoes to taste)
✓ Frozen low-fat entree
✓ Chicken burger (3 oz. ground chicken seasoned to taste and grilled) on ½ bun with lettuce, tomato, onion, mustard, and fat-free mayonnaise
✓ 1 c. pasta with ¾ c. fat-free Marinara Sauce 📄 and 1 t. Parmesan cheese
✓ A Legal Cheat (no more than once a week): A Wendy's burger on a sourdough bun, 1 slice of your favorite pizza, or 3 oz. of lean steak with ½ a baked potato

(*Note:* If you chose a lunch with chicken, turkey, or tuna, select one of the vegetarian dinner choices.)

SNACK

Choose from:
✓ ½ c. nonfat frozen yogurt with ¾ c. diced fruit
✓ A Legal Cheat (no more than once a week): Triple Chocolate Cheat or Glorious Goo Cheat (see p. 187)

EQ 2 (Low-Medium)

BREAKFAST

½ c. fruit juice or ¾ c. mixed berries
Choose from:
✓ 1 Banana Chocolate Chip Muffin 📄
✓ 1 oz. cereal

1 c. skim milk

SNACK

Choose from:
✓ 10 flavored mini rice cakes
✓ Master Snack List (Chapter 30, p. 341)

LUNCH

1 c. Vegetable Soup 📄 or canned fat-free vegetable soup
Choose from:
✓ Tuna salad (3 oz. water-packed tuna mixed with fat-free mayonnaise, chopped celery and onion, and any other vegetables and seasonings you like) on 1 slice bread
✓ Smoked turkey breast sandwich (3 oz. turkey, 1 slice bread, lettuce, tomato, onion, mustard, fat-free mayonnaise)
✓ 1 c. low-fat turkey or bean chili with 2 tortillas cut in wedges and baked until crisp
✓ Joe's scramble (sauté 2 oz. ground chicken with chopped onions and spinach; scramble in 3 egg whites) and 1 slice toast

SNACK

Choose from:
✓ 2 fat-free cookies
✓ Master Snack List (Chapter 30, p. 341)

DINNER

Mixed green salad with Poppyseed Dressing 📋 or bottled fat-free dressing
Choose from:
✓ Black bean burritos (2 corn tortillas, ½ c. canned black beans, 3 oz. browned ground turkey, and salsa, onions, and tomatoes to taste)
✓ Frozen low-fat entree
✓ Chicken burger (3 oz. ground chicken seasoned to taste and grilled) on ½ bun with lettuce, tomato, onion, mustard, and fat-free mayonnaise
✓ 1 c. pasta with ¾ c. fat-free Marinara Sauce 📋 , 3 oz. chicken, turkey, or seafood, and 1 t. Parmesan cheese
✓ A Legal Cheat (no more than once a week): A Wendy's burger on a sourdough bun, 2 slices of your favorite pizza, or 3 oz. of lean steak with a baked potato

SNACK

Choose from:
✓ ½ c. nonfat frozen yogurt with ¾ c. diced fruit
✓ A Legal Cheat (no more than once a week): Triple Chocolate Cheat or Glorious Goo Cheat (see p. 187)

EQ 3 *(Medium-High)*

BREAKFAST

½ c. fruit juice or ¾ c. mixed berries
Choose from:
✓ 1 Banana Chocolate Chip Muffin 📋
✓ 1 oz. cereal

1 c. skim milk

SNACK

Choose from:
✓ 10 flavored mini rice cakes
✓ Master Snack List (p. 341)

LUNCH

1 c. Vegetable Soup 📋 or canned fat-free vegetable soup
Choose from:
✓ Tuna salad (6 oz. water-packed tuna mixed with fat-free mayonnaise, chopped celery and onion, and any other vegetables and seasonings you like) on 2 slices bread
✓ Smoked turkey breast sandwich (6 oz. turkey, 2 slices bread, lettuce, tomato, onion, mustard, fat-free mayonnaise)
✓ 1½ c. low-fat turkey or bean chili with 2 tortillas cut in wedges and baked until crisp
✓ Joe's scramble (sauté 4 oz. ground chicken with chopped onions and spinach; scramble in 5 egg whites) and 2 slices toast

SNACK

1 c. skim milk
Choose from:
✓ 2 fat-free cookies
✓ Master Snack List (Chapter 30, p. 341)

DINNER

Mixed green salad with Poppyseed Dressing 🗐 or bottled fat-free dressing
Choose from:
✓ Black bean burritos (2 corn tortillas, ½ c. canned black beans, 3 oz. browned ground turkey, and salsa, onions, and tomatoes to taste)
✓ Frozen low-fat entree
✓ Chicken burger (3 oz. ground chicken seasoned to taste and grilled) on ½ bun with lettuce, tomato, onion, mustard, and fat-free mayonnaise
✓ 1 c. pasta with ¾ c. fat-free Marinara Sauce 🗐 , 3 oz. chicken, turkey, or seafood, and 1 t. Parmesan cheese
✓ A Legal Cheat (no more than once a week): A Wendy's burger on a sourdough bun, 2 slices of your favorite pizza, or 3 oz. of lean steak with a baked potato

SNACK

Choose from:
✓ ½ c. nonfat frozen yogurt with ¾ c. diced fruit
✓ A Legal Cheat (no more than once a week): Triple Chocolate Cheat or Glorious Goo Cheat (see p. 187)

EQ 4 (High)

BREAKFAST

½ c. fruit juice or ¾ c. mixed berries
Choose from:
✓ 1 Banana Chocolate Chip Muffin 🗐
✓ 1 oz. cereal

1 c. skim milk

SNACK

Choose from:
✓ 10 flavored mini-rice cakes
✓ Master Snack List (Chapter 30, p. 341)

LUNCH

1 c. Vegetable Soup 🗐 or canned fat-free vegetable soup
Choose from:
✓ Tuna salad (6 oz. water-packed tuna mixed with fat-free mayonnaise, chopped celery and onion, and any other vegetables and seasonings you like) on 2 slices bread
✓ Smoked turkey breast sandwich (6 oz. turkey, 2 slices bread, lettuce, tomato, onion, mustard, fat-free mayonnaise)
✓ 1½ c. low-fat turkey or bean chili with 2 tortillas cut in wedges and baked until crisp

✓ Joe's scramble (sauté 4 oz. ground chicken with chopped onions and spinach; scramble in 5 egg whites) and 2 slices toast

1 piece fresh fruit

SNACK

Choose from:
✓ 2 fat-free cookies
✓ Master Snack List (Chapter 30, p. 341)

DINNER

Mixed green salad with Poppyseed Dressing 🗎 or bottled fat-free dressing
Choose from:
✓ Black bean burritos (4 corn tortillas, 1 c. canned black beans, 3 oz. browned ground turkey, and salsa, onions, and tomatoes to taste)
✓ Frozen low-fat entree with a roll
✓ Turkey burger (3 oz. ground turkey seasoned to taste and grilled) on a bun with lettuce, tomato, onion, mustard, and fat-free mayonnaise
✓ 1½ c. pasta with 1½ c. fat-free Marinara Sauce 🗎 , 3 oz. chicken, turkey, or seafood, and 1 t. Parmesan cheese and 1 slice sourdough bread
✓ A Legal Cheat (no more than once a week): A Wendy's burger on a sourdough bun, 2 slices of your favorite pizza, or 3 oz. of lean steak with a baked potato

SNACK

Choose from:
✓ ½ c. nonfat frozen yogurt with ¾ c. diced fruit
✓ A Legal Cheat (no more than once a week): Triple Chocolate Cheat or Glorious Goo Cheat (see p. 187)

SUPPLEMENT YOURSELF

■ Simplify your life with a multi-vitamin and mineral supplement—but don't use this as an excuse to derail your healthy diet.

Vegetable Insurance

As you get comfortable with your new way of eating, you can dodge many a food sabotage by keeping plenty of "safe" nibbles on hand in which you can indulge at whim—vegetables, that is! Make up a big batch of Vegetable Soup 🗎 and have a small cup when you're feeling empty inside; keep Poppyseed Dressing 🗎 in the refrigerator so you can have a fat-free salad whenever you feel like it; and always have plenty of raw vegetables on hand for snacking.

Legal Cheats

"Cheating" on anything—your taxes, a diet, a tennis game—is usually an illegitimate way of expressing legitimate anger. After watching one client after another go seriously off track in response to anger with their jobs, loved ones, or the eating plan itself, I decided to legalize cheats. It's an old theory—if you legalize it, you can control the content. There are plenty of foods that feel like cheats without sabotaging your health. Some actually supply important nutrients. But don't worry about that. In unmanageable moments, just take all your ill intentions and funnel them into these foods:

✓ Whole cracked crab for taking out aggression with your teeth. Imagine that the crab claws belong to the source of your anger as you tear them apart and suck them dry.
✓ A Wendy's burger on a sourdough bun (no special sauce or cheese).
✓ Pizza—a low-fat frozen brand, or buy a vegetarian slice and pat off the grease with a paper napkin.
✓ Lean steak—top round, top loin, round tip, tenderloin, sirloin, or eye of round.
✓ Triple Chocolate Cheat: 1 fat-free brownie, 4 oz. chocolate frozen yogurt, and 2 t. Fat-Free Fudge Sauce 📄 .
✓ Glorious Goo Cheat: 1–2 meringues or 1-oz. slice fat-free pound cake topped with ¼ c. marshmallow creme and 2 t. Fat-Free Fudge Sauce 📄 or fruit syrup.
✓ Banana Chocolate Chip Muffin 📄 .

The number of cheats you allow yourself depends on circumstance and your own emotional makeup. Annette needed three a week when she first started out; she had at least that many angry eating obstacles to overcome. As she became confident with her eating plan and released some of her aggression through aerobic boxing, she needed to cheat less frequently.

Every cheat represents excess calories, and every excess calorie can slow down your weight loss, or turn into body fat if you're eating at maintenance

WORK YOURSELF OUT

Exercise is an indispensable ally in weight loss, a great motivator, and an outlet for stress and anger. Take advantage of these benefits by choosing activities that you truly love:

■ Anger outlets: football, rugby, racquetball, hockey, aerobic boxing, martial arts.
■ Anything you like, whenever you like to do it. It matters more that you do something—anything—at least three times a week than that you follow a rigidly structured training regimen.

levels. But none of these legal cheats is serious enough to interfere with the healthy eating process. They are blips rather than blockades on your personal path to fitness. Use your legal cheats to nip self-sabotage in the bud.

✳

In a world of unexpected developments, the ability to dance and dodge a bit can be a real lifesaver. But if it's your life, health, and self you really want to save, just remember: Don't dodge your healthy destiny. Eat By Design for the happiness and peace of mind and body you truly deserve.

Artful Dodger Assertions

- I am the only person who can take care of my health and well-being.
- I deserve a strong, healthy body and mind.
- Small steps create continual success.
- I trust myself and the principles of healthy eating.
- My last meal is less important than my next one.
- Food is not an outlet for anger.
- Scales don't measure my self-worth.
- I have a healthy food plan for my new life, and it begins today.
- Change in my body is exciting and positive.
- I use my heart, my head, and my stomach to make the right eating choices.
- Every day I learn more and strengthen my resolve.
- I enjoy the process of making choices, and I choose well.

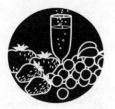

19

THE PASSIONFLOWER'S PERSONAL PRESCRIPTION

Welcome to the wonderful world of fine low-fat dining. Eating By Design holds a bounty of new taste sensations as you explore the most exciting avenue of contemporary cuisine: good food that makes you look and feel good. Join many of the nation's top chefs as you experiment with new ways of cooking and eating that allow you to eat well all the time, without sacrificing your good looks or health.

Eating is a pleasure to which you are condemned for a lifetime, so your Personal Prescription helps you to become a *healthy* epicure by emphasizing the taste experience and identifying your satisfaction cues. This sensible approach to sensual gratification allows you to pursue a low-fat, high-style life with a passion. We have entered a new era of elegant dining for beautiful people, in which you can truly have it all.

✳

Flavor Without Fat: A New Dimension of Taste Sensation

The Passionflower's Pantry

The Eating By Design pantry provides a palette of low-fat and fat-free flavors and textures with which to experiment. As you incorporate these ingredients into your culinary creations, you'll find yourself reaching less and less for the butter, oil, and cream, and more and more for flavors and tastes. Stock your refrigerator and pantry with the following high-flavor, low-fat elements of eating well, then let your sensual self run wild.

Sensualist Staples (see Master Market List for brand names)

_____ Fresh seafood

_____ Free-range chicken breasts

_____ Freshly baked bread (sourdough, herbed, onion, or other fat-free type)

_____ Wolferman's low-fat crumpets

_____ Fat-free crackers

_____ Wild, arborio, and basmati rice

_____ Flavored pastas: sun-dried tomato, spinach-basil, lemon-pepper, etc. (egg- and oil-free)

_____ Instant polenta

_____ French lentils

_____ Polenta, risotto, or pasta chips

_____ Reggiano Parmesan cheese

_____ Defatted chicken, beef, and vegetable broth

_____ Clam juice

_____ Canned low-sodium plum tomatoes

_____ Tomato paste

_____ Artichoke hearts (not marinated)

Creamy Things

_____ Nonfat milk, buttermilk, yogurt

_____ Goat cheese

_____ Nonfat sour cream

_____ Light whipped cream

_____ Evaporated skim milk

Harvest Bounty

_____ Onions, shallots, scallions

_____ Garlic

_____ Fresh vegetables: carrots, celery, tomatoes, sweet potatoes, sweet and hot peppers, asparagus, artichokes, wild mushrooms, baby vegetables

_____ Mixed greens, radicchio, endive

_____ Fresh herbs: basil, oregano, thyme, sage, rosemary, arugula, marjoram, dill, chives

_____ Fresh fruits: papayas, mangos, pineapple, kiwis, strawberries, raspberries, bananas, persimmons, pears

_____ Fresh-squeezed juices

_____ Lemons, limes

Flavor Jolts

_____ Vinegars: balsamic, wine, rice, cider, raspberry, herb-infused

_____ Mustards: Dijon, 3-grain, honey, flavored, etc.

_____ Salsas and chutneys
_____ Capers
_____ Sherry, white wine, red wine
_____ Spices
_____ Imported bay leaves

Sweet Temptations
_____ Frozen yogurt
_____ Low-fat cookies
_____ Biscotti
_____ Amaretti cookies
_____ Fat-free dessert sauces and pure fruit syrups
_____ Pure maple syrup
_____ Dutch process cocoa

Luxuries and Exotica
_____ Sun-dried tomatoes (not packed in oil)
_____ Dried porcini or shiitake mushrooms
_____ Dried cherries, cranberries, apricots, pears
_____ Whole or pureed chestnuts
_____ Caviar
_____ Smoked salmon (Nova Scotia)

Quenchers
_____ Arrowhead spring water
_____ Sparkling mineral water (no fruit juice)
_____ Whole bean coffee
_____ Paradise tea (flavored with exotic fruit essences)

The Sensual Kitchen

Now that your Passionflower's pantry is stocked, set to enjoying it. Experiment with the following foods and cooking techniques for sensual flavor without fat. For more ideas, see the Low-Fat Cooking Techniques in Part Four. Read on for a meal plan incorporating high-flavor, low-fat foods into a portioned Passionflower day.

- Roasted garlic
- Onions caramelized in stock
- Roasted red and yellow sweet peppers
- Wild mushrooms and shallots sautéed in chicken stock
- Winter squash and sweet potatoes

- Smoky flavors: smoked salmon, chicken, and turkey breast; chipotle chiles; mesquite-grilled meats, vegetables, and fruits
- Fresh and dried fruits in salsas, chutnies, and relishes paired with meats, seafood, and poultry
- Wine and stock reductions
- Fat-free and low-fat sauces
- Continental Breakfast Toast Spread: Blend equal parts fat-free ricotta cheese with raspberry or strawberry preserves, guava jam, English marmalade, specialty honey, California wine jelly, or your sweet spread of choice. Use your creativity to mix and match flavors. Keep covered in the refrigerator and spread on sourdough toast for an elegant Continental breakfast.
- Piquant Dipping Sauce: Mix fat-free mayonnaise, Dijon mustard, Worcestershire sauce, capers, and fresh lemon juice to taste. Use to dip artichokes, spread on sandwiches, or top grilled meats or fish.

❋

Passionflower Meal Plan*

EQ 1 (Low)

BREAKFAST

½ c. exotic fruit juice (passionfruit, etc.)
Choose from:
✓ 1 slice Stuffed Blueberry French Toast 📋 with 1 t. pure maple syrup and ½ c. vanilla or cappuccino nonfat yogurt
✓ 1 slice sourdough toast with 2 T. Continental Breakfast Toast Spread (above) and café latte with ½ c. evaporated skim milk

LUNCH

1 c. Carrot Ginger Soup 📋 or consommé
Choose from:
✓ 1 wedge Cilantro Pesto Vegetable Torte 📋 with ¾ c. strawberries tossed with balsamic vinegar
✓ 1 serving Spring Salmon Salad 📋 with 1 slice country bread spread with roasted garlic
✓ Bagel with 1 oz. smoked salmon or trout, 2 T. fat-free cream cheese, sliced red onion, and capers; ½ papaya or mango

DINNER

Choose from:
✓ Mixed baby greens tossed with raspberry vinegar and Dijon mustard
✓ 1 steamed artichoke with 1 T. Piquant Dipping Sauce (above)

---

* 📋 = See recipe in Chapter 33.

Choose from:

✓ 1 California Pizza (Shrimp and Chèvre or Artichoke and Sun-Dried Tomato)
✓ 3 oz. mesquite-grilled free-range baby chicken marinated in lemon, rosemary, and garlic with ½ c. Vegetable Risotto 🗐 or wild rice with baby vegetables
✓ 3 oz. wine-poached fresh seafood with ½ c. Vegetable Risotto 🗐 or wild rice with baby vegetables

Choose from:

✓ 1 slice Chocolate Cheesecake 🗐
✓ Tiramisu 🗐
✓ ½ c. fresh raspberries or strawberries floating in a glass of champagne

EQ 2 (Low-Medium)

BREAKFAST

½ c. exotic fruit juice (passionfruit, etc.)
Choose from:

✓ 1 slice Stuffed Blueberry French Toast 🗐 with 1 t. pure maple syrup and ½ c. vanilla or cappuccino nonfat yogurt
✓ 1 slice sourdough toast with 2 T. Continental Breakfast Toast Spread (see p. 192) and café latte with ½ c. evaporated skim milk

LUNCH

1 c. Carrot Ginger Soup 🗐 or consommé
Choose from:

✓ 1 wedge Cilantro Pesto Vegetable Torte 🗐 with ¾ c. strawberries tossed with balsamic vinegar
✓ 1 serving Spring Salmon Salad 🗐 with 1 slice country bread spread with roasted garlic
✓ Bagel with 1 oz. smoked salmon or trout, 2 T. fat-free cream cheese, sliced red onion, and capers; ½ papaya or mango

DINNER

Choose from:

✓ Mixed baby greens tossed with raspberry vinegar and Dijon mustard
✓ 1 steamed artichoke with 1 T. Piquant Dipping Sauce (p. 192)

Choose from:

✓ 1 California Pizza (Shrimp and Chèvre or Artichoke and Sun-Dried Tomato)
✓ 6 oz. mesquite-grilled free-range baby chicken marinated in lemon, rosemary, and garlic with ½ c. Vegetable Risotto 🗐 or wild rice with baby vegetables
✓ 6 oz. wine-poached fresh seafood with ½ c. Vegetable Risotto 🗐 or wild rice with baby vegetables

Choose from:

✓ 1 slice Chocolate Cheesecake 🗐
✓ Tiramisu 🗐
✓ ½ c. fresh raspberries or strawberries floating in a glass of champagne

EQ 3 (Medium-High)

BREAKFAST

½ c. exotic fruit juice (passionfruit, etc.)
Choose from:
✓ 1 slice Stuffed Blueberry French Toast 📄 with 1 t. pure maple syrup and
  1 c. vanilla or cappucino nonfat yogurt
✓ 1 slice sourdough toast with 2 T. Continental Breakfast Toast Spread (see p. 192) and café
  latte with 1 c. evaporated skim milk

LUNCH

1 c. Carrot Ginger Soup 📄 or consommé
Choose from:
✓ 1 wedge Cilantro Pesto Vegetable Torte 📄 with ¾ c. strawberries tossed with balsamic
  vinegar
✓ 1 serving Spring Salmon Salad 📄 with 1 slice country bread spread with roasted garlic
✓ Bagel with 1 oz. smoked salmon or trout, 2 T. fat-free cream cheese, sliced red onion, and
  capers; ½ papaya or mango

DINNER

Choose from:
✓ Mixed baby greens tossed with raspberry vinegar and Dijon mustard
✓ 1 steamed artichoke with 1 T. Piquant Dipping Sauce (p. 192)

Choose from:
✓ 2 California Pizzas (Shrimp and Chèvre or Artichoke and Sun-Dried Tomato)
✓ 6 oz. mesquite-grilled free-range baby chicken marinated in lemon, rosemary, and garlic
  with 1 c. Vegetable Risotto 📄 or wild rice with baby vegetables
✓ 6 oz. wine-poached fresh seafood with 1 c. Vegetable Risotto 📄 or wild rice with baby
  vegetables

Choose from:
✓ 1 slice Chocolate Cheesecake 📄
✓ Tiramisu 📄
✓ ½ c. fresh raspberries or strawberries floating in a glass of champagne

EQ 4 (High)

BREAKFAST

½ c. exotic fruit juice (passionfruit, etc.)
Choose from:
✓ 1 slice Stuffed Blueberry French Toast 📄 with 2 t. pure maple syrup and 1 c. vanilla or
  cappuccino nonfat yogurt
✓ 2 slices sourdough toast with 4 T. Continental Breakfast Toast Spread (see p. 192) and café
  latte with 1 c. evaporated skim milk

<u>LUNCH</u>

1 c. Carrot Ginger Soup 📄 or consommé
Choose from:
✓ 1 wedge Cilantro Pesto Vegetable Torte 📄 with ¾ c. strawberries tossed with balsamic vinegar
✓ 1 serving Spring Salmon Salad 📄 with 1 slice country bread spread with roasted garlic
✓ Bagel with 1 oz. smoked salmon or trout, 2 T. fat-free cream cheese, sliced red onion, and capers; ½ papaya or mango

<u>DINNER</u>

Choose from:
✓ Mixed baby greens tossed with raspberry vinegar and Dijon mustard
✓ 1 steamed artichoke with 1 T. Piquant Dipping Sauce (p. 192)

Choose from:
✓ 2 California Pizzas (Shrimp and Chèvre or Artichoke and Sun-Dried Tomato)
✓ 6 oz. mesquite-grilled free-range baby chicken marinated in lemon, rosemary, and garlic with 1 c. Vegetable Risotto 📄 or wild rice with baby vegetables
✓ 6 oz. wine-poached fresh seafood with 1 c. Vegetable Risotto 📄 or wild rice with baby vegetables

Choose from:
✓ 1 slice Chocolate Cheesecake 📄
✓ Tiramisu 📄
✓ ½ c. fresh raspberries or strawberries floating in a glass of champagne

PASSIONFLOWER POINTERS

- Always watch your portions!
- If you must have multicourse meals, skip between-meal snacks. While large, widely spaced meals are not optimal for your energy or blood sugar, this boundary is crucial to controlling your calorie count.
- Don't skip breakfast. Though many people are too sleepy to get much sensory pleasure from their morning meal, breakfast is important to your health—look forward to it as you wind up your evening meal.

SUPPLEMENT YOURSELF

Guard against the immune-attacking effects of overindulgence and late party nights with a daily dose of B complex and vitamin C.

✳

Seek Your Inner Satiety Cues

I know, you're probably thinking: These portions tailored to my EQ are all very well and good, but what if when I'm all done my sensual self still wants *more?* Here are some tricks for slow, luxurious eating to maximize your pleasure within your portion boundaries.

- Always remember: Eating just to satisfaction now will guard your gusto for future pleasures.
- Start meals with uncreamed soup, like a clear consommé or vegetable puree. Studies show that this cuts mealtime consumption by up to 25%.
- Make your taste buds take a break. Wait at least five minutes between each course to let real hunger catch up to perceived hunger.
- Look for early warning signs that you're full, such as:
  —A crowded stomach. Can you comfortably suck in your breath? Do your clothes feel tight? Could you wear your most revealing outfit right now?
  —Greater interest in what's coming next than in what's on your plate. You can still crave contrasting flavors long after you're full. If the rest of your entree looks like too much but dessert sounds great, clear away your plate and have just a bite of the next course, to satisfy your taste buds' curiosity.
- Use closure cues to put an unequivocal end to each meal, such as:
  —Coffee, espresso, or tea (limit caffeinated choices to twice per day).
  —A bit of something sweet. At the end of a nourishing meal, a little bit of sugar signals fullness to your appetite center, and can prevent a lot of fat calories. Enjoy a piece of exotic fruit, or a bite of dessert. Don't try to fool yourself with artificial sweeteners; your appetite knows better.
- Never, ever eat something that you don't like. Your unfulfilled sensory appetite will drive you to eat again.

Derive More Pleasure from Less

As a Passionflower, you must gratify demanding taste buds and an eager appetite. But food flows past your palate and into your body, with all excess stored as fat. In the battle to make every bite count, your allies are intense flavors, mental concentration, and variety. Your enemies are lackluster foods, careless eating, and boredom.

- Indulge your cravings, either in healthy preparations or tiny amounts (see sidebar).

- Maximize each meal's variety by sharing dishes, taking bites, having half portions.
- Explore the widest world of healthy foods.
- Sit down to eat in a beautiful environment.
- Luxuriate in all the rituals and sensations of eating. Light candles, cut flowers, lay out your best china and flatware, present beautiful plates of contrasting colors and garnishes, pipe in music. Smell deeply. Chew slowly. Taste keenly.
- Make mealtimes purely pleasurable experiences. Avoid personal conflicts and worrisome thoughts.
- Seek out the best in everything: the freshest seafood, the wildest mushroom, the juiciest papaya, the oldest barrel-aged balsamic vinegar.
- Build a library of gourmet low-fat cookbooks and magazines. This collection serves two purposes:
  —Recipes and tips: Develop a repertoire of ravishing dishes that satisfy your appetite for the best. Resolve to try new recipes on a regular basis—once a week, or at least once a month. Scan for fat-reducing tips and ideas you can use right now.
  —Fantasy: Feast your eyes on the recipes and photographs when your senses are hungry but your stomach is not. Plan elaborate menus for special occasions. Luxuriate in the bountiful possibilities for future pleasure.

QUENCHING YOUR CRAVINGS

Denying your appetite makes a Passionflower pout. It's better to carefully evaluate what you want and have it, in a healthy preparation or small portion. Beware fat-free products that don't satisfy your appetite; it's better to have a bite of the real thing than overdo on an unsatisfactory substitute.

Quench a craving for:	With:
Salt	1 T. caviar
	4 olives
	1 oz. smoked salmon
	1 oz. feta or gorgonzola cheese
Sweet	Perfectly ripe fruit, plain or tossed with liqueur or balsamic vinegar
	A taste or half serving of a decadent dessert
	1 biscotti or 2 amaretti cookies
Cream	4 oz. frozen nonfat yogurt
	1 oz. goat cheese
Chocolate	4 oz. nonfat frozen chocolate yogurt with Wax Orchards fat-free topping
	1 piece chocolate (a turtle, Baci kiss, truffle, etc.)

- Invest in the best-quality cookware, such as professional nonstick anodized aluminum, to spark your creative spirit.
- Chat with your favorite restaurateurs. Find out what they can do without butter and oils; more importantly, find out what they can do well. Cast your vote in favor of further recipe development if you find their healthy options wanting.

There's one major caveat on the pursuit of variety: Eating many different things in one meal can cause you to eat a lot more. One study showed that people eating a meal of four contrasting courses ate 60% more than those eating a single-course meal. This is because your senses get bored—the second cookie tastes less sweet than the first, the second pretzel less perfectly crunchy and salty—but they are restimulated by a new food sensation. Remember your boundaries!

✳

Seek Pleasure Outside of Your Palate

Once you've used your sharpened satiety cues to know that you're full, there's only one sound strategy: STOP EATING. But does that mean pleasure must cease? Certainly not!

When Melissa craved sensual stimulation between meals, I gave her a "perfume prescription"—to open one of her bottles of perfume and inhale deeply, a kind of weight management aromatherapy. There are many roads to rapture that don't involve chewing and swallowing. Try some of the following when you don't need fuel:

- Spa services: massage, facials, mud baths, etc.
- A massage shower head.
- Beautiful aromas, from scented bath products to potpourri, fresh cut flowers, and windowsill herb gardens.
- A leisurely candlelit bath.
- Music—try a lush Romantic like Ravel, voluptuous jazz tenor saxophone, the dulcet tones of Bach harpsichord, or some smooth soul.
- Silk sheets and pajamas.
- Love.

Love Is the Drug

Love can be one of the healthiest sensual activities. It burns calories, stimulates feel-good chemicals, and keeps your mouth busy. Technically, you should be able to leave your palate far behind in the heat of passion.

But food and seduction have been associated since long before *9½ Weeks*, and sometimes the instinct to fuel your fun with a luscious treat is irresistible. Good eating habits don't have to stop at the bedroom door—just indulge in healthy foods for love that will leave you light and ready to go:

- Champagne with red raspberries or strawberries, or peach nectar ice cubes in suggestive shapes.
- Hand-fed champagne grapes.
- Oysters—their zinc boosts potency.
- Ginseng tea, a calorie-free aphrodisiac.
- Suggestive sundaes: a pear half drizzled with fat-free fudge sauce and topped with light whipped cream and a cherry for him, a chocolate-dipped banana (a great source of potassium) for her.
- Soft and juicy fruits, like papaya and mango. Fruit is one of nature's naturally sweet pleasures, and sometimes it can be hard to squeeze in your recommended servings before bedtime.
- Honey for your honey.
- Fat-free fudge sauce—warm it up and dribble it on. Chocolate is an age-old seduction tool and symbol of lovers.

WORK YOURSELF OUT

Some feel-good physical activities for pleasureful calorie-burning:

- Bike rides or walks in beautiful places.
- Moonlight swims or skinny dips.
- Aqua aerobics in the hot tub.

✳

There is a big world within and outside you for all five of your senses to appreciate. May Eating By Design make food a healthy element of your rich palette of pleasures.

Daily Passions

- I live low-fat in high style
- I love my body inside and out and do everything I can to make it feel good.
- I slow down and seek out my inner satisfaction cues.
- I am in touch with my pleasure centers.
- I fully experience the moment when I eat.
- I am passionate about eating well.
- Restraint in the present means pleasure in the future.

- I like my flavors pure, clean, and uncoated by fat.
- I have many opportunities for pleasure and passion in my life.
- No bite is ever the last I will have in my life.
- An overfull stomach feels unpleasant.
- I choose light, flavorful foods that make me feel good all over.
- I will wait a few minutes for satisfaction to set in.

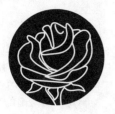

20

THE BLUE ROSE'S PERSONAL PRESCRIPTION

Your Personal Prescription centers around a piece of good news: You can strike a balance between mind, body, and mood that enables you to comfort your psyche while nourishing a healthy body and happy state of mind. In fact, a healthy diet can actually stimulate biochemical responses that help control your appetite and lift your mood.

Recent research indicates that the same chemical imbalances that cause sadness and feeling down can also cause overeating. This suggests treating both problems together, with a Personal Prescription for low-fat, high-carbohydrate mini-meals that feed the flow of soothing neurotransmitters in your brain. The result is enhanced health, energy, and cheer, to shift the tint of your world-viewing glasses from blue to rose.

✳

Serotonin Stew

The Blue Rose Meal Plan is formulated to facilitate the steady release of serotonin, the mood-boosting neurotransmitter. The glucose necessary to serotonin stimulation is most easily obtained from simple carbohydrates like sugars and milk. But before you go out to celebrate with a box of Twinkies, beware! Sugar contains empty calories prone to add pounds, especially in combination with the typically high-fat content of cookies, cakes, and ice cream. Fat also reduces the serotonin-stimulating power of glucose. And eating too much sugar can lead to fatigue and mood swings in some people, wiping out any benefit of the serotonin.

The Eating By Design solution is to derive glucose more slowly and gradually from complex carbohydrates like breads, pasta, cereals, and grains, without added fat. And what should you put on your bread for maximum serotonin benefits? Yes to jam or jelly; no to fatty spreads like butter, margarine, or mayonnaise. Like fat, protein also inhibits serotonin production, so eat it only as indicated in the meal plan.

Only a small amount of simple or complex carbohydrate—about one to two ounces—is needed to trigger serotonin, and eating more won't increase the beneficial effect. So the best strategy for good mood, calorie control, and strong satisfaction cues is a series of small mini-meals throughout the day. Your meal plan calls for eight meals over a fourteen-hour day. That sounds like plenty of food, doesn't it? Such is the magic of Eating By Design.

The delicate chemical balance of the Blue Rose makes it extremely important not to skip meals. The more paralyzed or hopeless you feel, the more you need a steady source of fuel to stabilize your emotions and your blood sugar.

In addition to fourteen hours a day of mood-boosting food, the Blue Rose Meal Plan is rich in folic acid and selenium, deficiencies of which are linked to depression.

My success with Danielle was reliant on her relationship with a professional therapist to work out emotional issues and, in her case, medicate with an antidepressant. Don't substitute any eating plan for professional medical care.

❋

Blue Rose Meal Plan*

EQ 1 (Low)

MEAL I (7:00 A.M.)

Choose from:
✓ 1 oz. puffed wheat or vitamin-fortified cereal
✓ Fat-free toaster pastry
✓ 1 packet instant flavored oatmeal

1 c. skim milk

MEAL II (9:00 A.M.)

1 piece fresh fruit

---

* 📄 = See recipe in Chapter 33.

MEAL III (11:00 A.M.)

Choose from:
✓ 1 packet low-fat ramen noodles
✓ Low-fat pasta, couscous, or rice cup-of-soup
✓ Serotonin Snack (p. 207)

MEAL IV (1:00 P.M.)

Choose from:
✓ 1 serving Tuscan Bean Salad 📄
✓ Salad bar (mixed greens, assorted vegetables, ½ c. beans, and fat-free dressing)
✓ ½ pita stuffed with assorted vegetables and fat-free dressing
Raw vegetables

MEAL V (3:00 P.M.)

Choose from:
✓ ½ baked potato with salsa
✓ Serotonin Snack (p. 207)

MEAL VI (5:00 P.M.)

Choose from:
✓ ½ bagel with 1 T. fat-free cream cheese
✓ Serotonin Snack (p. 207)

MEAL VII (7:00 P.M.)

½ c. pasta with ½ c. fat-free Marinara Sauce 📄 and 3 oz. seafood or chicken breast
Steamed greens or spinach salad with fat-free dressing

MEAL VIII (9:00 P.M.)

Serotonin Snack (p. 207)

EQ 2 (Low-Medium)

MEAL I (7:00 A.M.)

Choose from:
✓ 1 oz. puffed wheat or vitamin-fortified cereal
✓ Fat-free toaster pastry
✓ 1 packet instant flavored oatmeal

1 c. skim milk

MEAL II (9:00 A.M.)

1 piece fresh fruit

MEAL III (11:00 A.M.)

Choose from:
✓ 1 packet low-fat ramen noodles
✓ Lowfat pasta, couscous, or rice cup-of-soup
✓ Serotonin Snack (p. 207)

MEAL IV (1:00 P.M.)

Choose from:
✓ 1 c. Winter Squash Soup 📖
✓ 1 c. fat-free vegetable soup or chili

Choose from:
✓ 1 serving Tuscan Bean Salad 📖
✓ Salad bar (mixed greens, assorted vegetables, ½ c. beans, and fat-free dressing)
✓ ½ pita stuffed with assorted vegetables and fat-free dressing

Raw vegetables
1 piece fresh fruit

MEAL V (3:00 P.M.)

Choose from:
✓ ½ baked potato with salsa
✓ Serotonin Snack (p. 207)

MEAL VI (5:00 P.M.)

Choose from:
✓ ½ bagel with 1 T. fat-free cream cheese
✓ Serotonin Snack (p. 207)

MEAL VII (7:00 P.M.)

1 c. pasta with ¾ c. fat-free Marinara Sauce 📖 and 3 oz. seafood or chicken breast
Steamed greens or spinach salad with fat-free dressing

MEAL VIII (9:00 P.M.)

Serotonin Snack (p. 207)

EQ 3 (Medium-High)

MEAL I (7:00 A.M.)

Choose from:
✓ 1 oz. puffed wheat or vitamin-fortified cereal
✓ Fat-free toaster pastry
✓ 1 packet instant flavored oatmeal

1 c. skim milk

MEAL II (9:00 A.M.)

1 piece fresh fruit

MEAL III (11:00 A.M.)

Choose from:
✓ 1 packet low-fat ramen noodles
✓ Low-fat pasta, couscous, or rice cup-of-soup
✓ Serotonin Snack (p. 207)

MEAL IV (1:00 P.M.)

Choose from:
✓ 1 c. Winter Squash Soup 📖
✓ 1 c. fat-free vegetable soup or chili

Choose from:
✓ 1 serving Tuscan Bean Salad 📖
✓ Salad bar (mixed greens, assorted vegetables, ½ c. beans, and fat-free dressing)
✓ ½ pita stuffed with assorted vegetables and fat-free dressing

Raw vegetables
½ c. nonfat yogurt with ¾ c. fresh fruit

MEAL V (3:00 P.M.)

Choose from:
✓ 1 baked potato with salsa
✓ 2 Serotonin Snacks (p. 207)

MEAL VI (5:00 P.M.)

Choose from:
✓ ½ bagel with 1 T. fat-free cream cheese
✓ Serotonin Snack (p. 207)

MEAL VII (7:00 P.M.)

1 c. pasta with ¾ c. fat-free Marinara Sauce 📖 and 6 oz. seafood or chicken breast
Steamed greens or spinach salad with fat-free dressing

MEAL VIII (9:00 P.M.)

Serotonin Snack (p. 207)

EQ 4 (High)

MEAL I (7:00 A.M.)

Choose from:
✓ 1 oz. puffed wheat or vitamin-fortified cereal
✓ Fat-free toaster pastry
✓ 1 packet instant flavored oatmeal

1 c. skim milk

MEAL II (9:00 A.M.)

1 piece fresh fruit

MEAL III (11:00 A.M.)

Choose from:
✓ 1 packet low-fat ramen noodles
✓ Low-fat pasta, couscous, or rice cup-of-soup
✓ Serotonin Snack (p. 207)

MEAL IV (1:00 P.M.)

Choose from:
✓ 1 c. Winter Squash Soup 📄
✓ 1 c. fat-free vegetable soup or chili

Choose from:
✓ 1 serving Tuscan Bean Salad 📄
✓ Salad bar (mixed greens, assorted vegetables, ½ c. beans, and fat-free dressing)
✓ ½ pita stuffed with assorted vegetables and fat-free dressing

Raw vegetables
½ c. nonfat yogurt with ¾ c. fresh fruit

MEAL V (3:00 P.M.)

Choose from:
✓ 1 baked potato with salsa
✓ 2 Serotonin Snacks (p. 207)

MEAL VI (5:00 P.M.)

Choose from:
✓ 1 bagel with 2 T. fat-free cream cheese
✓ 2 Serotonin Snacks (p. 207)

MEAL VII (7:00 P.M.)

1 c. pasta with ¾ c. fat-free Marinara Sauce 📄 and 6 oz. seafood or chicken breast
Steamed greens or spinach salad with fat-free dressing

MEAL VIII (9:00 P.M.)

Serotonin Snack (p. 207)

SUPPLEMENT YOURSELF

Round out your mood-enhancing diet with supplements of:

- Folic acid (a B vitamin), deficiency of which is linked to depression.
- Selenium (a trace mineral), which promotes feelings of well-being.

Serotonin Snack Attack

You may have once considered the snack attack your mortal enemy in the weight management battle. When every blip on your moodometer demands to be fed, snacks can indeed add up to extra body fat. But frequent carbohydrate mini-meals are crucial to maintaining a steady state in your body and mind. So go ahead and snack. Just stick to the schedule in your meal plan, and pick high-carbohydrate pick-me-ups from the list below for the benefits of serotonin.

Serotonin Snacks

1 oz.* fat-free cookies
1 oz.* gingersnaps
1 oz.* vanilla wafers
1 oz.* biscotti
1 oz.* tea biscuits
1 oz.* animal crackers
2 graham crackers
1-oz. slice fat-free cake
1 fat-free toaster pastry
1 small fat-free muffin
2 large or 10 mini sweet flavored rice cakes
1 fat-free granola bar
1 oz. dry cereal or fat-free granola
1 low-fat frozen waffle with 2 t. maple syrup
Herbal tea with honey

✳

Take Action to Mobilize Motivation

Act Now, Think Later

When gloom has you in its claws and is gnawing away at your self-esteem, you can't afford to wait for motivation—you need to *create* it by taking that first step, then follow through with small but positive actions. Here are seven mini-steps to feed your motivation for healthy eating. Try one each day for a week. Watch your motivation grow.

DAY ONE: Eat a carbohydrate breakfast. See how much brighter the day looks with serotonin on your side.

---

*1 oz. is generally 2 medium cookies.

DAY TWO: Go shopping for at least two of the serotonin snacks listed on the previous page. Buy some small plastic bags and pack your snacks into personal portions. Tomorrow, take one with you for the morning, one for the afternoon.

DAY THREE: Buy three different kinds of pasta and two low-fat or fat-free vegetarian sauces. Have a pasta dinner tonight. Measure your portions.

DAY FOUR: Try a low-fat, high-carbohydrate lunch.

DAY FIVE: Take a walk or have a brief workout.

DAY SIX: Clean your cupboards of unhealthy temptations. Throw or give them away.

DAY SEVEN: Follow the Blue Rose Meal Plan all day long.

Each day, focus on the action at hand. Try to eat healthfully for the rest of the day, but don't worry too much about the details. Keep a brief log of how you feel each day after taking action. At the end of the week, read over your log.

You might need to renew your motivation periodically. Go back on this seven-step plan any time you go off track. Keep all your logs on hand to read over whenever you wonder why you bother to Eat By Design.

Move Your Mood

Another way to add impetus to your healthy eating plan is to move—literally. For Danielle, a brief daily workout had disproportionate physical and psychological benefits. The very act of moving seemed to stir her mood, enhancing her energy and giving her a sense of being alive and present in her body. Exercise is also a natural appetite regulator that helps to reinforce the body's fullness signals to the brain. It burns calories and boosts the metabolism, providing a crucial edge to your weight management efforts. And why not indulge in a little natural high? Exercise releases endorphins, biochemical feel-good stimulants.

I recommend exercising every day, preferably in a regular schedule that you can stick to regardless of your mood swings. You can also use exercise as a spontaneous remedy to feelings of anger and despair. If a mood is clouding up your horizon, move it along.

WORK YOURSELF OUT

> - Take advantage of the natural boost to mood and self-esteem that exercise brings—do something small every day, even if only for fifteen minutes. If your dread of a long jog is keeping you on the couch, go for a brisk walk instead.
> - Seek out exhilarating exercise like dance, aerobics, biking, or other uplifting undertakings.

Mediate Your Mood

One of the greatest gifts I could offer Danielle was assurance that her feelings were real and required attention. It wouldn't have been constructive to say, "Oh it's ridiculous to worry-about your script being bad; you just had a major box office smash!" Danielle was worried and had to face that emotional fact. I was also sympathetic to her self-loathing about being fat. Who cares that you haven't committed murder or started an international war? Something about the very basic and personal nature of eating makes it all the more painful when the process goes awry.

But accepting your moods isn't enough. Once you've met your feelings face-to-face, you need to respond. Different moods might require different responses to get on with the process of being the good and valuable person you are. Any response that makes you feel good and in control—including eating, if it's a healthy food in moderation—is valid for mediating your mood.

When a mood swoops down and threatens to take your happiness hostage, make a small move affirming that the sensitive person beneath your feelings is active and alive—whether it's choosing a healthy snack that soothes your mood or saying an affirmation that focuses on your strong points, inner worth, and potential.

Mood Mediators

Here are some responses to move you from feeling to action:

Mood:	Food Mediator:	Nonfood Mediator:
Boredom	—Something small that takes a long time to eat: fructose-sweetened hard candies, air-popped popcorn, fat-free mini-pretzels.	—Watch a movie, on the VCR or at the theater; or read a book.

Mood:	Food Mediator:	Nonfood Mediator:
Anger	—Something crunchy: raw vegetables, mini rice cakes, fat-free granola, fat-free pretzels or chips.	—Take a bike ride, run, or walk.
Loneliness	—Something comforting, like a cup of fat-free soup.	—Call a friend or write a letter.
Sadness or hopelessness	—Something sweet: fat-free or low-fat cookies, graham crackers, granola bar, sweetened rice cakes.	—Choose an affirmation to write on a note card and post on your bathroom mirror, refrigerator, dashboard, or office desk. Write your own, or pick one from the end of this chapter.

Keep Up the Treatment

As far as we know, depression and the overeating that might be associated with it are chronic chemical conditions, without a permanent cure. Just as fitness requires ongoing attention to your eating habits, depression must be continually treated with a combination of diet, exercise, therapy, and perhaps medication. It's hard to imagine feeling down when you're up, so it's easy to throw caution to the wind when you're feeling good. But a false sense of security can sideswipe your healthy eating plan.

To realize the mood and weight management benefits of your Personal Prescription, you have to follow it all the time. Don't skip a carbohydrate snack just because you're feeling great. Don't abandon the meal plan because you lost five pounds and are happy with your weight. The five pounds will be back before you know it, and you will be desolate. Instead, readjust your Eating Quotient as necessary for maintenance, and enjoy a healthy mind and body.

On the other hand, don't criticize yourself for small mistakes, or feel trapped by the meal plan. It's there to help you, not to control you. By following these guidelines, you are in control of your own personal balance, adjusting your own attitude away from the blue and toward a happier, healthier you.

Blue Rose Affirmations

Plant these thoughts all over your kitchen to help mobilize your mind and body for craving control:

- I eat the right foods to feel good.
- I am in control of my food chemistry.
- I know the difference between mood and food.
- I take action when I feel low.
- The world is a bright place with a happy, healthy place for me.
- Good health enhances my happiness.
- I know how to satisfy my hungers with healthy foods.

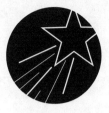

21

THE SHOOTING STAR'S PERSONAL PRESCRIPTION

Congratulations! By coming this far in Eating By Design, you've made an exciting step toward a better and more beautiful you. If you started on a bit of whim, take it as an omen that *this* is the plan that's going to work for you, for good. Your excellent choice in selecting a proven program incorporating deep nutritional truths with the latest knowledge about metabolism, the role of fats in the body, and the secrets of a stimulating healthy diet shows that you are aware, well-informed, and committed to being the best that you can be.

Your Personal Prescription programs plenty of variety and stimulus into your meal plans to insure you the spice of life worthy of a Shooting Star. Eating well is nothing more than making the right choices from a sensational array of thrilling foods. Just let my Personal Prescription steer you while you tap into your high-energy enthusiasm to gallop into good health. Right now, in this moment, begin to be fantastically fit.

✳

Set the Stage for Success

Most Shooting Stars have Scarlett O'Hara's strong will—without her willpower concerning food. Elise was a classic example. She didn't like to be told what to do, and when she began the Diet Designs program, she was mortally terrified that I was going to tell her exactly what to eat and when. "There's no surer way to make me cheat," she said. "It seems the minute I know what I'm supposed to do, a secret force wants to do the opposite. If you tell me to have fish, I can't live another minute without a bite of pasta! And if you tell me to eat the same thing twice in one week? Dear heaven, you might as well send me directly to the pastry shop!"

In devising Elise's meal plan, I emphasized fun, spice, spontaneity, and sweets—and than I gave her lots and lots of tips for keeping her Shooting Star on a steady course. Here are my very best strategies for Eating By Design with a dramatic twist, followed by meal plans that make easy work of following your EQ.

Breakfast

Since mornings are rushed and you're always happy to cut a calorie here and there, breakfast is probably way down on your list of priorities. But your morning meal is indispensable to launch you on your day and control your hunger for hours to come. It's a small concession with a big payoff. I make it easy in your meal plan. Either:

✓ Grab toast or a bagel and a cappuccino, or
✓ Concoct a mix-and-match one-bowl buffet: Combine different cereals, fruits, and yogurt flavors to taste. Mix up crunchy cereals like fat-free granola, Grape-Nuts, or Kashi Medley; creamy vanilla, tangy lemon, or luscious fruit yogurt; and fun fruits like bananas, berries, or papaya.

Lunch and Dinner

Always start your meal with a mixed green salad or fat-free soup to help you slow down when you get to the big stuff. Select from the choices on your meal plan, feeling free to switch items between lunch and dinner if it pleases you better. Improvise! You're a Shooting Star!

Make Fat-Free or Low-Fat Choices

I've long despaired of trying to tell a Shooting Star exactly how much to eat. Counts get forgotten, measurements fudged in the heat of the moment. But you *can* control the fat content of your food. Limiting fat intake cuts calories and the risk of heart disease, stoke, and cancer. Instead of wasting your energy on portion tallies you're likely to forget or ignore, channel your choices to low-fat foods. You might move as fast as greased lightning, but the lubrication doesn't need to come from your diet. Check these choices for a glance at how easy it is to cut calories by cutting fat.

Fat-Calorie Shortcuts

Compare:
High fat
Low fat

	Serving	Calories	Fat
Danish pastry	1	**235**	**13 g**
Fat-free muffin	1	150	0 g
Beef tenderloin	4 oz.	**275**	**12 g**
Chicken breast	4 oz.	187	4 g
Big Mac	1	**560**	**32 g**
Turkey burger	4 oz. w/ bun	250	3 g
Superpremium ice cream	4 oz.	**175**	**12 g**
Nonfat frozen yogurt	4 oz.	76	0 g

NOTE: Beware "light" labels, which only mean the product has half the fat or one third fewer calories than the original.

Don't add fats or oils in cooking or at the table. Use herbs, spices, lemon and lime juice, vinegar, mustard, salsa, fat-free dressing, tomato, onion, garlic, ginger, Tabasco, Worcestershire, soy sauce, barbecue sauce, or hot additions from the Tongue-Tingling Arsenal (coming up) for extra flavor. Spread with fat-free cream cheese or ricotta or fruit-sweetened preserves instead of butter or margarine.

As you dart from one drama to the next, this low-fat principle is the single most important element of your Personal Prescription. No matter how you might improvise with your meal plan, be true to the low-fat rule.

Hot Thrills

Intensity, spice, and color are the drama in a healthy diet. There are no calories in the fire of red pepper, no cholesterol in the vibrant contrast between bright green arugula and ripe red cherry tomatoes, no fat in the savory licorice bite of fresh basil. You'll find these delicacies in your meal plan to keep your diet spiced up to the smoke point:

✓ A quesadilla made with fat-free cheese, a no-lard whole wheat tortilla, sliced fresh or canned jalapeño or serrano pepper, and salsa, cooked in a nonstick skillet until the cheese melts.

✓ Low-fat ramen noodles spiked with sliced scallions, grated fresh ginger, and Chinese five-spice power.

✓ Blender Gazpacho 🗎 with a dash of red pepper flakes.*

✓ Pasta tossed with oil-free Marinara Sauce (homemade 🗎 or bottled) bolstered with any combination of minced fresh garlic, chopped fresh basil and oregano, hot sauce, minced jalapeño, and red pepper flakes.

✓ Quick cupboard chili:

- Stock your pantry with cans of turkey or vegetarian chili; black, kidney, or pinto beans; corn; and low-sodium tomatoes.

- Combine at will with serranos, jalapeños, chipotles, cayenne powder, or the chile of your choice and heat.

- Top with one or more of these options: grated fat-free cheese, sliced scallions, diced fresh tomato, crumbled baked tortilla chips, fat-free sour cream.

✓ Penne with Turkey and Chili Pepper Cream Sauce 🗎 .

✓ Shrimp Fajitas 🗎 .

THE TONGUE-TINGLING ARSENAL

Add fat-free warmth and glow to any dish with:

✓ Hot sauce, from the medium-hot Louisiana Tabasco to Half Way to Pure Hell, Trinidad Mild, and Pili Sauce, to the hottest, like West Indies Creole Sauce, Spitfire Pepper Sauce, Inner Beauty Real Hot Sauce, Melinda's XXXXtra Reserve '94, Vic's Fire, and Pure Hell
✓ Chili peppers—fresh, canned, dried, or pickled
✓ Spice blends
✓ Vinegars, all varieties, plain and flavored
✓ Mustards, all varieties, plain and flavored
✓ Relishes
✓ Chutnies
✓ Salsas
✓ Horseradish
✓ Garlic and ginger

Sodium alert: Many of these condiments have high salt content; be sparing if you're watching your sodium intake!

Breads

This common gobble has snuffed out the slim intentions of many a Shooting Star. Put boundaries on your bread intake by selecting fat-free versions of sourdough, whole wheat, pumpernickel, rye, bagels, and pita, and limiting yourself to one serving per level of your EQ per day.

---

* 🗎 = See recipe in Chapter 33.

Booze

Too many parties can pour too many empty calories into your diet. Limit alcoholic beverages to wine no more than 3–4 times per week, and count each glass as a snack in your EQ.

Sweets for the Sweet

Let's face it. Food is a source of pleasure, and sometimes you just have to indulge yourself—it's in your nature! I personally believe that life should be a constant joy, and that part of that joy comes from special treats.

Have these low-fat treats as snacks (remember to limit each to about 100 calories) or as special indulgences for special occasions. If you choose a low-fat splurge, resist the urge to eat more than you would of its higher-fat original!

✓ Dip fruit, graham crackers, or low-fat cookies in fat-free fudge sauce. For an extra thrill, freeze it on waxed paper first.
✓ Fat-free cake, brownies, Danish, coffee cake, or cookies
✓ Fat-free pudding, prepared, or made from mix with skim milk
✓ Mocha or Lemon Mousse 📄
✓ Caramel rice cakes
✓ Frozen grapes
✓ Frozen fruit bars
✓ Fruit salad with fresh mint and a squeeze of lime
✓ Fat-free taffy (5–8)*
✓ Gummy bears (10–15)*
✓ Jellybeans (10–15)*
✓ Licorice twists (3)*

Beware "sugar-free" sweets that contain sorbitol, fructose, or fruit juice concentrate—these are just as high in calories as the originals.

Red Lights

Some foods have a way of being available and seemingly irresistible even when you're not hungry and have no intention of eating. When you see these red lights, STOP. Do not connect hand to mouth. Get off the fast track to calorie collision.

---

*These snacks are on the nonnutritive side. Limit them to one per day and count as a snack from the Complex Carbohydrate Group in your EQ.

- Fried chips with salsa or dip.
- Cheese and crackers
- Peanuts or mixed nuts
- Candy bars
- Cookies
- Doughnuts
- Desktop candy bowls
- Restaurant bread baskets
- Alcoholic beverages

Signposts

Because action so quickly follows impulse for the Shooting Star, it's wise to have a travel plan for any contingency. When the eating impulse strikes,

GO TO:

- The frozen yogurt store
- A chicken rotisserie
- The salad bar
- The healthy snack section of the supermarket
- The vegetable crisper

- The fat-free granola box
- Your own healthy meal

DO NOT STOP AT:

- The ice cream store
- A burger joint
- The buffet
- The take-out counter of the supermarket
- Your spouse's leftover submarine sandwich
- The candy jar
- Another person's plate

FAST FUN

If you find the golden arches or another symbol of fast food fun beckoning to you consider your options:

- You *could* order a double cheeseburger, fries, and a shake—for about 1,200 calories, or the entire daily allotment for EQ 1.

OR

- You could follow the Fast Food Guidelines in Chapter 30 and make this meal a normal part of your healthy lifestyle—no regrets, no remorse.

Eat When You're Hungry

It sounds obvious, but many people neglect their hunger and simply eat when they see food (the infamous "see food diet").

- DO eat when you're hungry, keeping in mind that low-fat foods might stick with you for shorter intervals than higher-fat fare, requiring a more frequent snacking schedule.
- DON'T eat when you're not hungry, even if it's mealtime.
- If you're not hungry in the morning, you're probably eating too much at night. Likewise, if you're hungry late at night, you're probably not eating enough during the day. Adjust your eating schedule to keep you satisfied during your waking hours.

Second-Guess

Give your synapses time to fire before you fuel up by asking yourself two questions:

- "Am I hungry?"

If yes, then proceed. If no, ask yourself why you want to eat.
- "Is this a healthy low-fat food?"

If yes, go ahead. If no, find an alternative that is, or ask yourself why you must have this particular food. Do you really want it, or are you about to eat it just because it's there?

You Are More Fascinating than Your Food

Though your meal plan contains all kinds of wonderful foods to choose from, remember: Food is only fuel to power *you* to center stage. When I first met Elise, I was concerned that her frequent restaurant meals for business, often as many as three a day, would present an obstacle to her success. She proved herself a true Shooting Star when she told me this was the least of her worries.

"Are you kidding? This is my time to shine, to hook the client and reel him in! I can't waste it on eating. I have so much to tell, such an impression to make! I order something small, an appetizer, and nibble on it just enough for effect and to keep me going through the meeting and the property tour. Darling, I have eaten in some of the best restaurants in the world, and there's one thing I know—when I am 'on,' I am far more fascinating than any piece of food!"

Remember Elise's philosophy as you explore your meal plan. Your warmth, glow, and zest for life always outshine the food you make, serve, and eat. The only fascinating foods are those that make you healthy and beautiful—and even they aren't as fascinating as the person they nourish.

✳

The Shooting Star Meal Plan

| EQ 1 (Low) |

BREAKFAST

Choose from:
✓ Mix-and-match one-bowl buffet: 1 oz. crunchy cereal, ½ c. nonfat yogurt. ¾ c. fresh fruit
✓ ½ c. juice, 1 slice toast or ½ bagel with 1 T. fat-free cream cheese and 1 t. pure fruit preserves, cappuccino with 1 c. skim milk

LUNCH

Mixed green salad with fat-free dressing
Choose from:
✓ 1 c. pasta with ¾ c. oil-free marinara or fresh tomato sauce
✓ 1 serving low-fat vegetarian ramen noodles
✓ 1 c. vegetarian quick cupboard chili (see p. 215)
✓ Quesadilla (1 whole wheat tortilla, 1½ oz. fat-free jack or cheddar cheese)

SNACK 1

Choose from:
✓ 1 oz. string cheese
✓ ½ c. fat-free, sugar-free pudding

SNACK 2

Choose from:
✓ 15 frozen grapes
✓ ¾ c. fruit salad
✓ ½ c. chocolate-dipped fruit (see p. 216)

DINNER

1 c. Blender Gazpacho 📄 or other uncreamed soup
Choose from:
✓ 1 serving Penne with Turkey and Chile Pepper Cream Sauce 📄
✓ 1 serving Chicken or Shrimp Fajitas 📄
✓ 2 wedges thin-crusted pizza with poultry or seafood

Steamed or grilled vegetables
½ c. Mocha or Lemon Mousse 📄 , or choose from Sweets for the Sweet snack list (p. 216)

EQ 2 (Low-Medium)

BREAKFAST

Choose from:
✓ Mix-and-match one-bowl buffet: 1 oz. crunchy cereal, ½ c. nonfat yogurt, ¾ c. fresh fruit
✓ ½ c. juice, 1 slice toast or ½ bagel with 1 T. fat-free cream cheese and 1 t. pure fruit preserves, cappuccino with 1 c. skim milk

SNACK

Choose from:
✓ 1 oz. fat-free pretzels
✓ 1 oz. baked cheese puffs

LUNCH

Mixed green salad with fat-free dressing
Choose from:
✓ 1 c. pasta with ¾ c. oil-free marinara or fresh tomato sauce and 3 oz. chicken or seafood
✓ 1 fast food sandwich or chef's salad (see Chapter 30)
✓ 1 c. turkey quick cupboard chili (see p. 215)
✓ Quesadilla (1 whole wheat tortilla, 1½ oz. fat-free jack or cheddar cheese, 3 oz. chicken or shrimp)

SNACK 1

1 oz. string cheese with 1 oz. fat-free crackers

SNACK 2

Choose from:
✓ 15 frozen grapes
✓ ¾ c. fruit salad
✓ ½ c. chocolate-dipped fruit (see p. 216)

DINNER

1 c. Blender Gazpacho 📋 or other uncreamed soup
Choose from:
✓ 1 serving Penne with Turkey and Chile Pepper Cream Sauce 📋
✓ 1 serving Chicken or Shrimp Fajitas 📋
✓ 2 wedges thin-crusted pizza with poultry or seafood

Steamed or grilled vegetables
½ c. Mocha or Lemon Mousse 📋 , or choose from Sweets for the Sweet snack list (p. 216)

EQ 3 (Medium-High)

BREAKFAST

Choose from:
✓ Mix-and-match one-bowl buffet: 1 oz. crunchy cereal, 1 c. nonfat yogurt, ¾ c. fresh fruit
✓ ½ c. juice, 1 slice toast or ½ bagel with 1 T. fat-free cream cheese and 1 t. pure fruit preserves, cappuccino with 2 c. skim milk

SNACK

Choose from:
✓ 1 oz. fat-free pretzels
✓ 1 oz. baked cheese puffs

LUNCH

Mixed green salad with fat-free dressing
Choose from:
✓ 1½ c. pasta with ¾ c. oil-free marinara or fresh tomato sauce and 3 oz. chicken or seafood
✓ 1 fast food sandwich or chef's salad (see Chapter 30)
✓ 1½ c. turkey quick cupboard chili (see p. 215)
✓ Quesadilla (1 whole wheat tortilla, 1½ oz. fat-free jack or cheddar cheese, 3 oz. chicken or shrimp)

SNACK 1

1 oz. string cheese with 1 oz. fat-free crackers

SNACK 2

Choose from:
✓ 15 frozen grapes
✓ ¾ c. fruit salad
✓ ½ c. chocolate-dipped fruit (see p. 216)

DINNER

1 c. Blender Gazpacho 📄 or other uncreamed soup
Choose from:
✓ 1 serving Penne with Turkey and Chile Pepper Cream Sauce 📄
✓ 1 serving Chicken or Shrimp Fajitas 📄
✓ 2 wedges thin-crusted pizza with poultry or seafood

Steamed or grilled vegetables
½ c. Mocha or Lemon Mousse 📄 , or choose from Sweets for the Sweet snack list (p. 216)

EQ 4 (High)

BREAKFAST

Choose from:
✓ Mix-and-match one-bowl buffet: 1 oz. crunchy cereal, 1 c. nonfat yogurt, ¾ c. fresh fruit
✓ ½ c. juice, 1 slice toast or ½ bagel with 1 T. fat-free cream cheese and 1 t. pure fruit preserves, cappuccino with 2 c. skim milk

SNACK 1

1 piece fresh fruit

SNACK 2

Choose from:
✓ 1 oz. fat-free pretzels
✓ 1 oz. baked cheese puffs

LUNCH

Mixed green salad with fat-free dressing
Choose from:
✓ 1½ c. pasta with ¾ c. oil-free marinara or fresh tomato sauce and 3 oz. chicken or seafood
✓ 1 fast food sandwich or chef's salad (see Chapter 30)
✓ 1½ c. turkey quick cupboard chili (see p. 215)
✓ Quesadilla (1 whole wheat tortilla, 1½ oz. fat-free jack or cheddar cheese, 3 oz. chicken or shrimp)

SNACK 1

1 oz. string cheese with 1 oz. fat-free crackers

SNACK 2

Choose from:
✓ 15 frozen grapes
✓ ¾ c. fruit salad
✓ ½ c. chocolate-dipped fruit (see p. 216)

DINNER

1 c. Blender Gazpacho 📄 or other uncreamed soup
Choose from:
✓ 1 serving Penne with Turkey and Chile Pepper Cream Sauce 📄
✓ 1 serving Chicken or Shrimp Fajitas 📄
✓ 2 wedges thin-crusted pizza with poultry or seafood

Steamed or grilled vegetables
½ c. Mocha or Lemon Mousse 📄 , or choose from Sweets for the Sweet snack list (p. 216)

WORK YOURSELF OUT

- Buy fabulous workout clothes that make you look great as you pursue the best body.
- Check out the action at public jogging or bike paths.
- Bike or walk to fun destinations—your favorite bookstore or boutique, a museum, a new film.
- Take upbeat aerobics, jazz, and funk workout classes.
- Go out dancing every weekend.

SUPPLEMENT YOURSELF

- For fast and easy vitamin treatment, try a liquid formulated for daily use.

※

Dining in the Spotlight

Social Butterfly

Ever out and about, the Shooting Star is constantly landing in social occasions stocked with so much tempting *food.* As a Shooting Star, you probably don't like to share the spotlight with anything, including a meal—but you need a way to take Eating By Design principles public with you, to guard against undereating at a social meal and overeating in private, or diving into the food when the social event proves less stimulating than you had hoped.

Eat for Show

An elegant and effective solution to the temptations of social life is to eat a small meal or snack immediately before an event, then "eat for show": Pick or sip your way daintily through small bites of everything, or choose something very simple and low-fat—a cup of uncreamed soup, a vegetable salad, a bowl of mixed fruit, or a cappuccino with nonfat milk. Your delicacy will be much envied and admired. If quizzed on the secret to your control, you might smile mysteriously, or let your healthy character declare, "It's just the way I *am!*" It is, isn't it?

SCRIPT FOR AN EVENING OUT

Prologue, getting dressed
Enjoy a cup of fat-free vegetable noodle soup. Put on your most fabulous dress, preferably one just a little tight in the waistline.

Act I, appetizers
Sip on a glass of tomato juice laced with Tabasco and lemon.

Act II, dinner
Nibble on just a few bites each of the chicken (it has a rich sauce), the vegetables (they're smothered in butter), the rice (ditto).

Act III, dessert
Feel the gentle reminder of your closely fitting dress keeping you on track. Pass up the chocolate torte in favor of a steaming espresso.

Curtain Call, back home
Brew an herbal tea to unwind; lights out in the kitchen (unscrew the bulb if you must).

Party Portions

Social occasions tend to feature a wider selection of foods than normal meals. You can enjoy the bounty without ballooning outward by taking small samples of several things. Here are some tips for party portion control:

- If hors d'oeuvres are passed, try no more than one piece of each. Don't stand or sit near limitless eating opportunities such as bowls of chips or blocks of cheese. Station yourself near the vegetable tray, and skip the dip.
- For buffets, limit yourself to one trip with one plate. Look at your fully loaded dish—is it a lot more lavish than your usual meal? If so, dispose of the excess before you sit down.
- For plated meals, such as a sit-down dinner party, decide what and how much on your plate to eat, then discreetly douse the rest with enough black pepper, salt, or hot sauce to make it inedible. Alternatively, ask for your plate to be cleared as soon as you've eaten your allotment.
- Don't waste calories on anything you don't love. Use a discerning eye—why have a meatball when you see darling little quiches across the room?
- Limit your alcohol consumption—it contains empty calories, and the power to impair your good eating judgment. Count each drink as one snack.
- Drink lots and lots of water throughout the event.

All these pointers apply equally when you're hosting a social event, with one postscript: What do you do when the last guest departs and you're left with a suddenly empty house, lots of dirty dishes, and mounds of leftovers just begging to be eaten by the tired and harried host? Here are some options:

- Flee!—out of the house or to bed, depending on the hour. Hire someone else to clean up or do it in the morning, when the flush of the party has faded. (Note: You should throw away any food left out overnight to prevent the risk of food-borne illness.)
- Package and put away leftovers first, so you won't be tempted to nibble while you clean up everything else.
- Reflect on the social successes of the evening.
- Think of how much more interesting those leftovers will be tomorrow or the next day, when you're fresh and energized.

✳

Now you know the secret: You can be beautifully trim and still eat thrilling food, while following scientific nutrition principles that will keep your star burning bright for years to come. Eating can be a fun and flexible aspect of your ever-exciting life.

Remember, food isn't the only factor in fulfilling your potential for health and beauty. Exercise, relaxation, sleep, and lots of water will all contribute to good looks that radiate from the inside out. All the accoutrements of grooming—hair and skin care, makeup, and wardrobe—are at your disposal to perfect your image. And an appreciative audience awaits to share the fruits of your efforts. You continually create yourself. Never give up.

Shooting Star Lines

- I feel pretty (handsome), witty, and far too fabulous to be waylaid by food.
- I have a huge array of exciting, healthy foods to choose from.
- Lowfat food is *divine.*
- I eat good food to fuel my flame and burn ever brighter.
- I love to have all eyes on me and know that I look and feel my personal best.
- I like to feel light, lively, and sparkling.
- I make fascinating conversation when my mouth isn't full.
- My stomach is just too small to hold large platefuls of food.

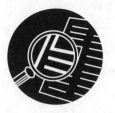

22

THE PERFECTIONIST'S PERSONAL PRESCRIPTION

Your Personal Prescription is about using control to your advantage to pursue the ongoing *process of perfection.* On the surface, your self-control makes you my very best client, willing and able to do it right. You eagerly embrace the details, schedules, and rules that accompany the healthiest eating plan. I'll provide you with plenty of those, helping you to build a routine out of the right foods and portion sizes, so you always know exactly what to do to achieve your goals.

But your reliance on routine can also deprive you of essential nutrients, make you extra-sensitive to small slipups, and leave you victim to dietary burnout. So the second half of your Personal Prescription explores your options—letting you realize that you can safely vary your routine and discover a new world of eating enjoyment that will enhance your body and your health. Tips for efficient cooking, weekly meal planning, and addressing your own eating anxieties all help you to literally lighten up. Remember—perfection is a process, and you can pursue it every day by Eating By Design.

✳

The Right Routine

There's not a thing wrong with routine. In fact, our physical bodies are completely governed by regular cycles and are more than happy to be fed on a set schedule. The trick is to establish the *right* routine—the right foods, portions, and times—and then vary it, within safe and healthy boundaries, just enough to keep you interested and properly nourished.

Purge the Pantry

Within hours after beginning the Diet Designs program, Amy had completely reconstructed her kitchen, creating a healthy space where she could make no mistakes. For a Perfectionist, organization is the key to any major change. Planning and preparedness—your great strengths—are at the center of your Personal Prescription. Use your highly developed organizational skills to arrange and systematize a harmonious center of healthy eating operations with three easy steps.

1. Come Clean

First, come clean in your kitchen by tossing out everything that stands between you and Eating By Design. Hit the pantry, the refrigerator, the freezer, and come clean with all your secret nooks and crannies. Old treats will become temptations; trash them while you still have the chance.

COMING CLEAN: WHAT TO TOSS

Refrigerator:

- Butter and margarine
- Cream, sour cream, whole milk
- Bacon, lunch meats, hot dogs
- Regular cheese
- Mayonnaise
- High-fat salad dressings and sauce

Freezer:

- High-fat and high-sodium frozen desserts, meals, pizzas, and sauced vegetables
- Ice cream
- Your homemade chocolate chip cookie dough, stashed for a rainy day

Pantry:

- Oils
- Canned sauces and sauce mixes
- Creamed soups
- Cereals, breads, and crackers containing fat, salt, and sugar
- Baking mixes, chocolate, packaged frosting
- Fruit preserves with sugar
- Sodas and drink mixes
- Salt and seasoned salt
- Regular soy and teriyaki sauce
- ALL the junk food: chips, candy, cookies, packaged popcorn. Be merciless. Cry if you must; you won't be the first.

WHEN YOU WAVER, CONSULT THE LABEL

> Use the information on food labels to assess the contents of any nutritionally dubious package. Give the boot to any food containing more than 8 grams of fat, 15 grams of sugar, or 550 milligrams of sodium per serving. Also be suspicious of long ingredient lists filled with words you don't know—junk alert!

2. Stock Up

Now, use the Master Market List and Equipment List (Chapter 30) to stock your healthy kitchen.

- Make photocopies of your shopping lists, check off what you already have, and use a highlighter to mark items you definitely want to buy. Plan at least an hour for your first trip to the market: you'll probably find yourself fascinated by labels, comparing fat grams, ingredients, and prices.
- Buy every sort and size of storage container you can think of—Tupperware, canisters, mason jars, Ziploc bags, etc.—to keep your food portioned, fresh, and neat.
- Be sure you have a complete set of measuring cups and spoons and a food scale. You'll have plenty of opportunity for precision and perfection in your portioning!
- After your initial stock-up, continue to use copies of the Master Market List as an inventory and shopping list. As time goes on, you'll probably develop favorite items or brands and cross off some things you never use. Consider typing up your own edited version of the list to keep it short and personal.

3. Organize

For easy access to your new supplies:

- Put all your pastas, grains, and legumes in one cupboard in clear glass or plastic jars that let you see their contents.
- Stack cans of soup, broth, and tomatoes nearby.
- Fill canisters with flours and powdered fructose for baking.
- Put bins for onions, garlic, and potatoes in a cool, dark place. Don't store onions and potatoes in the same container; they encourage each other to rot.
- Arrange your spices and seasonings in a decorative rack.
- Designate a snack cupboard.
- Use wire racks to organize your refrigerator and freezer.
- Label every container that's not clearly marked with contents and date.
- Organize your pots and pans so they're easy to find and use. A hanging system keeps them neat and visible.

Map Out Your Meals

Perfectionists never travel without a road map—so why should you eat without a meal map?

One of Amy's favorite aspects of Diet Designs was the weekly meal plan telling her exactly what she was going to eat and when. She liked eating lunch knowing what she was going to have for dinner. "It helps me stop eating when I know what I have to look forward to," she said.

Below is the Eating By Design Meal Map, a weekly schedule that you can photocopy and fill in so that you always know what you're going to be eating. Make your choices from the Perfectionist Meal Plan for your EQ, which follows the Meal Map.

MEAL MAP LEGEND

- The Meal Map gives you the same breakfast, snack, dressing, sauces, and dessert throughout the week, so you can work your way through a package or potful without waste.
- **Lunch and Dinner:**
  Select one main carbohydrate meal and one main protein meal a day, to be sure you get a good dose of both these essential nutrients on a daily basis. Most people prefer a carbohydrate lunch and protein dinner, which is how I've organized the Perfectionist Meal Plan—but you can switch them as you like.
- **For Snack and Dessert of the Week:**
  See the Perfectly Portioned Snack List in this Chapter or the Master Snack List in Chapter 30.
- **Weekly Prep:**
- Once a week, make sauces and dressing in advance, switch your breakfast, snack, and dessert choices for variety, and stock up on the week's staples.
- Make or buy an oil-free pasta sauce and a fat-free dressing, enough to last the week. Don't miss the Marinara Sauce with variations 📄 in Chapter 33—it's my most efficient and versatile recipe.*
- If you like, make a gourmet sauce to top poultry and seafood (see Chapter 33).
- Portion sauces into individual servings and store in plastic containers or bags.
- Buy your Snack of the Week and portion it into small Ziploc bags.
- Buy the fixings for your Breakfast of the Week. Preportion cereal into bags if you like an extra-easy morning.
- Inventory staples such as pasta, rice, and potatoes, and stock up if you're low.
- Stock the freezer with turkey and vegetarian burgers, skinless chicken breasts, and fish fillets. Or if you prefer these foods fresh, buy a few days' worth and restock midweek.

*See recipe in Chapter 33.

Simple, structured, and consistent—the Eating By Design Meal Map is perfect!

WORK YOURSELF OUT

- Pick a Workout of the Week, just as you do your breakfast, snack, etc. Be sure to rotate aerobic, strength, and flexibility activities from one week to the next for proper cross-training (see the Master Exercise Plan in Chapter 31).
- Make a daily habit of working out, with one day of rest a week to let muscle tissue repair.
- Pick the time of day that works best for you, then stick to it. I recommend first thing in the morning, to start your day with a sense of achievement—jump-starting the process of perfection.

✳

Eating By Design Meal Map, Week of _____

	Workout 7:00 A.M.	Breakfast 8:00 A.M.	Snack 10:00 A.M.	Lunch 12:00 P.M.	Snack 3:00 P.M.	Dinner 6:00 P.M.	Dessert by 8:00 P.M.
MON.	Workout of the Week ———	Breakfast of the Week ———	Fresh Fruit		Snack of the Week ———		Dessert of the Week ———
TUES.	⇩	⇩	⇩		⇩		⇩
WED.	⇩	⇩	⇩		⇩		⇩

	Workout 7:00 A.M.	Breakfast 8:00 A.M.	Snack 10:00 A.M.	Lunch 12:00 P.M.	Snack 3:00 P.M.	Dinner 6:00 P.M.	Dessert by 8:00 P.M.
THUR.	Workout of the Week _____	Breakfast of the Week _____	Fresh Fruit		Snack of the Week _____		Dessert of the Week _____
FRI.	⇩	⇩	⇩		⇩		⇩
SAT.	⇩	⇩	⇩		⇩		⇩
SUN.	⇩	⇩	⇩		⇩		⇩

❋

The Perfectionist Meal Plan*

Choose from the meal plan for your EQ below and fill in your Eating By Design Meal Map.

EQ 1 (Low)

BREAKFAST

½ c. orange juice
Choose from:
✓ ½ bagel with 1 T. fat-free cream cheese and ½ c. fruit-sweetened nonfat yogurt
✓ 1 oz. cereal or fat-free granola with 1 c. skim milk
✓ Low-fat crumpet with 2 t. pure fruit preserves and ½ c. fruit-sweetened nonfat yogurt
✓ Low-fat waffle with ½ c. nonfat cottage cheese and 2 t. pure fruit syrup

SNACK

1 piece fresh fruit

LUNCH

Mixed green salad with fat-free dressing
Choose from:
✓ 1 c. pasta with ¾ c. sauce of the week
✓ 1 medium or ½ large baked potato topped with steamed or broth-sautéed vegetables and 1½ oz. fat-free cheese
✓ Steamed or grilled vegetable plate with 1 c. rice, pasta, grains, or legumes

SNACK

Choose from the Perfectly Portioned Snack List (p. 238)

DINNER

Choose from: 3 oz. of grilled, broiled, baked, or poached
✓ Skinless chicken breast
✓ Skinless turkey breast
✓ Seafood

Choose from: 1 serving of
✓ Tomato-Fennel Sauce 🗏
✓ Dijon-Shallot Sauce 🗏
✓ Raspberry Sauce 🗏
✓ Pesto Sauce 🗏
✓ Marsala Cream Sauce 🗏

½ c. rice, pasta, grains, or legumes
Steamed vegetables

---

*   🗏   = See recipe in Chapter 33.

DESSERT

Choose from:
✓ 4 oz. nonfat frozen yogurt
✓ Perfectly Portioned Snack List (p. 238) or Master Snack List (Chapter 30)

EQ 2 (Low-Medium)

BREAKFAST

½ c. orange juice
Choose from:
✓ ½ bagel with 1 T. fat-free cream cheese and ½ c. fruit-sweetened nonfat yogurt
✓ 1 oz. cereal or fat-free granola with 1 c. skim milk
✓ Low-fat crumpet with 2 t. pure fruit preserves and ½ c. fruit-sweetened nonfat yogurt
✓ Low-fat waffle with ½ c. nonfat cottage cheese and 2 t. pure fruit syrup.

SNACK

1 piece fresh fruit

LUNCH

Mixed green salad with fat-free dressing
Choose from:
✓ 1½ c. pasta with ¾ c. sauce of the week
✓ 1 medium or ½ large baked potato topped with steamed or broth-sautéed vegetables and 1½ oz. fat-free cheese
✓ Steamed or grilled vegetable plate with 1½ c. rice, pasta, grains, or legumes

SNACK

Choose from the Perfectly Portioned Snack List (p. 238)

DINNER

Choose from: 6 oz. of grilled, broiled, baked, or poached
✓ Skinless chicken breast
✓ Skinless turkey breast
✓ Seafood

Choose from: 1 serving of
✓ Tomato-Fennel Sauce 📄
✓ Dijon-Shallot Sauce 📄
✓ Raspberry Sauce 📄
✓ Pesto Sauce 📄
✓ Marsala Cream Sauce 📄

1 c. rice, pasta, grains, or legumes
Steamed vegetables

DESSERT

Choose from:
✓ 4 oz. nonfat frozen yogurt
✓ Perfectly Portioned Snack List (p. 238) or Master Snack List (Chapter 30)

EQ 3 (Medium-High)

BREAKFAST

Choose from:
✓ 1 bagel with 2 T. fat-free cream cheese and 1 c. fruit-sweetened nonfat yogurt
✓ 2 oz. cereal or fat-free granola with 2 c. skim milk
✓ 2 low-fat crumpets with 4 t. pure fruit preserves and 1 c. fruit-sweetened nonfat yogurt
✓ 2 low-fat waffles with 1 c. nonfat cottage cheese and 4 t. pure fruit syrup.

SNACK

1 piece fresh fruit

LUNCH

Mixed green salad with fat-free dressing
Choose from:
✓ 1½ c. pasta with ¾ c. sauce of the week
✓ 1 medium or ½ large baked potato topped with steamed or broth-sautéed vegetables and 1½ oz. fat-free cheese
✓ Steamed or grilled vegetable plate with 1½ c. rice, pasta, grains, or legumes

SNACK

Choose from the Perfectly Portioned Snack List (p. 238)

DINNER

Choose from: 6 oz. of grilled, broiled, baked, or poached
✓ Skinless chicken breast
✓ Skinless turkey breast
✓ Seafood

Choose from: 1 serving of
✓ Tomato-Fennel Sauce 📄
✓ Dijon-Shallot Sauce 📄
✓ Raspberry Sauce 📄
✓ Pesto Sauce 📄
✓ Marsala Cream Sauce 📄

1 c. rice, pasta, grains, or legumes
Steamed vegetables

DESSERT

Choose from:
✓ 4 oz. nonfat frozen yogurt
✓ Perfectly Portioned Snack List (p. 238) or Master Snack List (Chapter 30)

EQ 4 (High)

BREAKFAST

Choose from:
✓ 1 bagel with 2 T. fat-free cream cheese and 1 c. fruit-sweetened nonfat yogurt
✓ 2 oz. cereal or fat-free granola with 2 c. skim milk
✓ 2 low-fat crumpets with 4 t. pure fruit preserves and 1 c. fruit-sweetened nonfat yogurt
✓ 2 low-fat waffles with 1 c. nonfat cottage cheese and 4 t. pure fruit syrup.

SNACK

1 piece fresh fruit

LUNCH

Mixed green salad with fat-free dressing
Choose from:
✓ 2 c. pasta with ¾ c. sauce of the week
✓ 1 large baked potato topped with steamed or broth-sautéed vegetables and 1½ oz. fat-free cheese
✓ Steamed or grilled vegetable plate with 2 c. rice, pasta, grains, or legumes

SNACK

Choose from the Perfectly Portioned Snack List (p. 238)

DINNER

Choose from: 6 oz. of grilled, broiled, baked, or poached
✓ Skinless chicken breast
✓ Skinless turkey breast
✓ Seafood

Choose from: 1 serving of
✓ Tomato-Fennel Sauce 🗒
✓ Dijon-Shallot Sauce 🗒
✓ Raspberry Sauce 🗒
✓ Pesto Sauce 🗒
✓ Marsala Cream Sauce 🗒

1½ c. rice, pasta, grains, or legumes
Steamed vegetables

DESSERT

Choose from:
✓ 4 oz. nonfat frozen yogurt with ¾ c. diced fruit
✓ 1 piece fresh fruit and 1 item from the Perfectly Portioned Snack List (p. 238) or Master Snack List (Chapter 30)

SUPPLEMENT YOURSELF

> Steady reliance on favorite foods can deprive you of your RDAs. Perfect your nutritional profile with a good daily multivitamin and mineral supplement every morning after breakfast.

Home Economics

You can use your propensity for planning and organization to keep your cooking neat, quick, and economical:

- Buy food in the smallest packages appropriate to your household. While this sometimes seems more expensive, it's economical in the long run if the alternatives are overeating or throwing it away. Individual servings of soup, sauces, and dressing are increasingly available. Freeze extra portions of larger packages for later use.
- Buy cooked chicken and turkey and low-fat cheeses at the deli counter in individual portion sizes. Ask your server to weigh and wrap servings separately.
- Cook several portions of pasta, grains, and legumes at a time. Store the leftovers in individual servings in the refrigerator or freezer.
- Cut vegetables in the morning, arrange in a steamer basket, and put water in the pan below. In the evening, simply turn on the burner for instant steamed vegetables. Keep frozen vegetables on hand for emergencies.
- Grill or broil poultry and seafood, or do a quick stir-fry in stock.
- Use vacuum jars to store unrefrigerated perishables such as snacks and baked goods.
- Save vegetable trimmings for stocks.
- Keep a windowsill herb garden that lets you harvest as needed. Or freeze store-bought herbs and use straight from the freezer.
- Don't ever cook extra "just in case." Weigh and measure *before* you cook.

Perfectionists tend to finish what's on the plate or in the package out of a basic puritan impulse. Your sense of good form rebels against the notion of waste, whether it's time, effort, or food. But remember: Food is as wasted in your fat cells as it is in the trash can—and poses a bigger threat to your well-being.

Create Your Own Comfort Zone

Once you've mastered your meal plan at home, one of the most important assurances you can offer yourself as a Perfectionist is an advance plan for dining out that saves you from making difficult, on-the-spot decisions outside of your private comfort zone. Any restaurant menu can be analyzed in advance. Just call and have a menu mailed or faxed, then circle simple salads, pastas, and entrees without buttery or oily sauces. Consult your EQ and decide what you'll order before even walking through the door.

See the restaurant recommendations in Chapter 30. As always, feel free to ask for dishes to be split in half and prepared without oil. If you prefer, phone ahead with your special requests. Advance planning allows you to carry your comfort zone with you at all times.

You can employ the same strategy when dining at catered events or other people's homes. Most hosts are more likely to be concerned for your comfort than offended by your requests, and will be happy to accommodate you.

Whenever you find yourself outside of your comfort zone, remember that, barring a food allergy, it's unlikely that eating any given food once will ruin your life. Your digestive system will dispatch with it before you even know what hit you.

FOOD ALLERGIES: HOW LIKELY?

Many of my Perfectionist clients are concerned that they might be allergic to certain foods. Allergies are indeed dangerous, and it's important to identify and avoid anything that causes an allergic reaction. But true food allergies are rare, afflicting fewer than one percent of American adults. Here are a few food allergy facts:

- An allergy is present when the body mistakenly produces antibodies to fight a perceived threat, resulting in anything from a rash to shock. The most common food allergies are to shellfish, eggs, milk, wheat, nuts, and soybeans.
- More common are intolerances, or the absence of certain digestive enzymes, which can result in unpleasant but not medically threatening discomfort—stomach aches, bloating, gas, diarrhea. Common intolerances are for milk (correctable by taking the digestive enzyme lactase) and gluten.
- Also fairly common are reactions to additives such as MSG and sulfites. There is as yet little scientific evidence to explain or predict these reactions.
- Even the standard accepted tests for food allergies are known to show false positive results. There are also many completely unproven testing methods in circulation. The only conclusive test is a carefully controlled elimination diet.

If you suspect a food allergy or intolerance, consult a physician. Explore your options and feel sure before eliminating any healthful food that you enjoy from your diet.

✳

Do It by the Book

Calculate Your Calories, Count Your Cheese Puffs, and Log Your Lunches

Studies show that dieters tend to underestimate their eating by up to 1,000 calories a day! When we analyzed Amy's typical day of mega-muffin, tuna sandwich, yogurt, pasta, and Tofutti, we found that she often exceeded her optimal daily intake by that amount, and came up woefully short on the fresh fruits and vegetables so crucial to health and longevity.

The solution? *Do it by the book.* Weigh, measure, or count everything that crosses your lips. Don't presume you know a cup of pasta or an ounce of pretzels by sight. Calculate before you consume. Then, write it down.

One of my clients came into her consultation with a full computer spreadsheet of everything she'd eaten, with calories and fat grams in separate columns, for the entire week. We identified her strengths and weaknesses in a flash, which made fine-tuning a breeze. Even if you're maintaining your weight, you might be missing your optimal daily nutritional mix.

The Perfectly Portioned Snack List

To achieve perfection in your snack portioning, count—your cheese puffs, rice cakes, etc. Here are the proper counts for perfect portions of some favorite Eating By Design snacks.

6	Laura Scudder's fat-free pretzels, small (not mini)
10	Rold Gold fat-free pretzel "thins"
30	Louise's fat-free potato chips
22	Guiltless Gourmet tortilla chips
32	fat-free cheese puffs
20	Auburn Farms fat-free crackers
5	Health Valley fat-free crackers
9	Snackwell's fat-free wheat crackers
4	dried apricot halves
1	large fat-free rice cake with 1 T. nonfat ricotta cheese and 2 t. pure fruit jam
1	frozen fruit bar
1	Häagen-Dazs low-fat yogurt bar
½	cup fat-free pudding

The Perfectionist's Primer

The best way to do it by the book is—well, with a book, Photocopy the forms below or use your own computer program and assemble them in a three-ring binder. This is your Perfectionist's Primer for Eating By Design.

1. Refer to your Eating Quotient in Chapter 13 to find your daily allotments of calories, fat, protein, and carbohydrate. Fill in below.
   Eating Quotient　　　　　　———————
   Calories　　　　　　　　　　———————
   Fat (grams)　　　　　　　　———————
   Protein (grams)　　　　　　———————
   Carbohydrate (grams)　　　———————

2. Use the ledger below or your own computer spreadsheet program to log your intake every day. Read nutrition labels or refer to a good food counts book (see References and Recommended Reading in Appendix) to record your calories, fat, protein, and carbohydrate grams, and tally them up for each day.

3. At the end of the week, cross-check your actual intake with your daily allotments above. Target problem days and times—is the discrepancy in your plan, your portions, or something else that made you wander off course? Use this weekly self-check to perfect your plan.

DAILY INTAKE LOG
Week of _____

FOOD & PORTION	CALORIES	FAT	PROTEIN	CARBS
MON. Breakfast: Lunch: Dinner: Snacks: **Totals:**				
TUES. Breakfast: Lunch: Dinner: Snacks: **Totals:**				
WED. Breakfast: Lunch: Dinner: Snacks: **Totals:**				
THURS. Breakfast: Lunch: Dinner: Snacks: **Totals:**				
FRI. Breakfast: Lunch: Dinner: Snacks: **Totals:**				
SAT. Breakfast: Lunch: Dinner: Snacks: **Totals:**				
SUN. Breakfast: Lunch: Dinner: Snacks: **Totals:**				

Write Your Own Rules

No matter how many rules and guidelines I give you to structure your diet, everybody has a few special obstacles requiring personal rules to move closer to perfection. For example, here are some common healthy eating obstacles, with their Eating By Design solutions:

OBSTACLE:	**RULE:**
I overeat late at night.	I may not eat after 8:00 P.M.
I can't open a package of cookies without eating the whole thing.	I must pack cookies into snack portions as soon as I open the package. I may not have more than one portion a day.
I love steak.	I will eat steak no more than once a month, and will highlight it in my food diary to be sure I don't slip up.
I hate to cook vegetables.	I will eat 2 cups of vegetables a day, even if they're frozen or from the salad bar.
I eat last night's leftover frozen yogurt for breakfast.	I will buy frozen yogurt in individual servings and throw away any leftover every night.

Sit down and write out ten rules that will help you stick to your healthy eating plan and add them to your book. Refer to them and write additional rules as often as you need to. Remember, a stitch in time saves nine.

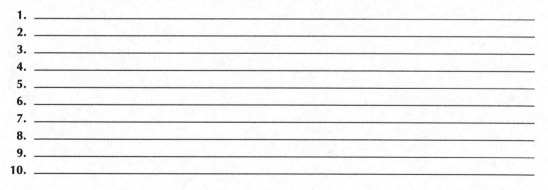

1. _____
2. _____
3. _____
4. _____
5. _____
6. _____
7. _____
8. _____
9. _____
10. _____

✳

The planning and preparation are over. You have a well-stocked and organized kitchen and inventory lists to keep it that way. You have a Meal Map to plan each week of Eating By Design in advance. And you have your Perfectionist's Primer to log all the details and track your progress.

So what now? Just sit back and relax. Laugh. Live a little. Perfection is a process—and meanwhile, you're Eating By Design.

✳

Credos for Controlled Consumption

Use your strong will and love of order to keep your routine on the right track:

- I will be *persistent* in *planning.*
- I will be *meticulous* in *measuring.*
- I will be *fussy* about *fat.*
- I will *insist* on *interval eating.*
- I will be *painstaking* in *portioning.*
- I will be *obstinate* against *overeating.*

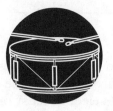

23

THE SOLOIST'S PERSONAL PRESCRIPTION

As a Soloist, you certainly have a mind of your own. The aim of your Personal Prescription is to turn your strong mind to the task of caring for your body—without distracting from the other interests and concerns that populate your busy inner world. Every element is calculated to respect and care for your Soloist self as an autonomous being, while providing for the special attention that can sometimes slip from a Soloist's self-care habits.

Because the Soloist approach to food is generally convenience-driven, the key to renovating your diet is incorporating *healthy* convenient choices into your already-established habits, therefore cutting back on the salt and fat that plague packaged foods. These easy, high-energy options will naturally trim down your body, to make sure that those thick walls you build to protect your privacy aren't made of body fat. So go ahead and march to a different drummer—with a new spring to your step.

✳

Project Preparation

Survey the Literature

The logical Soloist is easily persuaded with an argument grounded in fact. Fortunately, all the facts support the efficacy of eating well in promoting health, energy, and longevity. Treat your body to the best information you can find on its inner workings. Begin by reading Part Two from start to finish. Then, turn to References and Recommended Reading in the Appendix to go in-depth on topics of particular interest to you—perhaps the latest research on antioxidants and phytochemicals, or the role of genetics in fat processing and storage.

To build a basic library covering both the latest breakthroughs and the classic axioms of nutrition and physiology, I recommend you select at least one of each of the following from the list:

1. A text or reference book.
2. A comprehensive food counts book.
3. A subscription to a journal for the latest scholarly work.
4. A subscription to a newsletter, for reader-friendly nutritional news.

Optional: Enlist an Ally

Jay's aversion to talking about his dieting efforts left him without the moral support most people, even Soloists, need in order to stick to a new eating plan. Just as the Lone Ranger had Tonto and Don Quixote had Sancho Panza, I suggested that Jay share his healthy eating ambitions with an ally. He enlisted the support of his assistant, one of the few people he saw on a regular basis. It turned out his new ally was eager to lose a few pounds himself.

To ease your transition to Eating By Design, consider picking a trusted buddy—friend, significant other, whomever—to undertake your Personal Prescription with you (remember, you can each tailor the plan to your individual needs using the Eating Quotient). Here are some things to do *à deux* with your healthy eating ally:

Once a week:
- Go on a "healthy foods only" grocery shopping trip.
- Cook a healthy dinner together.
- Bike, run, hike, play tennis, rollerskate, swim, ski, or any other sporting activity.
- Have a regular session to report your progress to each other. Praise each other's achievements for the week, whether at work, school, in relationships, or Eating By Design. Come clean about any slipups; this is a safe space in which to share and forgive yourself. Follow with a movie on the VCR and some air-popped popcorn.

Once a month:
- Take each other's measurements, and/or go to the health club for a body fat test.
- Clean out each other's kitchens of unhealthy foods.

If you choose to go it alone, that's fine—your Personal Prescription is perfectly tailored for solo dining. Just be sure to give yourself all the positive reinforcement you deserve.

✳

Stock Up for Solitary Dining

Though you may share meals, a home, even a life with someone, chances are your solo style causes you to eat alone a lot. A simple system for stocking your kitchen with single-portion or long-lasting foods makes it easy to eat well without waste or the nutritional hazards of standard convenience foods.

Solo Staples (See Master Market List for brand names)

Keep your shelves and refrigerator stocked with the following items:

_____ Cereal variety packs (unsweetened)
_____ Individual flavored oatmeal packets
_____ Individually wrapped low-fat breakfast bars
_____ Small cartons of nonfat milk
_____ Small cartons of fruit-sweetened yogurt
_____ Individual fresh or frozen chicken breasts or fish filets
_____ Sliced roasted or smoked turkey from the deli (healthier than packaged lunch meats)
_____ Egg- and oil-free dried pasta
_____ Low-fat or fat-free pasta sauces
_____ Canned soups
_____ Low-fat ramen noodles, couscous, pasta, or soup cups
_____ Individual cans of tuna
_____ Potatoes
_____ ReadyPak mixed salad greens
_____ Fresh veggies from the salad bar
_____ Fat-free dressing

Living from the Low-Fat Freezer

The technology of freezing food revolutionized American eating habits, making it easier than ever to eat without fuss or bother. Unfortunately, until recently, the nutritional value of freezer fare left much to be desired.

But lately, frozen food has taken a turn for the better both in terms of nutrition and aesthetics. As a solo diner, the freezer is your friend, as long as you don't fill it with fat, sugar, and sodium. Be sure to follow the Eating By Design Convenience Foods Guidelines in the sidebar when making your frozen choices.

_____ Low-fat, low-sodium frozen entrees
_____ Frozen vegetables
_____ Frozen fruit juice concentrates
_____ Low-fat waffles or pancakes
_____ Nonfat egg substitute
_____ Frozen nonfat yogurt
_____ Frozen yogurt bars and fruit bars
_____ Fudgsicles

FIVE REASONS TO EAT FROM THE LOW-FAT FREEZER

- Individual portion sizes.
- Food lasts indefinitely.
- Nutrient preservation—frozen vegetables that haven't undergone transport and refrigeration can contain more vitamins than fresh.
- Maximum variety and minimum waste.
- Easy shopping and preparation.

EATING BY DESIGN
CONVENIENCE FOODS GUIDELINES

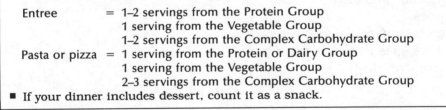

Use the following guidelines to select and serve healthy refrigerated or frozen entrees.

- Keep entrees below 400 calories, 10 grams of fat, 15 grams of sugar, and 550 milligrams of sodium.
- Avoid any brand that contains hydrogenated or cottonseed, palm, or coconut oils.
- Use the following guidelines to plug your dish into the Eating By Design Mosaic:

    Entree   = 1–2 servings from the Protein Group
                              1 serving from the Vegetable Group
                              1–2 servings from the Complex Carbohydrate Group
    Pasta or pizza = 1 serving from the Protein or Dairy Group
                              1 serving from the Vegetable Group
                              2–3 servings from the Complex Carbohydrate Group
- If your dinner includes dessert, count it as a snack.

Quick Pick-ups

Take-out food is a Soloist's best friend. Take-out fat and additives are a Soloist's worst enemy. Follow these take-out guidelines to keep your meals fresh, spontaneous, and within the Eating By Design parameters:

- Supermarket or deli:
  - ✓ Sushi 6-pack

✓ Individual servings of *low-fat* enchiladas, burritos, pasta, spa salads (check the nutrition label against the Convenience Food Guidelines).

✓ Half pints of low-fat deli salads (pasta, grains, legumes, vegetables, poultry, seafood). **AVOID** mayonnaise, oil, cheese.

✓ Turkey or chicken breast sandwich with lettuce, tomato, onion, mustard; **AVOID** mayonnaise, cheese.

✓ Roasted chicken with skin removed; buy the breast meat only.

✓ Salad bar: Greens, vegetables, limited quantities of beans or cottage cheese, a spoonful of raisins, plain vinegar or your own fat-free dressing. **AVOID** composed salads with oil or mayonnaise, cheese, nuts, seeds, bacon bits, croutons.

- Take-out restaurants:

  ✓ Chicken rotisseries: Skinless breast meat only. Accompany with salsa or honey-mustard dip; corn tortillas, rice, beans, or roll; corn on the cob or vegetable salad. **AVOID** coleslaw, cheese, sour cream, guacamole.

  ✓ Chinese: Any chicken, seafood, or vegetable dish with steamed white or brown rice, or vegetables lo mein.

  AVOID:
  —Breaded (orange or lemon chicken, sweet & sour)
  —Crispy
  —Fried noodles
  —Sesame sauce
  —Peanuts, cashews

Microwave Menus

Not all convenience food comes from the freezer or the take-out counter. You can be a home convenience cook with the help of your microwave oven, which offers quick preparation, easy one-dish cleanup, and a fat-free cooking method that retains maximum moisture and nutrients. You can cook just about anything in the microwave; most ovens come with a book listing cooking times for a variety of foods. Just keep in mind the important tips below, then try a few of these nutritionally nuclear ideas.

- Most cooking instructions presume a 600–700 watt oven. If yours is in the lower 400–500 watt range, add cooking time as necessary.
- Use only microwave-safe dishes. No metals or foil!
- Cover food with vented plastic wrap or a lid to ensure even cooking and keep moisture in.
- Stir food halfway through the cooking time. Place thicker foods on the outside edge of the dish, where things cook faster.

- Pay attention to resting times; the food actually finishes cooking after you take it out of the oven.

Start with these simple labor-saving recipes to get the hang of high-speed low-fat cooking.

Nuclear Omelette: Cook chopped vegetables of your choice, covered, on high for 2 minutes, stirring halfway through. Add ½ c. nonfat egg substitute and season to taste. Cook uncovered for 1–2 minutes. Stir and cook for 1–2 minutes more. Let rest for 1 minute.

Baked Potato or Yam: For crispier skin than the usual microwaved spud, pierce potato with a fork and cook on high on a paper towel for 3–5 minutes, then wrap in a paper towel and let rest for 5 minutes.

Winter Squash: This natural source of antioxidant vitamins is a delicious antidote to processed foods. Pierce the skin in several places with a knife, place on a paper towel, and cook on high for 1–2 minutes. Cut in half, remove seeds, and continue cooking until tender, about 5 minutes.

Hi-Tech Frozen Vegetables: Both freezer and microwave technology work to preserve the vitamins in vegetables—an added bonus to the convenience factor! Cook vegetables straight from the freezer in a covered dish with 2 tablespoons of water. Follow the cooking times on the package, or use a general guideline: Cook 6 minutes, stirring halfway through; let stand for 2 minutes more.

Other healthy foods that fare well in the microwave: Oatmeal, canned and dried low-fat soups, all kinds of fresh vegetables, chicken breasts or fish filets cooked in a fat-free sauce (try marinara or barbeque), leftover Chinese food or pasta (add a splash of water if it looks dry), popcorn.

Now you're stocked up with a wide range of solo meal options that will make you healthy without hassle. Put these options into action with the Soloist Meal Plan.

✳

The Soloist Meal Plan*

EQ 1 (Low)

BREAKFAST

½ c. orange juice
½ c. nonfat yogurt or cottage cheese
Choose from:
✓ Mini-pack cereal or individual oatmeal packet with ½ c. skim milk
✓ 1 Blueberry or Raspberry Muffin 📄 or other fat-free muffin
✓ Low-fat breakfast bar
✓ Nuclear Omelette (p. 248)

LUNCH

Choose one:
From the deli or supermarket
✓ Salad bar: lettuce, assorted vegetables, ½ c. cottage cheese, fat-free dressing
✓ ½ pint low-fat deli salad
✓ ½ turkey sandwich without mayonnaise
✓ Individual low-fat enchilada, burrito, pasta, or spa salad

From home
✓ 1 serving Chicken Caesar Salad 📄
✓ 2 c. canned or dried low-fat soup

SNACK

Choose from the Solo Snacks (p. 253)

DINNER

Choose one:
Take-out
✓ Rotisserie or supermarket roasted chicken: ½ skinless breast, ½ c. rice or beans, ½ cob of corn
✓ Sushi 6-pack
✓ Chinese entree with ½ c. rice

Make at home
✓ 1 serving Nachos 📄
✓ Frozen low-fat entree
✓ 1 c. pasta with ¾ c. oil-free Marinara Sauce 📄 and 1 t. Parmesan cheese

Steamed fresh or frozen vegetables

SNACK

Choose from the Solo Snacks (p. 253)

---

* 📄 = See recipe in Chapter 33.

EQ 2 (Low-Medium)

BREAKFAST

½ c. orange juice
½ c. nonfat yogurt or cottage cheese
Choose from:
✓ Mini-pack cereal or individual oatmeal packet with ½ c. skim milk
✓ 1 Blueberry or Raspberry Muffin 📄 or other fat-free muffin
✓ Low-fat breakfast bar
✓ Nuclear Omelette

SNACK

Choose from the Solo Snacks

LUNCH

Choose one:
From the deli or supermarket
✓ Salad bar: lettuce, assorted vegetables, ½ c. cottage cheese, fat-free dressing, and roll
✓ ½ pint low-fat deli salad
✓ ½ turkey sandwich without mayonnaise and 1 c. uncreamed soup
✓ Individual low-fat enchilada, burrito, pasta, or spa salad

From home
✓ 1 serving Chicken Caesar Salad 📄
✓ 2 c. canned or dried low-fat soup

SNACK

Choose from the Solo Snacks

DINNER

Choose one:
Take-out
✓ Rotisserie or supermarket roasted chicken: ½ skinless breast, 1 c. rice or beans, ½ cob of corn
✓ Sushi 6-pack
✓ Chinese entree with 1 c. rice

Make at home
✓ 2 servings Nachos 📄
✓ Frozen low-fat entree
✓ 1½ c. pasta with ¾ c. oil-free Marinara Sauce 📄 and 1 t. Parmesan cheese

Steamed fresh or frozen vegetables

SNACK

Choose from the Solo Snacks

EQ 3 (Medium-High)

BREAKFAST

½ c. orange juice
1 c. nonfat yogurt or cottage cheese
Choose from:
✓ Mini-pack cereal or individual oatmeal packet with ½ c. skim milk
✓ 1 Blueberry or Raspberry Muffin 🗒 or other fat-free muffin
✓ Low-fat breakfast bar
✓ Nuclear Omelette

SNACK

Choose from the Solo Snacks

LUNCH

Choose one:
From the deli or supermarket
✓ Salad bar: lettuce, assorted vegetables, 1 c. cottage cheese, fat-free dressing, and roll
✓ 1 pint low-fat deli salad
✓ Turkey sandwich without mayonnaise and 1 c. uncreamed soup
✓ Individual low-fat enchilada, burrito, pasta, or spa salad

From home
✓ 1 serving Chicken Caesar Salad 🗒
✓ 2 c. canned or dried low-fat soup

SNACK

Choose 2 from the Solo Snacks

DINNER

Choose one:
Take-out
✓ Rotisserie or supermarket roasted chicken: ½ skinless breast, 1 c. rice or beans, ½ cob of corn
✓ Sushi 6-pack
✓ Chinese entree with 1 c. rice

Make at home
✓ 2 servings Nachos 🗒
✓ Frozen low-fat entree
✓ 1½ c. pasta with ¾ c. oil-free Marinara Sauce 🗒 and 1 t. Parmesan cheese

Steamed fresh or frozen vegetables

SNACK

Choose from the Solo Snacks

EQ 4 (High)

BREAKFAST

½ c. orange juice
1 c. nonfat yogurt or cottage cheese
Choose from:
✓ Mini-pack cereal or individual oatmeal packet with ½ c. skim milk
✓ 1 Blueberry or Raspberry Muffin 📄 or other fat-free muffin
✓ Low-fat breakfast bar
✓ Nuclear Omelette

SNACK

Choose from the Solo Snacks

LUNCH

Choose one:
From the deli or supermarket
✓ Salad bar: lettuce, assorted vegetables, 1 c. cottage cheese, fat-free dressing, and roll
✓ 1 pint low-fat deli salad
✓ 1 Turkey sandwich without mayonnaise and 1 c. uncreamed soup
✓ Individual low-fat enchilada, burrito, pasta, or spa salad

From home
✓ 1 serving Chicken Caesar Salad 📄
✓ 2 c. canned or dried low-fat soup

SNACK

Choose from the Solo Snacks

DINNER

Choose one:
Take-out
✓ Rotisserie or supermarket roasted chicken: ½ skinless breast, 1 c. rice or beans, 1 roll or 2 tortillas, ½ cob of corn
✓ Sushi 6-pack
✓ Chinese entree with 1½ c. rice

Make at home
✓ 2 servings Nachos 📄
✓ Frozen low-fat entree
✓ 2 c. pasta with 1½ c. oil-free Marinara Sauce 📄 and 2 t. Parmesan cheese

Steamed fresh or frozen vegetables

SNACK

Choose from the Solo Snacks

SOLO SNACKS

These come in small packages for easy solo snacking:

✓ Individual bag of pretzels, low-fat chips, apple chips, mini rice cakes
✓ Smartpop
✓ Granola bar
✓ 1 piece fresh fruit
✓ Mini box of raisins
✓ Cup of soup
✓ Frozen yogurt bar or fruit bar
✓ Fudgsicle
✓ 4 oz. soft-serve frozen nonfat yogurt
✓ Carton of fruit-sweetened nonfat yogurt
✓ Individual string cheese

WORK YOURSELF OUT

- Install a piece of exercise equipment in your home.
- Take up solo activities like hiking, biking, swimming, running, jumping rope, weight lifting, exercise videos or television shows.

SUPPLEMENT YOURSELF

- A superpotent multiple vitamin and mineral supplement helps fill in any gaps left by your Soloist lifestyle.

✳

Come Out of the Closet—It's Hip to Be Healthy

As you whisper to the waiter about oil-free preparation, raise your little finger when the flight attendant yells out, "Who has the low-cal plate?," or rustle the wrapper off your fat-free breakfast bar under the conference room table, remember: It's socially desirable to eat right. Doing so will only raise you in the esteem of others, giving the clear message that your self is worth caring for. In fact, the latest nutritional news makes a great subject for small talk. Even utter strangers are willing to compare fat grams at the drop of a hat.

Though eating is at one level a very personal activity—it is, after all, *your* body—it is also a social occasion across cultures. Nearly everyone has some inner conflicts about the way they eat, but your healthy outer self is proof positive that you do it well. Breaking bread need not always be a private issue.

Come out of the closet with your healthy eating habits with the confidence that you're doing the right thing.

DINING ALONE IN PUBLIC WITH PANACHE

If you're a little shy about solo dining, take a few tips from the timid but hungry:

- Try to pick a restaurant where you're familiar with the menu—one of the national chains covered in Chapter 30, or a local spot where you've been before. You'll have fewer questions to ask and choices to make.
- Pick a corner table or sit at the counter.
- Take something to read—newspapers are great when there's plenty of space; magazines and books slip into a briefcase and make more compact companions.

✳

Independence is a cherished human value, built right into the foundation of our government. As a Soloist, you can use your great personal strength to declare your independence from the tyranny of ill health and poor eating habits that has gripped our society.

However, evidence suggests that those who live alone are more susceptible to disease, especially later in life. Guard against the potential toll of your individuality by committing to self-care with all the autonomous power of the Soloist.

Soloist Reflections

- I care for my own health with good food choices.
- Eating well increases my sense of independence and autonomy.
- My home is a healthy haven.
- Food is my fuel, not my friend. Excess or unhealthy food is a false friend.
- I need and deserve fresh, whole foods full of nutrients and natural energy.
- Eating good food on a regular schedule enhances my work and projects.
- I feel best outside of my cocoon, free to fly without excess baggage.
- I am attractive in many ways, and I become more attractive the better I feel.
- Body fat is not a good barrier against the world.
- I have the power to change my body.

Make a tape of these affirmations, and play them back when you want to hear a friendly voice.

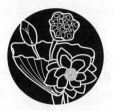

24

THE LOTUS EATER'S PERSONAL PRESCRIPTION

This Personal Prescription is the medicine you need if food has become a prop, a hit, or a high for you. It's time to take treatment. If you're leaning on some other substance, be forewarned that, as for my client Jenni, it could become food anytime in your future. Forearm yourself by learning the signs, signals, and solutions for food using.

Eating By Design will help you return food to its rightful role as fuel; then watch your health, energy, and self-esteem return with renewed power. Your Personal Prescription provides concrete information to help you treat yourself with a recovery diet and offers several behavioral techniques for breaking your food habit.

✳

Help Yourself

Though I firmly believe that every food user needs and deserves outside help (see my discussion in Part One), you also have great power to help yourself. Personal empowerment is not a mystical force of which you've somehow been unfairly deprived. It's really nothing more than a set of behaviors, turning inner thoughts into outer actions. Breaking your behaviors down into small, discrete actions helps you take control, to fuel yourself without using. Your Personal Prescription for Eating By Design is merely the sum of these actions.

The Recovery Diet

The Lotus Eater Meal Plan is a "recovery diet" designed to break the cycle of compulsion with some simple principles:

- No sugar, refined flours or grains, caffeine, or alcohol. All of these foods can be addictive.
- Carbohydrates and protein are carefully balanced to keep you steadily satisfied. Lotus Eaters tend to be carb cravers, which can trigger overeating and binges. Protein provides preventive medicine.
- The foods of the meal plan are simple, solid, and satisfying. Snack foods, even fat-free brands, are too tempting during recovery.
- You have just two or three easy-to-prepare options for each meal. Your goal for now is to take your focus off food.
- The plan emphasizes things you can get or store in small packages, to keep your boundaries clear.

In the meal plans below, I've indicated the exact portions for each EQ. Eventually, you should become exacting in your portion control—but perfect portions are really not necessary just now. Don't be too concerned with amounts at first. The important thing is to break your food using habit.

✳

Lotus Eater Meal Plan*

EQ 1 (Low)

BREAKFAST

½ c. fruit-sweetened nonfat yogurt with ¾ c. diced fruit

SNACK

Choose from Lotus Eater Snack List in this chapter

LUNCH

Choose from:
✓ 1 serving Chopped Chicken or Shrimp Salad 📋
✓ 1 c. fat-free lentil soup and ½ turkey sandwich (1 slice 7-grain bread, 3 oz. turkey breast, lettuce, tomato, onion, mustard, fat-free mayonnaise)
✓ Turkey Burger 📋 or low-fat vegetarian burger on ½ whole wheat bun with lettuce, tomato, onion, mustard, and fat-free mayonnaise, and a mixed green salad with fat-free dressing

SNACK

Choose from Lotus Eater Snack List in this chapter

DINNER

Choose from:
✓ 1 c. whole wheat pasta with ¾ c. oil-free Marinara Sauce 📋 and 3 oz. chicken or turkey breast or seafood
✓ 3 oz. grilled, broiled, baked, or poached chicken or turkey breast or seafood with 1 c. brown or wild rice

Steamed vegetables

SNACK

Choose from Lotus Eater Snack List

---

* 📋 = See recipe in Chapter 33.

EQ 2 (Low-Medium)

BREAKFAST

Choose from:
✓ ½ c. fruit-sweetened nonfat yogurt with ¾ c. diced fruit
✓ 1 serving Veggie Scramble 📋 and ½ c. fruit juice

SNACK

Choose from Lotus Eater Snack List in this chapter

LUNCH

Choose from:
✓ 1 serving Chopped Chicken or Shrimp Salad 📋
✓ 1 c. fat-free lentil soup and ½ turkey sandwich (1 slice 7-grain bread, 3 oz. turkey breast, lettuce, tomato, onion, mustard, fat-free mayonnaise)
✓ Turkey Burger 📋 or low-fat vegetarian burger on ½ whole wheat bun with lettuce, tomato, onion, mustard, and fat-free mayonnaise, and a mixed green salad with fat-free dressing

SNACK

Choose from Lotus Eater Snack List

DINNER

Choose from:
✓ 1 c. whole wheat pasta with ¾ c. oil-free Marinara Sauce 📋 and 3 oz. chicken or turkey breast or seafood
✓ 3 oz. grilled, broiled, baked, or poached chicken or turkey breast or seafood with 1 c. brown or wild rice

Steamed vegetables
1 piece fresh fruit

SNACK

Choose from Lotus Eater Snack List

EQ 3 (Medium-High)

BREAKFAST

Choose from:
✓ ½ c. fruit-sweetened nonfat yogurt with ¾ c. diced fruit
✓ 1 serving Veggie Scramble 🗏 and ½ c. fruit juice

1 c. skim milk

SNACK

Choose from Lotus Eater Snack List in this chapter

LUNCH

Choose from:
✓ 2 servings Chopped Chicken or Shrimp Salad 🗏
✓ 1 c. fat-free lentil soup and turkey sandwich (2 slices 7-grain bread, 6 oz. turkey breast, lettuce, tomato, onion, mustard, fat-free mayonnaise)
✓ Turkey Burger 🗏 or low-fat vegetarian burger with 1½ oz. fat-free cheese on whole wheat bun with lettuce, tomato, onion, mustard, and fat-free mayonnaise, and a mixed green salad with fat-free dressing

SNACK

Choose 2 from Lotus Eater Snack List

DINNER

Choose from:
✓ 1 c. whole wheat pasta with ¾ c. oil-free Marinara Sauce 🗏 and 3 oz. chicken or turkey breast or seafood
✓ 3 oz. grilled, broiled, baked, or poached chicken or turkey breast or seafood with 1 c. brown or wild rice

Steamed vegetables
1 piece fresh fruit

SNACK

Choose from Lotus Eater Snack List

EQ 4 (High)

BREAKFAST

Choose from:
✓ ½ c. fruit-sweetened nonfat yogurt with ¾ c. diced fruit
✓ 1 serving Veggie Scramble 🗐 and ½ c. fruit juice

2 slices whole wheat toast
1 c. skim milk

SNACK

Choose from Lotus Eater Snack List in this chapter

LUNCH

Choose from:
✓ 2 servings Chopped Chicken or Shrimp Salad 🗐
✓ 1 c. fat-free lentil soup and turkey sandwich (2 slices 7-grain bread, 6 oz. turkey breast, lettuce, tomato, onion, mustard, fat-free mayonnaise)
✓ Turkey Burger 🗐 or low-fat vegetarian burger with 1½ oz. fat-free cheese on whole wheat bun with lettuce, tomato, onion, mustard, and fat-free mayonnaise, and a mixed green salad with fat-free dressing

1 piece fresh fruit

SNACKS

Choose 2 from Lotus Eater Snack List

DINNER

Choose from:
✓ 1 c. whole wheat pasta with ¾ c. oil-free Marinara Sauce 🗐 and 3 oz. chicken or turkey breast or seafood
✓ 3 oz. grilled, broiled, baked, or poached chicken or turkey breast or seafood with 1 c. brown or wild rice

Steamed vegetables
1 piece fresh fruit

SNACK

Choose from Lotus Eater Snack List

SUPPLEMENT YOURSELF

- Chromium picolinate might enhance your metabolism of carbohydrates and keep you out of the craving cycle—take 200–300 mcg per day.

Lotus Eater Snack List

The following snacks are specially selected to maximize your satisfaction and minimize the dangers of bingeing. Choose from them as indicated in your meal plan:

✓ ¼ c. nonfat cottage cheese with ¼ c. diced fruit
✓ 1 piece fresh fruit
✓ Sugar-free frozen fruit bar
✓ Fruit-sweetened granola bar
✓ ½ whole wheat bagel with 2 T. fat-free ricotta and 1 t. pure fruit jam
✓ 1 oz. string cheese

RECOVERY RULES

- Don't skip meals. Low blood sugar can set you off on a binge.
- Stick to the Lotus Eater Snack List for now. Many of the snacks in the Master Snack List are likely to act as trigger foods and are inappropriate for recovery.
- Free foods:
  ✓ Raw vegetables. Try carrots, celery, peppers, green beans, turnips, water chestnuts, snap peas, radishes, mushrooms, cucumber, summer squash, broccoli, cauliflower, lettuce and greens, or sprouts.
  ✓ Defatted chicken broth.
  ✓ Sugar-free chewing gum.

TRAPPED IN THE SUGAR CYCLE

Many food users turn to sweets when seeking a quick hit—like Jenni with her hard candies, the last holdout of her addictive eating habit. But this hit can be the first bite of a binge. Eating any concentrated form of sugar can cause the body to release a flood of insulin into the bloodstream. Under normal circumstances, insulin's job is to usher glucose, the basic sugar obtained from digesting all different kinds of food, out of the bloodstream and into the body's cells, where it provides fuel for cellular functions. But when you eat sweets, which break down very rapidly into a tidal wave of glucose (the "hit"), your body panics and releases extra insulin, which in turn sweeps too much sugar out of your blood and leaves you feeling tired, drained, and craving another candy bar ("the letdown"). This cycle can go on ad infinitum, driving you to eat more and more in a futile search for satisfaction.

Beyond the Recovery Diet

The Lotus Eater Meal Plan is designed to set you on the road to recovery. Eventually, for your physical health, aesthetic gratification, and to keep you from feeling deprived, you should reintroduce variety into your diet. I recommend working with your therapist to determine when you're ready to take that step.

Once you're ready, begin slowly to rotate new dishes into your day. Choose foods and serving sizes from the Eating By Design Mosaic, and follow your EQ for the number of servings to have from each group each day. It's that easy. As long as you stick with your Eating By Design portions and proportions, you can eat whatever you like. For life.

Bulimics should be especially careful about reintroducing foods that once triggered binges, going slowly and trying small amounts. Anorexics should focus on perceiving food as a unit of energy, not a creator of body fat. Remember that the calories from bread or chicken breast are just as good for you and no more fattening than those from fruit or vegetables. Work with your therapist throughout the process to develop a flexible plan you can envision sticking with for a good, long time.

✳

Become a Conscious Eater

Once you've become acquainted with your meal plan, the other side to treating yourself and breaking your habit lies in behavioral techniques that help to control your food compulsion. Your goal is to become a *conscious eater.* Consciousness is the difference between being in and out of control.

Study these methods and put them into practice as soon and as thoroughly as you can.

Slow Down and Savor

Food users have a tightly wound spring inside that can explode whenever you eat. You can loosen this tension and gain an appreciation for food by building some slow-downs into your routine:

- When hunger strikes outside of your scheduled meal or snack times, wait fifteen minutes before eating. This is the time it takes a normal blood sugar dip to cycle through your body. If you're still hungry, snack on 4 ounces of fruit-sweetened nonfat yogurt.
- Sit down.

- Pick designated places for meals and snacks: the kitchen or dining room table, or special spot at the office. Stick to these places and your scheduled times for eating everything except raw vegetables.
- Serve your food in small portions.
- Focus on chewing, tasting, and swallowing.
- Put down your fork or spoon and take a deep breath between every bite.
- Experience the process, the movement from the beginning, through the middle, to the end of your meal.
- Plan something fun for right after you eat to help move you away from the table.
- Drink eight 8-ounce glasses of water per day. This keeps your mouth busy and provides essential hydration to your cells.

Eat in Peace

It's easier to respect your own boundaries and honor your commitment to healthy eating when you're relaxed. Here are some mini-relaxation tips for mealtimes.

Before:
- Sit down, take a deep breath, close your eyes, and think about what you're about to eat. Why do you want it? What will it be like?

During:
- Remain seated.
- Chew and swallow every bite before reaching for the next one.
- Take a moment to focus on the flavors and textures of your food.

After:
- Do all the dishes and put everything away. The chaos of a messy kitchen is an open invitation to eat.

Get the Focus off Food

When you use food, it has a way of permeating your life, popping up in your mind or your mouth at inappropriate times. By giving yourself plenty of alternatives to eating that make you feel good, amuse you, or express your emotions, you can prevent food from using you. Identify your hobbies, interests, and favorite pasttimes and pursue them with a vengeance. Here are a few other suggestions:

- Keep a journal, logging your feelings and interactions with other people. Writing is a great expressive outlet, more creative and satisfying than eating.
- Knitting, needlepoint, and other handicrafts keep your hands busy and help to calm and focus your physical and mental energies.

- Aerobic exercise is an indispensable Lotus Eater activity. It has the power to give you an endorphin high while you work out, reduce your stress reaction for several hours afterward, and relax your entire system for better sleep and daytime functioning throughout the week.

WORK YOURSELF OUT

> There's nothing wrong with having habits as long as they're healthy. One such habit is a daily exercise session, emphasizing aerobic activity like jogging, biking, or a cardiovascular machine. Just remember:
>
> - Don't overwork any muscle group or body part in any given session.
> - Any action beyond your control has the potential to hurt you. Don't exercise more than 1½ hours a day, or use excessive exercise to "purge" after eating binges.

Stay Satisfied

Physical hunger can be a scary thing, symbolic of every unmet need in your life and threatening to your sense of security. The resulting anxiety can drive you to disastrous overcompensation in bingeing, an apparently methodical but ultimately self-destructive satisfaction of this need. Staying satisfied—by preventing the feeling of need to begin with—is a simple and effective way of circumventing a binge.

The trick to staying satisfied is simply to eat according to your meal plan. Don't skip meals or snacks—even if you've recently overindulged. Remember that eating is a natural need, and a well-fueled body is rarely, if ever, ravenously hungry. Your healthy self feels light and satisfied on a consistent basis.

If you have a slipup, remember that your "fat feelings" after an impulsive binge are exaggerated by the water retention caused by extra food in your body. So don't fast! Going without food just slows down your metabolism. The best way to erase the effects of overeating is to go back on your healthy eating plan, adding a little extra to your workout routine until you're back in balance.

✳

With any habit, the hardest part of breaking it is taking the first step. You've already done that. Now, let your Personal Prescription do its good work on your body and mind, with its all-natural medicine to set you free of fear and food traps. Remember that the Recovery Diet is always there for you. Revisit it any time you feel that food is slipping out of your control.

In the meantime, relax, think of other things, and enjoy the secure feeling of Eating By Design.

✳

Lotus Eater Affirmations

Use the following affirmations to help you through each day.

Morning:
- I'm happy and lucky to wake up a beautiful person in a beautiful world.
- Today, I will eat to fuel myself for healthy energy and good feelings.
- Today, I will make a special effort to experience every moment to the fullest.

Mealtimes:
- When I eat healthy foods, I feel them going to work fueling my body.
- This is a refueling stop in a day full of other interesting events and challenges.
- I eat slowly, deliberately, and with complete control.

In Moments of Temptation:
- I love myself and deserve to feel good.
- Food does not fill my inner emptiness.
- Health is a natural high.
- Food is fuel, not a substance.

In the Evening:
- Now is my time to relax and recharge for a new day tomorrow.
- Today was good, and tomorrow will be even better.
- Congratulations to me on making it through another day.
- The sun sets on this day, but never on my self-worth.

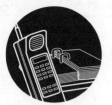

25

THE POWER PLAYER'S PERSONAL PRESCRIPTION

With all the efficiency experts in the world, why does nobody ever talk about the role of eating well in achieving your personal best? In the past, food for high-powered people has mostly served as a backdrop to meetings and negotiations. In the future, the cutting-edge achievers will be Eating By Design.

I've formulated your Personal Prescription to be a no-nonsense, effective tool for eating to develop your health potential and achieve the energy and appearance of a winner. The strategic elements include:

- Power nutrition for maximum mental performance.
- Snacking for stress relief.
- Delegating your dietary concerns to supportive people in your life.
- Negotiating business meals and travel with maximum elan and minimum distraction.

The bottom line for your body is improved mental and physical performance, less downtime for poor health, a built-in approach to stress management, and a physique as powerful and polished as your management style. Doesn't that seem like ample return on the small risk of taking your Personal Prescription on a test run?

❋

Food for Maximum Brainpower

Timing is everything, and no one knows this better than the Power Player. But most people don't know that this applies to eating as much as making deals.

Principles of Power Eating

Food is not a generic fuel. Everything you eat triggers complex chemical reactions in your body that affect your energy and mood. The implications of this fact go far beyond weight management and health. Food's unique biochemical properties can make or break your personal performance, giving an edge to those who eat to win. You can use the principles of power eating to give you the competitive advantage throughout your working day.

Here's inside information that the other side probably doesn't have:

- **Small, low-fat meals keep you alert** because they boost blood sugar, digest easily, and leave blood available to your brain and other organs. Large meals and fatty foods, by contrast, digest slowly and divert blood to the stomach and intestines, leaving you slow and dull. So, though a restaurant lunch meeting might seem like an efficient place to get in a big meal, your best bet for an alert afternoon is to keep it small and lean.

- **Interval eating throughout the day** supplies constant blood sugar for energy, soothes stress, may reduce cholesterol levels, and keeps you satisfied even with smaller meals. Later in the chapter, you'll find a special Power Player Snack List that makes it easy to stock up your office for interval eating.

- **Protein provides brain power** by releasing the amino acid tyrosine, which in turn stimulates two neurotransmitters, dopamine and norepinephrine, that promote mental clarity. So when you're ready for a brain boost, choose lean protein foods like chicken breast or seafood.

- **Carbohydrates soothe you** and slow down your mind by releasing the amino acid tryptophane, which stimulates the production of the neurotransmitter serotonin, a natural tranquilizer. Carbs are good for a quick boost in the morning and unwinding after a stressful day, but a baked potato at a business lunch can send you to sleep.

- **Timing is everything.** Your body is programmed to wake up full of energy and slow down progressively throughout the day. You can use your intake of protein and carbohydrates to reinforce or counter your internal rhythms, depending on the demands of your schedule:
  —**Breakfast** should be nourishing and healthy. Your brain is naturally energized for the first six hours after sleep, so power nutrition principles are not yet in play. My Power Player breakfasts are rich in fiber from fruits and whole grains for cholesterol control and cancer prevention. Bread or cereal also helps to keep your stomach calm all morning and absorb your coffee, if you choose to indulge.
  —Your **coffee break** should be just that—coffee, or work straight through

until lunchtime. Your brain should still be powered up from a good night's sleep and a healthy breakfast, and doesn't need food yet.

COFFEE, NECTAR OF THE WORKAHOLIC

It's true, caffeinated coffee does indeed clear the cobwebs and enhance mental performance. Recent research has cleaned up coffee's bill of health enough to permit moderate consumption—2 cups per day—by those who choose. A cup of coffee remains in your bloodstream for up to six hours, so it's smart to space out your cups by that long to keep you powered all day. Use regular or evaporated skim milk; the fat in cream, half-and-half, and nondairy creamers will add calories and cloud your mind. Coffee acts as a diuretic, so rehydrate with an equal amount of water. And beware: Caffeine is an addictive substance, and more than two cups a day can contribute to insomnia, headaches, anxiety, irritability, lethargy, and depression.

If you prefer tea, avoid drinking it with food; it can cut iron absorption.

—**Lunch** should feature lean protein. The lift of dopamine and norepinephrine help you to shift into a more motivated state of mind as your natural rhythms start to slow. Carbohydrates should be avoided, or limited and eaten after protein. My protein-only lunch options help you trump the competition with tyrosine; you save your carbohydrates for a snack later on.

—Your **afternoon snack** should be a carbohydrate if you tend to feel stressed and irritable during this stretch of the day; the serotonin helps you to refocus. If an important presentation or speaking engagement lies ahead, though, choose protein instead for mental sharpness. The Nibbles for Noshers list guides you to the right snack.

THE HUNGRY MIND

News Flash: Skipping meals or snacks can starve your brain cells. One recent study found that people who ate a midafternoon snack performed more accurate work with better concentration. Another study tracked women performing memory tasks under calorie deprivation and found them less attentive and focused than normal. The explanation could be too much attention to their hunger, or too little serotonin in their system. Either way, don't let the distractions of an erratic diet make you miss a deadline or blow a deal!

THE COCKTAIL PARTY

Cocktail parties present potential calorie disasters, and the combination of alcohol and starchy foods can make you snooze right through important networking opportunities. To stay snappy, make your cocktail shrimp (2–4 pieces; count as a protein snack) instead of alcohol, and have plenty of mineral water and raw veggies.

—**Dinner,** like lunch, should be primarily protein if you need to perform during or after. But if your working day is done, wind down with a high-carbohydrate meal like pasta. My meal plan provides both options.

—An **evening snack** of carbohydrates will help soothe you to sleep after a stressful day. Eating something sweet and starchy half an hour before bed releases serotonin to help lull you off to dreamland. Good bets are fat-free cookies, graham crackers, vanilla wafers, gingersnaps, a granola bar, cooked oatmeal with honey, or rice cakes—sweetened or topped with honey or fruit preserves. Avoid milk; its protein could reignite your brain. If you've already eaten your snack allotment for the day, have hot herbal tea with a teaspoon of honey to calm you with very few calories.

■ **Concentration peaks** about fifteen minutes after a healthy low-fat meal, so it's best to close the deal after the plates are cleared.

■ **Your optimal power eating schedule** might be different every day, depending on your agenda. Planning is essential to power nutrition!

EAT LIGHT TO STAY BRIGHT

Besides being crucial to weight management, portion control is important to staying alert. There is a direct correlation between the number of calories consumed in a sitting and the slowing of mental processes. To keep the upper hand, limit your power meals to 500 calories or less. At restaurants, where servings tend to be big, this will require some proactive portioning:

■ Learn to eyeball serving sizes by weighing or measuring at home; take this mental gauge with you to business meals and restaurants.
■ Ask for half portions.
■ Demand proper service from the restaurants you patronize. Dishes should be prepared as you request—without fat, with extra lemon, salsa, mustard, etc.—without fuss or complaint.
■ Ask for your plate to be cleared as soon as you've finished your allotted portion.

✳

Power Player Meal Plan*

Use the following meal plan to get the most from your brain while filling your body with high-achievement energy. Pay special attention to timing, fat content, and portion size.

EQ 1 (Low)

BREAKFAST

Choose from:
✓ 1 piece fresh fruit, 1 bagel with 2 T. fat-free cream cheese and 2 t. pure fruit preserves
✓ 1 piece fresh fruit and 1 large fat-free muffin (bran or whole grain)
✓ ½ banana sliced over hot oatmeal (2 oz. dry) drizzled with 2 t. honey

Caffe latte with 1 c. skim milk

LUNCH

Choose from:
✓ 3 oz. chicken or turkey breast or seafood, grilled, broiled, baked, or poached, with steamed or grilled vegetables
✓ Tuna or chicken salad (mixed greens and chopped vegetables topped with 3 oz. water-packed tuna or cooked chicken breast and fat-free dressing)
This is an easy lunch to pack from home or order from a deli
✓ 2 orders sashimi with cucumber salad and steamed vegetables
✓ 3 oz. seafood salad on mixed greens (no creamy dressing!) with cocktail sauce and lemon

Dessert: ¾ c. mixed berries or fruit

SNACK

Choose from the Nibbles for Noshers list in this chapter.

DINNER

For power performance at a dinner meeting, choose from:
✓ Any lunch option, beginning with clear soup or salad with fat-free dressing
✓ A high-protein appetizer, such as seafood cocktail, seared ahi tuna, or salad topped with grilled chicken or shrimp (3 oz.), followed by half an oil-free, vegetarian pasta entree

To unwind, order in a restaurant or prepare at home:
Mixed green salad with fat-free dressing
Choose from:
✓ 1 c. pasta, 1½ c. Spaghetti Squash 📄 , or ½ baked potato with ¾ c. Marinara, Primavera, or Puttanesca Sauce 📄 or Fresh Tomato, Basil, and Garlic Sauce 📄 and 1 t. Parmesan cheese
✓ 1 serving oil-free Vegetable Stir-Fry 📄

---

* 📄 = See recipe in Chapter 33.

BEDTIME SNACK

Choose from Bedtime Snacks in the Nibbles for Noshers list.

EQ 2 (Low-Medium)

BREAKFAST

Choose from:
✓ 1 piece fresh fruit, 1 bagel with 2 T. fat-free cream cheese and 2 t. pure fruit preserves
✓ 1 piece fresh fruit and 1 large fat-free muffin (bran or whole grain)
✓ ½ banana sliced over hot oatmeal (2 oz. dry) drizzled with 2 t. honey

Caffe latte with 1 c. skim milk

LUNCH

Choose from:
✓ 6 oz. chicken or turkey breast or seafood, grilled, broiled, baked, or poached, with steamed or grilled vegetables
✓ Tuna or chicken salad (mixed greens and chopped vegetables topped with 6 oz. water-packed tuna or cooked chicken breast and fat-free dressing)
This is an easy lunch to pack from home or order from a deli.
✓ 4 orders sashimi with cucumber salad and steamed vegetables.
✓ 6 oz. seafood salad on mixed greens (no creamy dressing!) with cocktail sauce and lemon.

Dessert: ¾ c. mixed berries or fruit.

SNACK

Choose from the Nibbles for Noshers list in this chapter.

DINNER

For power performance at a dinner meeting, choose from:
✓ Any lunch option, beginning with clear soup or salad with fat-free dressing
✓ A high-protein appetizer, such as seafood cocktail, seared ahi tuna, or salad topped with grilled chicken or shrimp (6 oz.), followed by half an oil-free, vegetarian pasta entree.

To unwind, order in a restaurant or prepare at home:
Mixed green salad with fat-free dressing
Choose from:
✓ 2 c. pasta, 3 c. Spaghetti Squash 🗐 , or 1 baked potato with 1½ c. Marinara, Primavera, or Puttanesca Sauce 🗐 or Fresh Tomato, Basil, and Garlic Sauce 🗐 and 2 t. Parmesan cheese.
✓ 2 servings oil-free Vegetable Stir-Fry 🗐 .

BEDTIME SNACK

Choose from Bedtime Snacks in the Nibbles for Noshers list.

EQ 3 (Medium-High)

BREAKFAST

Choose from:
✓ 1 piece fresh fruit, 1 bagel with 2 T. fat-free cream cheese and 2 t. pure fruit preserves
✓ 1 piece fresh fruit and 1 large fat-free muffin (bran or whole grain)
✓ ½ banana sliced over hot oatmeal (2 oz. dry) drizzled with 2 t. honey

Caffe latte with 1 c. skim milk

LUNCH

Choose from:
✓ 6 oz. chicken or turkey breast or seafood, grilled, broiled, baked, or poached, with steamed or grilled vegetables
✓ Tuna or chicken salad (mixed greens and chopped vegetables topped with 6 oz. water-packed tuna or cooked chicken breast and fat-free dressing)
This is an easy lunch to pack from home or order from a deli.
✓ 4 orders sashimi with cucumber salad and steamed vegetables.
✓ 6 oz. seafood salad on mixed greens (no creamy dressing!) with cocktail sauce and lemon.

Dessert: ¾ c. mixed berries or fruit.

SNACK

Choose 2 from the Nibbles for Noshers list in this chapter.

DINNER

For power performance at a dinner meeting, choose from:
✓ Any lunch option, beginning with clear soup or salad with fat-free dressing
✓ A high-protein appetizer, such as seafood cocktail, seared ahi tuna, or salad topped with grilled chicken or shrimp (6 oz.), followed by half an oil-free, vegetarian pasta entree.

To unwind, order in a restaurant or prepare at home:
Mixed green salad with fat-free dressing
Choose from:
✓ 2 c. pasta, 3 c. Spaghetti Squash 📄 , or 1 baked potato with 1½ c. Marinara, Primavera, or Puttanesca Sauce 📄 or Fresh Tomato, Basil, and Garlic Sauce 📄 and 2 t. Parmesan cheese.
✓ 2 servings oil-free Vegetable Stir-Fry 📄 .

1 slice sourdough French bread

BEDTIME SNACK

Choose from Bedtime Snacks in the Nibbles for Noshers list.

EQ 4 (High)

BREAKFAST

1 oz. cereal with ½ c. skim milk
Choose from:
✓ 1 piece fresh fruit, 1 bagel with 2 T. fat-free cream cheese and 2 t. pure fruit preserves
✓ 1 piece fresh fruit and 1 large fat-free muffin (bran or whole grain)
✓ ½ banana sliced over hot oatmeal (2 oz. dry) drizzled with 2 t. honey

Caffe latte with 1 c. skim milk

LUNCH

Choose from:
✓ 6 oz. chicken or turkey breast or seafood, grilled, broiled, baked, or poached, with steamed or grilled vegetables
✓ Tuna or chicken salad (mixed greens and chopped vegetables topped with 6 oz. water-packed tuna or cooked chicken breast and fat-free dressing)
This is an easy lunch to pack from home or order from a deli.
✓ 4 orders sashimi with cucumber salad and steamed vegetables.
✓ 6 oz. seafood salad on mixed greens (no creamy dressing!) with cocktail sauce and lemon.

Dessert: ¾ c. mixed berries or fruit.

SNACK

Choose 2 from the Nibbles for Noshers list in this chapter.

DINNER

For power performance at a dinner meeting, choose from:
✓ Any lunch option, beginning with clear soup or salad with fat-free dressing
✓ A high-protein appetizer, such as seafood cocktail, seared ahi tuna, or salad topped with grilled chicken or shrimp (6 oz.), followed by half an oil-free, vegetarian pasta entree.

To unwind, order in a restaurant or prepare at home:
Mixed green salad with fat-free dressing
Choose from:
✓ 2 c. pasta, 3 c. Spaghetti Squash 🗐 , or 1 baked potato with 1½ c. Marinara, Primavera, or Puttanesca Sauce 🗐 or Fresh Tomato, Basil, and Garlic Sauce 🗐 and 2 t. Parmesan cheese.
✓ 2 servings oil-free Vegetable Stir-Fry 🗐 .

2 slices sourdough French bread

BEDTIME SNACK

Choose from Bedtime Snacks in the Nibbles for Noshers list.

WORK YOURSELF OUT

- Work out before breakfast—exercise on an empty stomach burns a greater proportion of body fat.
- Cardiovascular activity is vital to the health of high-powered people under pressure. Take advantage of the high-tech exercise equipment available for the home: Stair-Master, Lifecycle, treadmills, ski machines, and rowing machines. Add hand-held weights to your aerobic session for extra benefits.
- Try aggressive sports like aerobic boxing, squash, racquetball, handball, football, or hockey to take out your tensions.

SUPPLEMENT YOURSELF

The following supplements will help to keep you cool under pressure:

- In the morning, a B vitamin complex to combat stress.
- In the evening, to help you sleep, try a calcium-magnesium powder such as Calmax, or valerian root capsules or drops.

✳

Don't Stomach Your Stress

As I've pointed out, stress is the Power Player's number one day-to-day health enemy. Stress can tear down your body's defense system, even its basic structures, as well as disrupt your healthy eating habits. I know better than to ask you to give up pressures, urgency, and "due yesterday" deadlines. But please: Keep your stress on your desk and out of your stomach.

Put the Stress on Snacks

Perhaps surprisingly, one of the best medicines against the detrimental effects of stress is *food*—healthy food, in small portions and at frequent intervals. Interval eating, the controlled version of Cynthia's constant M&M's snack attacks, is a great way to keep a body under pressure healthy. A slow, steady stream of fuel helps to repair stressed-out tissues and cells, boost metabolism, lower LDL cholesterol levels, and control gastric acid. Eating can also help you to get outside of your busy head, giving your brain a much-needed break. All of these benefits enhance your resistance to disease, helping you to weather the storms of stress without succumbing to sickness.

Here's how to turn anxious eating into interval eating for health and stress control:

- DO save some of your mealtime calories for extra snacks if you're prone to stress.
- DON'T skip meals or snacks when you're stressed out and plan to eat "later, when I'm less tense and worried." Your times of greatest anxiety are when you need fuel the most. This is not carte blanche to eat unlimited amounts every time you feel a twinge of nerves. But stress chips away at the body's resources, which you need to replenish with healthy food. And realistically, your relaxed time probably comes in the evening, when you need fuel the least.
- Keep your meals small and low-calorie. If you're snacking on healthy, nutritious foods, you need less at mealtimes to meet your basic nutritional needs. And, as I pointed out earlier, lighter meals leave you more alert.
- Clues that you need a relaxation break include hot face, cold hands, stiff neck or jaw muscles, dizziness, burning stomach, or short temper. Monitor your personal stress profile with an annual physical to check your blood pressure, cholesterol, and blood chemistry (including triglycerides, electrolytes, and glucose).

Nibbles for Noshers

Stress snacks should be healthy and wholesome, just like you would choose for a meal. Use protein to power up your mind, crunchy foods to take out aggressions or anxieties with your teeth, bready snacks to soothe stress or calm an acid stomach, and sweet snacks for sweet dreams.

Protein snacks *for brain drain:*
- ✓ 4 oz. nonfat yogurt, refrigerated or frozen
- ✓ 3 oz. nonfat cottage cheese with 2 t. pure fruit preserves
- ✓ 1 oz. mozzarella, 1½ oz. fat-free cheese, or 1 individual string cheese
- ✓ 1 oz. turkey jerky
- ✓ 1–2 oz. sliced turkey breast
- ✓ 4 pieces shrimp

Crunchy snacks *for aggression:*
- ✓ 1 oz. fat-free chips—potato, tortilla, pasta, polenta, bagel
- ✓ 1 oz. fat-free crackers or rye crisps
- ✓ 1 oz. fat-free pretzels

Bready snacks *to soothe stress or calm an acid stomach:*
- ✓ Half a baked potato, or baked potato skins with nonfat sour cream
- ✓ Half a bagel or English muffin, a slice of bread or toast, or a large rice cake with fat-free cream cheese or ricotta and/or pure fruit preserves
- ✓ Fat-free muffin
- ✓ Fat-free cookies (2), cake (1 oz.), or brownie (1)

Bedtime snacks *to soothe you to sleep:*
- ✓ 2 graham crackers
- ✓ 2 vanilla wafers
- ✓ 2 fat-free cookies
- ✓ 2 gingersnaps
- ✓ 1 granola bar
- ✓ Hot oatmeal (1 oz. dry) with honey
- ✓ 10 mini rice cakes
- ✓ 2 plain large rice cakes topped with 2 t. honey or pure fruit preserves

Your continued success balances precariously on your good health and energy. Invest in these intangible assets by making a decision and commitment today. In a world of uncertain returns, the payoff of a healthy eating plan is a sure thing.

✳

Take Charge

As a Power Player, you're probably used to taking charge. Now, transfer your take-charge business habits to your eating habits for immediate energy and long-term health.

A Prospectus for Strategic Eating

Eating By Design is an investment of time and effort. Realize maximum profit from your investment by breaking the project down into achievable steps.

I. **Schedule**
    A. Write your eating and exercise schedule directly on your daily calendar.
    B. Make eating appointments with yourself, blocking out any available quiet time to close the door, focus on your food, and eat in uninterrupted peace.
    C. Project your needs for times away from the office on calls, meetings, or business trips. Pack snacks and meals if you won't have access to the right foods.

II. **Delegate**
    A. Enlist the help of an assistant to keep you scheduled and stocked. Ask him or her to:
        1. Write out your eating schedule every day with portions and times.
        2. Remind you of meals and snacks at appointed hours.
        3. Shop and stock the office with fruits, vegetables, and snacks.

    4. Portion your snacks into individual servings.

    5. Call ahead with special orders for restaurant meals, catered events, and plane trips.

  B. Give a copy of this book to all your support staff. Ask them to read it carefully and help you any way they can; you'll reward them with a stable temperament and softer spirit.

III. Set Objectives

  A. Set daily, weekly, and monthly goals and write them into your calendar. For example:

    1. Today: Skip the martini at lunch.

    2. This week: Order all restaurant meals without butter or oil.

    3. This month: Drop 1% body fat.

IV. Negotiate

  A. If your eating goal or schedule seems impossible—you'll blow the deal if you don't share a cup of sake with your client, or you can't eat your healthy snack in the middle of a formal business presentation—trade it in for another goal of equivalent "value."

  B. Reward yourself when you meet your goals with trade books, computer software, electronic gadgets, a power suit, a new cellular phone.

Delegate Your Diet

Once I had encouraged Cynthia to formulate her strategic plan for healthy eating, I wondered how I could insure its implementation. How could I assert my advisory presence in the context of Cynthia's jam-packed days? I realized I needed to find the driving logistical force behind those days, the battery that kept Cynthia ticking along on schedule: her assistant. I immediately enlisted Marcie's aid. "M&M's no more!" she vowed, and agreed to schedule Cynthia's healthy eating into her appointment book right along with her professional obligations.

   Efficient and enthusiastic, Marcie stocked the office with fruits, vegetables, and healthy stress snacks; wrote Cynthia a daily schedule of what, when, and how much to eat and exercise; and called ahead to restaurants and event caterers to order meals to my specifications. By facilitating her eating as she did the rest of her day, Marcie was literally Cynthia's lifesaver. When she hit her body fat target and was sailing through sixteen-hour days, Cynthia sent me a fax: "Victory is mine!" Of course, it was signed with Marcie's initials.

Filofax Your Food

Here's a page from Cynthia's Filofax, dutifully updated by Marcie:

Time	Activity	Meal/Snack
7:00 A.M.	StairMaster	
8:00 A.M.	Breakfast meeting w/ R. Hughes	BREAKFAST:
	The Four Seasons	1 c. oatmeal, ½ banana
9:00 A.M.	Conference call with New York	
10:00 A.M.	Staff meeting	
11:00 A.M.	Marketing plan review	
12:00 P.M.	" "	
1:00 P.M.	Lunch w/ bankers	LUNCH: Grilled vegetable salad
	The Ivy	with 6 oz. chicken (appetizer
		size), ¾ c. mixed berries
2:00 P.M.	Visit plant	
3:00 P.M.	" "	
4:00 P.M.	" "	STRESS SNACK:
		Fat-free pretzels
5:00 P.M.	Wrap-up with Marcie,	
	return phone calls	
6:00 P.M.	Congressional fund-raiser	BRAIN BOOST SNACK:
	cocktail party	Shrimp cocktail, mineral water
7:00 P.M.	Home: pack	DINNER: 1 c. mushroom soup,
		1½ c. pasta primavera, salad
11:00 P.M.	Red-eye flight to New York	BEDTIME SNACK: 1 oz. fat-free
		caramel corn

NOTES:
✓ You resolved to take today off from diet sodas.
✓ Remember to take the Travel Tips guidelines to New York to help you follow your eating plan on your trip!

A written schedule for your meals keeps you from loading up on quick-fix junk or eating huge restaurant meals. Even more importantly, it insures that you're power eating for performance, enjoying the fruits of your efficiency with maximized alertness and ever-improving fitness.

The Body as Bank

Cynthia liked to negotiate with me when she began to feel that I was asking too much, just as she did with her suppliers when they got out of line. Once she was on her maintenance plan, I told her a little negotiation was fine, but that in this case, I wasn't the bank—her body was.

Your body needs to balance calorie deposits and energy expenditures, just like your company accounts. Over the long run, you balance your body with a healthy diet of portions appropriate to your size, and with an exercise program. In the short term, you can balance an occasional excess deposit with an extra energy expenditure, or a smaller deposit the next day. This transaction approach is particularly useful when the demands of your business life just won't fit into your EQ. Let's make a deal!

Here's a sample body balance sheet:

Transaction:	Deposits:	Withdrawals:
Equilibrium	Eat according to your EQ.	Exercise on schedule.
Standard deposit/withdrawal	Eat 6 oz. of steak instead of 3 oz. of chicken at a catered event (200 calories).	Cut out two snacks (200 calories) tomorrow.
Maximum deposit/withdrawal	Go to town at a business dinner with crab Louis, steak with béarnaise, fried onions, creamed spinach, dessert, and a bottle of wine.	Cut portions and one snack for two days and add an hour of aerobic exercise to your week.
Possible bank error	Gain 2 pounds.	Warning! This could be water—but have you been following your EQ?
EXCESS DEPOSIT!	Gain 5 pounds.	Return IMMEDIATELY to your EQ and skip the indulgences until you're back on track.

Travel Tips

Once you've mastered eating well at the office, you're bound to discover that you don't spend as much time there as you thought—clients throughout the country request your visits; international associates require your consultation. With all the demands on your health and energy that traveling entails, the worst thing you could do would be to abandon your healthy eating plan when you take off.

You need not stop Eating By Design just because you've crossed state lines or cleared customs. Well-chosen meals in motion can help speed you toward your destination and make you more productive once you get there. Add some simple mobile meal planning to the itinerary for any journey.

Mile-High Meals

- Order special meals when you make your flight reservation. Low-calorie, low-cholesterol, low-fat, low-sodium, diabetic, kosher, and vegetarian menus are all likely to have a nutritional edge on standard fare.
- Drink water throughout every plane trip, to combat the drying effect of low-oxygen cabin air. Begin with a liter before you take off. Once aloft, skip the mini-cocktails (deadly dehydrators) and ask for a mineral water instead.
- Pack snacks that travel well and provide quick bites of energy en route:
  - ✓ Fresh fruit
  - ✓ Fresh vegetables
  - ✓ Rice cakes
  - ✓ Bagels (a good chew helps pop your ears on descent)
  - ✓ Pretzels (often available on the plane)
  - ✓ Granola bars
  - ✓ Bottled water
  - ✓ Rehydrating beverages (Recharge, Body Fuel, Gatorade)
- When you're stranded in the airport, look for these healthy options instead of the usual snack bar fare:
  - ✓ A hot pretzel with mustard
  - ✓ Frozen nonfat yogurt
  - ✓ Air-popped popcorn
  - ✓ Dried fruit
  - ✓ Fresh fruit with nonfat yogurt
- Schedule your meals according to your destination time zone. This is especially important when traveling west to east—the recovery rate is slower in this direction.
- Combat the tissue-damaging effects of radiation, ozone, tobacco smoke, and stress with antioxidant supplements.
- At the hotel:
  —Leave the key to the mini-bar at the front desk, or call ahead asking that the bar be stocked only with mineral water, juices, and pretzels.
  —To recharge after a long trip, order fresh fruit, vegetables, and water from room service. An advance phone call can have this awaiting you on your arrival.
  —To unwind for bed, have a hot bath and a cup of herbal tea.

SKY-HIGH STATISTICS ON THE AVERAGE AIRPLANE MEAL

	Calories	Fat
1 oz. peanuts	164	14 g
12 oz. Coca-Cola	144	0 g
Salad with 2 T. ranch dressing	160	8 g
4 oz. dark-meat chicken	287	18 g
¼ c. gravy	35	2 g
½ c. noodles	106	2 g
Roll with 1 T. butter	150	13 g
2 shortbread cookies	150	8 g
	1,196 calories	65 g fat

It takes some powerful jet propulsion to keep all this afloat . . .

✳

That's all there is to it. Power nutrition is quick and painless—just a few pages with a few basic principles—but what a payoff!

Eat By Design to join the vanguard of health care for brain and body, and realize all the promise of your formidable personal power.

✳

A Week of Power Pointers

Write one of the following reminders at the top of your daily agenda every morning.

1. Health is power.
2. Eating well is an investment in my most important asset: me.
3. I eat according to power principles to edge out the competition.
4. I am in charge of my mind and body, and make good, informed decisions to fuel them well.
5. The better I eat, the better I perform.

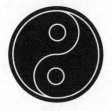

26

THE YIN-YANG'S PERSONAL PRESCRIPTION

Just as the possibilities for human potential are endless, there is an infinite array of propositions for how human beings ought to eat, endorsed by authorities ranging from the medical to the spiritual to the purely self-appointed. Some of these propositions come and go like dust in the wind; others contain seeds of truth that settle, adhere, and root in our consciousness. Your Personal Prescription is a simple distillation of those seeds of truth, a celebration of the natural bounty of foods that have nourished human life since the Garden of Eden.

✳

Mind-Body-Food

Before the Dawn of the New Age

Nutrition was one of the original holistic health practices, centuries before "holistic" was a buzzword and an industry had sprouted around the marketing of magical food elixirs. Since the dawn of humankind, feeding the body for internal balance and systemic vitality has been essential to the physical, mental, and spiritual well-being of the species. Every bite of good food suffuses your body with nutrients, your spirit with pleasure, and your mind with energy and intellectual stimulation. Furthermore, cooking and eating serve as settings for interaction with others and with the natural earth that likewise nourish your total self.

Eating is inherently an integrating activity: Your mind hears your body's hunger signals and decides what and when to eat; your body in turn signals satiety to the mind, then converts the fuel into a variety of neurotransmitters that affect your mental state. This food-centered dialogue between mind and body has been part of daily human life from the beginning.

Now, with nutritional news breaking a mile a minute, the "mind" element of the equation threatens to get too heavy and throw off the balance. My personal Prescription for the Yin-Yang says: *Don't* overthink your diet. *Do* tap in to your mind-body connection to be sure your diet is nourishing every part of you and stimulating your natural defenses. Following are some suggestions for sustaining a super, whole, harmonious you.

Superfoods: The Once and Future Supper

It's true—nature invests some foods with superpowers. These are not new inventions or technological advances, but the ancient essences of health that have nourished mankind for ages past. In fact, science suggests that it's the intrusion of modern processed foods on the traditional role of superfoods in our daily diet that has subjected us to a fatal epidemic of diet-related disease that threatens our survival into the future.

What are these superfoods? A beautiful bounty of fruits and vegetables that are naturally colorful, low in calories and fat, and full of nutrients for a healthy, balanced body and the prevention of long-term disease. In technical terms, these foods are packed with antioxidant vitamins and phytochemicals. In everyday language, they're delicious, nutritious, and the basis of a healthy mind-body-food plan.

Antioxidants and Phytochemicals: Nature's Pharmacy

We've always known that fruits and vegetables are good for you, but the details on exactly how and why have remained relatively fuzzy. A focus on the positive properties of vitamins and minerals has fueled a thriving supplement industry, and many people eat vitamin pills as hungrily as they do food. But recent evidence indicates that fruits and vegetables contain a host of compounds not yet isolated in the laboratory, suggesting that we haven't yet improved upon nature's pharmacy.

The two main contenders in this pharmacy are a group of vitamins known as antioxidants, and substances called phytochemicals, both of which seem to work against heart disease, cancer, and other illness associated with aging. The most important antioxidants are the vitamins C, E, and A (in the form of beta-carotene), which work, as the name suggests, to combat the detrimental effects of oxidation in the body. Oxidation, an inevitable by-product of living caused by normal breathing, athletic activity, stress, and smoking, causes the creation of "free radicals," or molecules containing an unpaired electron, in the body. The solo electron's innate instinct to mate drives free radicals to steal electrons from other molecules, eroding and breaking down cells, and so aging the body.

The antioxidant vitamins contain extra electrons, which they offer up to the free radicals. Happily bonded, the free radicals abandon their cellular raids, halting the oxidation process. Only long-term studies will prove whether high levels of antioxidants in the diet actually lengthen lifespan, but existing evidence certainly makes a case for eating foods naturally rich in these electron-generous substances.

Phytochemicals, the other class of natural pharmaceuticals in fruits and vegetables, are a group of substances such as flavanoids in garlic and onions that work in various ways to protect cells. Our understanding of how and why they do their lifesaving work is still too incomplete to manufacture supplements. There's no faking your phytochemical intakes; you simply have to eat food.

There's a reason why a colorful plate thrills your spirit and your soul—your mind is signaling to your body the maximum nutritive content that naturally colorful foods offer. So follow your spirit and eat for color—the more deeply orange or green a vegetable is, for example, the more vitamin A it has. That means green leaf lettuce wins out over pale, bland iceburg, and one small sweet potato has twice your RDA for vitamin A—quite an edge on its pale-faced cousin!

Prevention in a Pill?

The proven importance of vitamins and minerals to fighting disease and promoting a long, healthy life can make it tempting to take high-potency supplements that supply these substances in concentrated doses. While vitamins and minerals can be a "cheap insurance policy" against inadvertent omissions in a healthy diet, substances synthesized in the laboratory are of different molecular structure than those found in food. Scientific uncertainty regarding the usefulness and long-term effects of these molecularly altered nutrients makes a good case for relying on the tried and true method of nourishing our bodies: food.

If you build your diet around the superfoods discussed in this chapter, you will be able to meet your nutritional needs with the confidence that the vitamins and minerals you consume are being properly utilized by your body.

A Superfood Shopping Trip

To get a super start on Eating By Design, go to your organic produce purveyor or health food store to stock up on a colorful cornucopia of superfoods rich in antioxidants and phytochemicals. Favor these for a supercharged diet offering maximum protection against cancer, heart disease, and other illnesses associated with aging:

- Garlic and ginger. In addition to containing antioxidants and lots of fat-free flavor, these roots may act to lower bad LDL cholesterol, raise good HDL cholesterol, lower the risk of blood clots, prevent cancer, slow the growth of cancerous tumors once they form, fight bacteria, and boost immunity.
- The onion family.
- Broccoli and the cabbage family.
- Winter squash, sweet potatoes, carrots, and other dark yellow vegetables.
- Spinach, kale, and other green leafy vegetables.
- Sweet peppers.
- Papaya, mangoes, and other dark yellow fruits.
- Citrus fruits.
- Soybeans.
- Wheat germ and whole grains.

Look for pesticide- and chemical-free foods that offer pure nutrients without toxic threat. Avoid preservatives, artificial colors or flavors, hormones, and antibiotics. Go organic whenever you can. Because organic labeling is largely unregulated, make sure you're getting the purity you paid for:

- Shop at reputable stores, and ask the manager who the suppliers are.
- Find out when deliveries arrive and buy the same day for maximum freshness and nutritional value.
- For the greatest confidence, grow your own garden-fresh organic produce.
- Scrub produce carefully.
- Refrigerate preservative-free baked goods.

✳

Yin-Yang Meal Plan*

The Yin-Yang Meal Plan is a superfood diet placing complex carbohydrates, vegetables, and fruits at the center, with low-fat dairy, soy, poultry, and seafood in a surrounding circle. Sugars come mostly from natural fruit sources, and additives and preservatives are minimized. The result is a nutrient-rich, immune-boosting diet for longevity, skimmed of the high fat content of many health food regimes. Following the Yin-Yang Meal Plan for your EQ will naturally encourage your body to burn off excess fat and reach a lean and healthy balance.

---

* 🗒 = See recipe in Chapter 33.

EQ 1 (Low)

BREAKFAST

Choose from:
✓ Supersmoothie 📄
✓ Hot Kashi cereal (1 oz.) with ½ c. nonfat milk or soy beverage, and ¾ c. fresh fruit

SNACK

If you had a Supersmoothie for breakfast, choose from:
✓ 1 oz. whole grain pretzels
✓ 1 oz. plain brown rice cakes or other fat-free rice snacks

If you had cereal for breakfast, choose from:
✓ ¾ c. diced papaya with a squeeze of lime
✓ 1 c. fresh fruit juice *or* 2 c. fresh vegetable juice *or* 1½ c. mixed fruit and vegetable juice

LUNCH

Seaweed or spinach salad tossed with rice vinegar and soy sauce
Choose from:
✓ 1 Vegetable Roll-Up 📄
✓ 2 Black Bean Enchiladas 📄

SNACK

Choose from:
✓ Edensoy shake
✓ ½ baked yam
✓ ¾ c. strawberries
✓ ½ c. Brown Cow fruit-sweetened yogurt

DINNER

Choose from:
✓ 1 serving Linguine with Spinach and Lentils 📄
✓ ½ serving of Asian Tuna, Salmon, or Halibut 📄
✓ 3 oz. grilled chicken or turkey breast or seafood with ½ c. Three-Mushroom Sauce 📄

Choose any or all:
✓ Steamed beets and winter squash, cubed and sautéed in fresh orange juice until glazed
✓ Red and yellow peppers, broccoli florets, red onion, and plenty of garlic sautéed together in vegetable stock
✓ Diced vegetables stir-fried in chicken or vegetable broth with lots of minced ginger and garlic and soy sauce to taste

Choose from:
✓ 1 Banana Berry Bar 📄
✓ Frozen Rice Dream 📄
✓ 1 oz. dried fruit

EQ 2 (Low-Medium)

BREAKFAST

Choose from:
✓ Supersmoothie 📄
✓ Hot Kashi cereal (1 oz.) with ½ c. nonfat milk or soy beverage, and ¾ c. fresh fruit

SNACK

If you had a Supersmoothie for breakfast, choose from:
✓ 1 oz. whole grain pretzels
✓ 1 oz. plain brown rice cakes or other fat-free rice snacks

If you had cereal for breakfast, choose from:
✓ ¾ c. diced papaya with a squeeze of lime
✓ 1 c. fresh fruit juice *or* 2 c. fresh vegetable juice *or* 1½ c. mixed fruit and vegetable juice

LUNCH

Choose from:
✓ Dried natural low-fat cup-of-soup
✓ Seaweed or spinach salad tossed with ½ c. cooked soybeans tossed with rice vinegar and soy sauce

Choose from:
✓ 1 Vegetable Roll-Up 📄
✓ 2 Black Bean Enchiladas 📄

SNACK

Choose from:
✓ Edensoy shake
✓ ½ baked yam
✓ ¾ c. strawberries
✓ ½ c. Brown Cow fruit-sweetened yogurt

DINNER

Choose from:
✓ 2 c. Linguine with Spinach and Lentils 📄
✓ 1 serving of Asian Tuna, Salmon, or Halibut 📄
✓ 6 oz. grilled chicken or turkey breast or seafood with ½ c. Three-Mushroom Sauce 📄

Choose any or all:
✓ Steamed beets and winter squash, cubed and sautéed in fresh orange juice until glazed
✓ Red and yellow peppers, broccoli florets, red onion, and plenty of garlic sautéed together in vegetable stock
✓ Diced vegetables stir-fried in chicken or vegetable broth with lots of minced ginger and garlic and soy sauce to taste

Choose from:
✓ 1 Banana Berry Bar 📄
✓ Frozen Rice Dream 📄
✓ 1 oz. dried fruit

EQ 3 (Medium-High)

BREAKFAST

Choose from:
✓ Supersmoothie 📄
✓ Hot Kashi cereal (1 oz.) with ½ c. nonfat milk or soy beverage, and ¾ c. fresh fruit

SNACKS

Choose 2 from:
✓ 1 oz. whole grain pretzels
✓ 1 oz. plain brown rice cakes or other fat-free rice snacks
✓ ¾ c. diced papaya with a squeeze of lime
✓ 1 c. fresh fruit juice *or* 2 c. fresh vegetable juice *or* 1½ c. mixed fruit and vegetable juice

LUNCH

Choose from:
✓ Dried natural low-fat cup-of-soup
✓ Seaweed or spinach salad with ½ c. cooked soybeans tossed with rice vinegar and soy sauce

Choose from:
✓ 2 Vegetable Roll-Ups 📄
✓ 4 Black Bean Enchiladas 📄

SNACKS

Choose 2 from:
✓ Edensoy shake
✓ ½ baked yam
✓ ¾ c. strawberries
✓ ½ c. Brown Cow fruit-sweetened yogurt

DINNER

Choose from:
✓ 2 c. Linguine with Spinach and Lentils 📄
✓ 1 serving of Asian Tuna, Salmon, or Halibut 📄
✓ 6 oz. grilled chicken or turkey breast or seafood with ½ c. Three-Mushroom Sauce 📄

Choose any or all:
✓ Steamed beets and winter squash, cubed and sautéed in fresh orange juice until glazed
✓ Red and yellow peppers, broccoli florets, red onion, and plenty of garlic sautéed together in vegetable stock
✓ Diced vegetables stir-fried in chicken or vegetable broth with lots of minced ginger and garlic and soy sauce to taste

Choose from:
✓ 1 Banana Berry Bar 📄
✓ Frozen Rice Dream 📄
✓ 1 oz. dried fruit

EQ 4 (High)

BREAKFAST

Choose from:
✓ Supersmoothie 🗐
✓ Hot Kashi cereal (1 oz.) with ½ c. nonfat milk or soy beverage, and ¾ c. fresh fruit

SNACKS

Choose 2 from:
✓ 1 oz. whole grain pretzels
✓ 1 oz. plain brown rice cakes or other fat-free rice snacks
✓ ¾ c. diced papaya with a squeeze of lime
✓ 1 c. fresh fruit juice *or* 2 c. fresh vegetable juice *or* 1½ c. mixed fruit and vegetable juice

LUNCH

Choose from:
✓ Dried natural low-fat cup-of-soup
✓ Seaweed or spinach salad with ½ c. cooked soybeans tossed with rice vinegar and soy sauce

Choose from:
✓ 2 Vegetable Roll-Ups 🗐
✓ 4 Black Bean Enchiladas 🗐

1 orange or tangerine

SNACK

Choose 2 from:
✓ Edensoy shake
✓ ½ baked yam
✓ ¾ c. strawberries
✓ ½ c. Brown Cow fruit-sweetened yogurt

DINNER

Choose from:
✓ 2½ c. Linguine with Spinach and Lentils 🗐
✓ 1 serving of Asian Tuna, Salmon, or Halibut 🗐 with ½ c. soba noodles
✓ 6 oz. grilled chicken or turkey breast or seafood with ½ c. Three-Mushroom Sauce 🗐 and ½ c. quinoa, barley, or brown rice

Choose any or all:
✓ Steamed beets and winter squash, cubed and sautéed in fresh orange juice until glazed
✓ Red and yellow peppers, broccoli florets, red onion, and plenty of garlic sautéed together in vegetable stock
✓ Diced vegetables stir-fried in chicken or vegetable broth with lots of minced ginger and garlic and soy sauce to taste

Choose from:
✓ 1 Banana Berry Bar 🗐
✓ Frozen Rice Dream 🗐
✓ 1 oz. dried fruit

NATURAL SUPPLEMENTS TO THE SUPERFOODS

- Acidophilus, a culture occurring in some yogurts, helps the immune system by inhibiting the growth of yeast cells in the body. It also acts as a natural digestive aid. You can get a more concentrated dose in acidophilus liquid or capsules.
- Digestive enzymes such as papain and bromoline promote faster, more efficient digestion, especially of superfoods, which tend to be gaseous.

Power Juicing

What to sip alongside your superfood diet? The recent rash of new machinery and the potent anti-aging and protective nutrients dished up by vegetable and fruit cocktails make fresh juicing a good fad to follow. Turn to bartending for the nineties to sip from the fountain of youth.

WHY JUICE?

- An extremely concentrated source of nutrients, including antioxidants and other chemical compounds which protect against cancer, heart disease, and other effects of aging.
- Quick, convenient energy fix.
- Fresh juice generally has more nutrients than canned, bottled, or packaged.
- Endless creative combinations.
- A blast for the taste buds!

Beware of two limits on the virtues of juices: they are a more concentrated source of calories than their sources—especially fruit juices—and unless you have a juicer that leaves the pulp in, you lose the benefits of dietary fiber. Remember that the healthiest diet includes a wide variety of fruits and vegetables, prepared in many different ways.

- You can use a juicer or blender for most of the suggestions here. If you're investing in a new juicer, look for one that leaves the pulp—hence the fiber—in the juice.
- Turn a snack into a meal with the addition of protein powder and/or plain or sweetened nonfat yogurt.
- Spike the punch: add red pepper, Tabasco, or salsa to vegetable juices; cinnamon, nutmeg, or mint to fruit juices; lemon or lime juice or a dash of balsamic vinegar to either.
- Add fresh garlic or onion or vitamin powders for even greater antioxidant potency.

Here are some ideas for getting your feet wet:

Tomato Snap: Tomatoes, fresh spinach, jalapeño pepper.

Caffeine-Free Zinger: Pineapple, grapefruit, orange, fresh ginger root, sparkling mineral water.

Chocolate-Banana Shake (a complete breakfast; substitute for Supersmoothie in your meal plan): 1 banana, ½ c. skim milk, ½ c. vanilla nonfat yogurt, 1 t. cocoa powder, 2 t. honey, and ice cubes to taste.

For vitamin C (antioxidant): Citrus fruits, strawberries, sweet peppers.

For beta-carotene (antioxidant): Carrots, papaya, or anything orange or red.

For B vitamins (energy and immunity): Spinach, kale, turnip greens, brewer's yeast, wheat germ.

For potassium: Carrots, tomatoes, oranges, bananas.

Low-Fermentation Diets

The Yin-Yang Meal Plan is full of nutrients that will naturally support your immune system for natural health and defense against disease. However, certain depressed-immunity conditions respond to a more restrictive diet eliminating foods that ferment in the digestive process. These foods include sugars, wheat, many fruits, yeast, and vinegar. Digestive fermentation causes yeast in the body, which suppresses natural immunity functions. Low-fermentation diets have proven effective in treating conditions such as candidiasis, Epstein-Barr disease, chronic fatigue syndrome, and other viruses.

With an emphasis on whole foods and purity, low-fermentation diets offer the advantage of maximum disease protection and natural healthy energy, with the trade-off of a certain amount of tedium and difficulty in attaining proper nutritional balance. Because of these limitations, I don't include a low-fermentation diet in your Personal Prescription; if you'd like to explore the topic further, check your local library or health-food store.

I find that one month on a low-fermentation diet can serve to purify your system without exceeding the limits of patience, as in Susanna's case. Afterward, you should slowly reintroduce the full spectrum of foods in the Yin-Yang Meal Plan to assure complete nutrition and relieve boredom.

Funny Food Fads

I meet many people who have exceeded the boundaries of sensible nutrition to embrace an extremist diet that completely excludes or unduly emphasizes particular food groups. Some special diets have therapeutic purposes—people with diabetes or allergies, for instance, do need to avoid certain foods, eat particular combinations, and otherwise go beyond the basic precepts of a sensible low-fat diet. But barring medical necessity, most people ultimately find that ultraspecialized diets offer little pleasure and no tangible results superior to those of a low-fat diet based on a wide variety of foods. Worse, highly restrictive diets present the danger of both short- and long-term nutritional imbalance and deficiency. I recommend against any diet that excludes major food groups or requires strict combinations. Why restrict yourself, when the natural bounty of Eating By Design awaits to nourish and harmonize your body and mind?

✳

Never, never
Neglect your life though it's
Temporary:
Your present life, fleeting,
Is the only one that's yours.*

The highest intelligence is in yourself. You already know everything you need for health, if you can only hear it. Focus on yourself as a whole healthy person, and the universe will fall into line with your desires.

Yin-Yang Mantras

- My mind, body, and spirit work together to keep me energetic and well.
- The power to heal myself lies within me.
- The power to feed myself well lies within me.
- I eat from nature's bounty for inner and external beauty.
- My mind knows exactly how to feed my body for perfect health.
- I listen to myself. I hear myself. I am with myself in everything that I do, including eating.
- I select the very best foods that the earth has to offer.
- I believe in the nutritional lessons of human history.
- Good health is my destiny.

---

*Quotation from *A Zen Harvest: Japanese Folk Sayings*. Compiled and translated by Soiku Shigematsu. San Francisco: North Point Press, 1988.

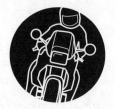

27

THE THRILL-SEEKER'S PERSONAL PRESCRIPTION

The Thrill-Seeker's Personal Prescription is filled with experimental eating that crosses culinary boundaries. You should also be guided by one critical principle: No matter how wildly you may risk curious flavor combinations or unlikely textural juxtapositions, never risk high-fat foods or heaping portions. Breakfast on slugs if you must; just don't drown them in butter sauce.

The world of healthy eating is limited only by your own imagination. Here's the key to unlock the first door.

✳

Explore the Wide World of Wonderful Foods

Experimental Eating

Eating should be an adventure, and your commitment to doing it right does not doom you to a lifetime of turkey sandwiches and rigid rules. Think of all the foods in the Eating By Design Mosaic as a palette of possibilities. Refer to the Low-Fat Cooking Techniques in Part Four for quick tips on creative cooking without added fats. Assemble a host of herbs, spices, and chiles. Now mix, match, and recombine to design your own dishes for maximum taste sensation and excitement. Eating By Design means never having to taste the same thing twice.

Fortunately, healthy fruits and vegetables are the most diverse foods on earth, full of interesting and varied flavors and textures. They add pizzazz to everything, and combine in the most strange and wonderful ways. Make them an important part of your experimental repertoire.

Here are some suggestions for thrilling eating to get you started. Feel free to throw in any other exciting ingredients that focus on flavor, without fat or chemicals.

✓ Naturally lean game meats (substitute for poultry in your meal plan): rabbit, buffalo, beefalo, ostrich, venison, quail, pheasant, Cornish game hen.
✓ Kitchen sink salad:
  1. Choose your own combination of lettuce, radicchio, endive, arugula, water chestnuts, hearts of palm, artichoke hearts, beets, turnip, jicama, pea pods, cooked asparagus, grilled eggplant, and any other vegetable of interest.
  2. Toss with fat-free dressing and herbs of choice.
  3. Garnish with a spoonful of chopped fresh fruit and/or crumbled oil-free bagel, potato, or corn chips.
✓ Anything-and-everything stir-fry:

1. Create your own oil-free stir-fry blend:
   —Chicken or vegetable stock
   —Soy sauce
   —Sherry
   —Rice vinegar
   —Hoisin sauce
   —Black bean paste
   —Plum preserves
   —Minced garlic and ginger
   —Chinese five-spice powder

2. Heat your sauté medium over high heat, toss in, and stir:
   —Diced chicken, turkey, or fish filet
   —Lobster, shrimp, scallops, squid, abalone
   —Chopped vegetables, greens, or sprouts
   (Hints: Cook chicken or seafood first and keep warm while you do the vegetables; cut everything the same size for uniform cooking time.)

3. Serve your creation over any mixture of:
   —White, brown, or wild rice
   —Flavored pastas in various shapes
   —Rice noodles
   —Soba noodles

Global Gusto

Whether exploring ethnic restaurants at home or Thrill-Seeking abroad, there's no need to let mysterious menus and cuisines steer you off your healthy course.

Simply turn your inquiring mind to the task of finding out what's in these exotic preparations.

If you're traveling to another country, use Bruce's trick of getting a cookbook for the region. Look for one with dishes named in their native language. Thumb through and compile your lists.

- "Yes" dishes should contain little or no added fat and focus on complex carbohydrates, vegetables, and lean meats and seafood.
- "No" dishes include anything fried or with large quantities of oil, butter, cream, nuts, or rich meats, and highly salted dishes.
- "Sometimes" dishes include pickled or smoked foods, small quantities of grilled beef, and favorites that are a little too high-fat for the "yes" list.

Take your list with you everywhere and stick to it, adding dishes as you collect reliable information about their ingredients.

You can conduct the same exercise for dining in ethnic restaurants at home. Here are some shortcut guidelines:

GLOBAL GUSTO LIST

Chinese

YES:
- Any chicken, seafood, or vegetable dish with steamed rice or noodles
  - Chow mein
  - Lo mein
  - Chop suey
  - Moo goo gai pan
  - Mu shu
  - Chicken or shrimp with broccoli, mushrooms, bean sprouts, etc.
- Steamed wontons (dumplings) or wonton soup
- Steamed or grilled fish

NO:
- Egg rolls or spring rolls
- Fried wontons
- Breaded, fried, or crispy anything (sweet and sour, lemon or orange chicken)
- Sesame sauce, peanuts, or cashews
- Beef or pork
- Spare ribs
- Fried rice or noodles
- Black bean sauce

Japanese

YES:
- Sushi
- Sashimi
- Chicken or seafood teriyaki
- Udon or soba noodles
- Yakitori

NO:
- California or salmon skin rolls
- Tempura
- Fried dumplings (gyoza)
- Fried noodles (yakisoba)
- Beef bowl

YES:
- Steamed or grilled fish
- Miso soup
- Cucumber salad dressed with vinegar only

NO:

Thai

YES:
- Hot and sour seafood, chicken, or vegetable soup without coconut
    Tom yum kai
    Tom yum koong
- Salads (no eggs or peanuts)
- Chicken larb
- Calamari, boiled or grilled
- Chicken or shrimp rad naa
- Any chicken, seafood, or vegetable dish with steamed rice or noodles
- Curries without coconut
- Steamed or grilled fish

NO:
- Coconut milk (in soup, curry, etc.)
- Fried egg roll, wonton, or tempura
- Crispy or fried anything
- Pan-fried noodles
    Pad thai
    Pad see-ew
- Chicken wings
- Spare ribs
- Satay
- Fried rice
- Sweet and sour
- Eggs
- Nuts

Indian

YES:
- Breads without fat
    Naan (can be stuffed with garlic or onion; not meat)
    Chapati
- Tandoor chicken or seafood with naan, chapati, or rice
- Curries without coconut
- Any chicken, seafood, or vegetable dish
- Dal (lentils)
- Bharta (eggplant dip)
- Raita (yogurt dip)
- Chutneys

NO:
- Breads with fat:
    Paratha
    Roti
- Ghee (butter) in anything
- Fried appetizers
    Samosas
    Pakoras
- Lamb or beef
- Cream or coconut milk
- Paneer (cheese, usually in vegetarian dishes)

California

YES:
- Ahi tuna tartare

NO:
- Crab cakes

YES:
- Chinese chicken salad (no fried noodles)
- Thin-crusted pizza
- Free-range chicken
- Grilled seafood or meats with exotic salsas
- Sourdough bread with rosemary, sun-dried tomatoes, etc.
- Grilled vegetables
- Goat cheese (limited amounts)
- Field or baby greens
- Coffee drinks with skim milk
- Fruit sorbet

NO:
- Cajun popcorn (deep-fried crayfish)
- Designer sausages
- Caesar salad
- Beurre blanc
- Focaccia
- Olive oil dip or sauce
- Coffee drinks with whole milk or ice cream
- Yogurt candy or chips
- Mega-muffins

In Asian restaurants, consider ending with a bowl of hot soup, as is customary instead of dessert. Always be light with soy sauce, teriyaki sauce, and pickled condiments. Avoid tofu unless you're vegetarian; chicken and seafood are lower-fat sources of protein.

When you're cooking at home, recreate the tastes of your travels with my recipes for Coconut Chicken 🗎 , Mu Shu Chicken 🗎 , or Thai Noodle Salad 🗎 .

THE WIDE WORLD OF FOOD

Here are a few more tips for eating well in the wide world:

- Be prepared for different eating customs abroad. If breakfast contains animal protein, for instance, cut back on protein somewhere else. Chances are the locals do too. Treat extra meals, such as high tea in England, as meals—i.e., skip dinner afterward—or have just a few bites and count it as a snack. The cuisines of most of the world are healthier than the American diet—*if* you eat according to local custom. Be aware and watch your portion size.
- Look for these healthy eating staples all around the globe:
  —Vegetables
  —Fruits
  —Potatoes and other root vegetables
  —Breads made without fat
  —Rice, pasta, and other grains
  —Clear soups
- Pack some healthy packaged snacks. The stress of traveling definitely calls for regular snacking, and the availability of healthy choices is unpredictable; much international street food is deep-fried.

Trial by Fire

Anyone who has seriously attempted cooking knows that it's not wimpy work. Bruce's fascination with the fish-blackening stove demonstrated the kind of primal pleasure that can be had in mixing it up with that basic element of nature—fire—that makes most food tasty and palatable.

Pure flame provides unsurpassed flavor to low-fat cooking. If you thrill to cooking on the grill, think of all the healthy foods that can derive smoky deliciousness from a trial by fire:

✓ Boneless, skinless chicken breast halves or sturdy cuts of fish, marinated in:
  —Lemon, garlic, and rosemary
  —Barbecue sauce
  —Sweet and sour sauce
  —White wine, honey, mustard, and tarragon
  —Worcestershire
  —Soy, ginger, garlic, and rice wine
  —Salsa
  —Flavored mustard or vinegar
  —Your favorite fat-free marinade or sauce
✓ Whole turkey breast; grill it with the skin on and peel it off afterward.
✓ All kinds of vegetables: onions, tomatoes, eggplant (sliced or whole), broccoli, summer squash, potatoes, sweet potatoes, mushrooms, asparagus, cooked winter squash halves, scallions, fennel, whole ears of corn.
✓ All kinds of fruit: apples, bananas, pears, papaya, peaches.
✓ Breads and pizzas.
✓ Experiment with the flavors of different wood chips: mesquite, hickory, oak, apple, etc.

NOTE: Be aware that grilling over an open flame can deposit carcinogenic compounds on food.

These ideas for experimental eating are incorporated into the following meal plan. Once you've got the hang of healthy choices and portions, do what you do best: Take the ball and run with it.

✳

Thrill-Seeker Meal Plan*

EQ 1 (Low)

BREAKFAST

Choose from:
- ✓ ½ English muffin topped with 1 T. fat-free ricotta, ¾ c. diced fruit, and 1 t. pure fruit jam and toasted under the broiler; 1 c. skim milk
- ✓ ½ c. leftover white or brown rice heated up with ½ c. skim milk, 1 t. honey, 1 oz. raisins, and a sprinkle of cinnamon
- ✓ Low-fat energy bar and ½ c. skim milk

LUNCH

Choose from:
- ✓ 1 serving Thai Noodle Salad 📋
- ✓ Kitchen sink salad (see p. 294)
- ✓ Anything-and-everything stir-fry (see p. 294; vegetarian, with 1 c. rice or noodles)

SNACK

Choose from:
- ✓ 1 piece fresh fruit or 1 oz. dried fruit
- ✓ Caffe latte with 1 c. skim milk
- ✓ 1 soft pretzel

DINNER

Choose from:
- ✓ 1 serving Coconut Chicken 📋 with steamed vegetables and ½ c. rice
- ✓ 1 serving Mu Shu Chicken 📋
- ✓ 1 Global Gusto entree (see p. 295; 3 oz. chicken or seafood, vegetables, 1 piece bread or ½ c. rice or noodles)
- ✓ 3 oz. grilled chicken or turkey breast or seafood with assorted grilled fruits and vegetables and ½ grilled potato

Choose from:
- ✓ 1 c. Asian-style soup and 1 piece fresh fruit
- ✓ 4 oz. nonfat frozen yogurt with ¾ c. diced fruit

---

* 📋 = See recipe in Chapter 33.

EQ 2 (Low-Medium)

BREAKFAST

Choose from:

✓ 1 English muffin-topped with 1 T. fat-free ricotta, ¾ c. diced fruit, and 1 t. pure fruit jam and toasted under the broiler; 1 c. skim milk

✓ 1 c. leftover white or brown rice heated up with 1 c. skim milk, 1 t. honey, 1 oz. raisins, and a sprinkle of cinnamon

✓ Low-fat energy bar and 1 c. skim milk

SNACK

Choose from:

1 piece fresh fruit or 1 oz. dried fruit

LUNCH

Choose from:

✓ 1 serving Thai Noodle Salad 📄 with 3 oz. shredded chicken breast

✓ Kitchen sink salad (see p. 294; add 3 oz. smoked turkey or chicken)

✓ Anything-and-everything stir-fry (see p. 294; with 3 oz. poultry or seafood and 1 c. rice or noodles)

SNACK

Choose from:

✓ 1 piece fresh fruit or 1 oz. dried fruit

✓ Caffe latte with 1 c. skim milk

✓ 1 soft pretzel

DINNER

Choose from:

✓ 1 serving Coconut Chicken 📄 with steamed vegetables and ½ c. rice

✓ 1 serving Mu Shu Chicken 📄

✓ 1 Global Gusto entree (see p. 295; 3 oz. chicken or seafood, vegetables, 1 piece bread or ½ c. rice or noodles)

✓ 3 oz. grilled chicken or turkey breast or seafood with assorted grilled fruits and vegetables and ½ grilled potato

Choose from:

✓ 1 c. Asian-style soup and 1 piece fresh fruit

✓ 4 oz. nonfat frozen yogurt with ¾ c. diced fruit

EQ 3 (Medium-High)

BREAKFAST

Choose from:
✓ 1 English muffin topped with 1 T. fat-free ricotta, ¾ c. diced fruit, and 1 t. pure fruit jam and toasted under the broiler; 1 c. skim milk
✓ 1 c. leftover white or brown rice heated up with 1 c. skim milk, 1 t. honey, 1 oz. raisins, and a sprinkle of cinnamon
✓ Low-fat energy bar and 1 c. skim milk

SNACK

1 piece fresh fruit or 1 oz. dried fruit

LUNCH

Choose from:
✓ 1 serving Thai Noodle Salad 📄 with 3 oz. shredded chicken breast
✓ Kitchen sink salad (see p. 294; add 3 oz. smoked turkey or chicken)
✓ Anything-and-everything stir-fry (see p. 294; 3 oz. poultry or seafood and 1 c. rice or noodles)

SNACK

Choose 2 from:
✓ 1 piece fresh fruit or 1 oz. dried fruit
✓ Caffe latte with 1 c. skim milk
✓ 1 soft pretzel

DINNER

Choose from:
✓ 2 servings Coconut Chicken 📄 with steamed vegetables and ½ c. rice
✓ 2 servings Mu Shu Chicken 📄 with 1 whole wheat tortilla
✓ 1 Global Gusto entree (see p. 295; 6 oz. chicken or seafood, vegetables, 1 piece bread or ½ c. rice or noodles)
✓ 6 oz. grilled chicken or turkey breast or seafood with assorted grilled fruits and vegetables and ½ grilled potato

Choose from:
✓ 1 c. Asian-style soup and 1 piece fresh fruit
✓ 4 oz. nonfat frozen yogurt with ¾ c. diced fruit

EQ 4 (High)

BREAKFAST

Choose from:
- ✓ 1 English muffin topped with 1 T. fat-free ricotta, ¾ c. diced fruit, and 1 t. pure fruit jam and toasted under the broiler; 1 c. skim milk
- ✓ 1 c. leftover white or brown rice heated up with 1 c. skim milk, 1 t. honey, 1 oz. raisins, and a sprinkle of cinnamon
- ✓ Lowfat energy bar and 1 c. skim milk

SNACK

1 piece fresh fruit or 1 oz. dried fruit

LUNCH

Choose from:
- ✓ 1 serving Thai Noodle Salad 📄 with 3 oz. shredded chicken breast
- ✓ Kitchen sink salad (see p. 294; add 3 oz. smoked turkey or chicken)
- ✓ Anything-and-everything stir fry (see p. 294; 3 oz. poultry or seafood and 1 c. rice or noodles)

SNACK

Choose 2 from:
- ✓ 1 piece fresh fruit or 1 oz. dried fruit
- ✓ Caffe latte with 1 c. skim milk
- ✓ 1 soft pretzel

DINNER

Choose from:
- ✓ 2 servings Coconut Chicken 📄 with steamed vegetables and 1 c. rice
- ✓ 2 servings Mu Shu Chicken with 2 whole wheat tortillas
- ✓ 1 Global Gusto entree (see p. 295; 6 oz. chicken or seafood, vegetables, 2 pieces bread or 1 c. rice or noodles)
- ✓ 6 oz. grilled chicken or turkey breast or seafood (p. 298) with assorted grilled fruits and vegetables and 1 grilled potato

Choose from:
- ✓ 1 c. Asian-style soup and 1 piece fresh fruit
- ✓ 4 oz. nonfat frozen yogurt with ¾ c. diced fruit

SUPPLEMENT YOURSELF

- Enhance your strength and tolerance for stress with a branched-chain amino acid formula.

Challenge and Charm

Bruce was always most excited about eating well when he was engaged in some kind of challenge or competition—wrestling with his stove, searching for the ultimate sushi octopus, peering behind the scenes at Chinese restaurants. The world could certainly benefit from some of your Thrill-Seeking energy for eating well. So go ahead. Lay down the gauntlet.

- **Challenge** the chef in a restaurant to meet your low-fat requirements. **Charm** your waitperson into making sure you get what you need.
- **Challenge** your local grocer to carry a wide variety of excellent fresh produce, poultry, and seafood, and to stock the latest low-fat food products. **Charm** him or her with a promise to spread the store's fame far and wide.
- **Challenge** your friends with a low-fat cook-off. Compete for the title of best low-fat chili, chocolate chip cookie, fruit dessert, or complete meal. **Charm** the assembled guests with a festive tasting of the results.

Don't Peak Out

The greatest enemy of a Thrill-Seeker's new eating habits is boredom. This is one mountain you can't climb only to descend back into the abyss. You need to shimmy up to the peak of your personal potential and *stay there*.

View your eating experiment as ongoing. Constantly change your scenery: Where you shop. What you buy. The restaurants you dine in. The foods in your pantry, refrigerator, and freezer. Your daily snacks. Recipes and menus. Where in the house you eat. What you eat with (serve your yogurt in a wine glass; use chopsticks for your salad).

When you tire of shrimp, switch to calamari. When pasta seems passé, try soba noodles. Transform your dining room into a Japanese garden for a month. Plant a patch of purple basil and make a purple pesto. Try steaming something you never steamed before. Cook something you always eat raw, like cucumbers. Buy a new spice and make a dinner entree and a dessert with it. Have a cup of vegetable soup for breakfast. Switch from potatoes to parsnips, chile peppers to chutnies. Dip into the ever-expanding assortment of new low-fat food products.

Change anything and everything except your low-fat ingredients and techniques, your attention to portion size, and a regular schedule of meals and snacks. The world of foods and ways to eat them is wide enough to keep you interested for the rest of your life.

✳

Go for a Natural High

Last Action Hero

Exciting as healthy food can be, you should be sure to complement your eating plan by pursuing thrills that also challenge your muscles and cardiovascular system (see sidebar). Activities such as skydiving, snowmobiling, race car driving, riding rollercoasters, and bungee jumping can also give you a natural high, but won't provide the same conditioning benefits.

WORK YOURSELF OUT

Improve your physique while you push the limits:

Activity	Approximate calories burned per hour:
▪ Hiking and backpacking	408
▪ Rock climbing	720
▪ Skiing the Alps	990
▪ Sailing the Caribbean	300
▪ Surfing Hawaii	480
▪ Windsurfing	600–900
▪ Mountain biking	300–720
▪ Rollerblading	480
▪ Whitewater rafting	600–900
▪ Scuba diving	360–750
▪ Waterskiing the Riviera	480
▪ Trekking in Nepal	336–420
▪ Competitive sports	420–660

The Weekend Warrior

In truth, few of us lead the life of Indiana Jones, or even of Bruce the photojournalist. Even highly adventuresome types are likely to find themselves going to work all week, perhaps escaping in a Jeep over the weekend for a two-day excursion. If you lead the stop-and-start life of a weekend warrior, you need to fine-tune your eating habits a bit so that you take in a few extra calories during your active days, and—even more important—cut back again during your sedentary week. It's also important that you don't abandon the good habits of the week just because you're off on a weekend adventure.

WEEKEND WARRIOR EXTRAS

- As a general rule of thumb, fuel up for an active day by adding one serving of complex carbohydrates per level of your EQ (see your EQ and the Eating By Design Mosaic in Part Two).

Don't overestimate the demands of what you're doing—a weekend of wine touring, for instance, probably doesn't require any additional intake. Listen to your body, and don't forget to pare back the extras when you return to workaday life.

It's also crucial that you train for your weekend exertions with a regular workout program during the week that includes plenty of cardiovascular conditioning and stretching to prevent muscle injury. See the Master Exercise Plan in Chapter 31 for a comprehensive workout plan.

THE LIGHTWEIGHT BACKPACK

Carry these foods to fuel outdoor adventures—they're all low in fat, packed with healthy energy, and easily transportable.

✓ Homemade trail mix; choose from fat-free granola and cereal, dried fruit, and toasted soybeans. Forgo traditional trail mixes, which are full of fat.
✓ Dried low-fat soups, such as Fantastic Foods or Nile Spice.
✓ Whole grain, fruit-sweetened, fat-free cookies and muffins.
✓ Low-fat ramen noodles, pasta, or couscous cups with vegetables, chicken, or shrimp.
✓ Canned tuna, salmon, or sardines packed in water.
✓ Fat-free crackers.
✓ Bagels.
✓ Fruit leather.
✓ Fresh celery, carrots, radishes, and snap peas.
✓ As much water as you can carry!

Running on Full

Thrill-Seekers are used to turning their energies outward, seeking their tests and trials in the outside world. But if you take a moment to look inward, you will probably find personal challenges that can be just as thrilling to conquer as a mountaintop, and ultimately more rewarding. Test your personal fortitude with the trial of Eating By Design and see if the reward isn't rich enough to make it part of your life.

Thrill-Seeker Reminders

Write the following reminders on slips of paper and stash them in unexpected places—the glove compartment, your luggage, camera bag, ski parka pockets—for surprise prompts to rise to your healthy eating challenge:

- Eating well is an exciting experiment in health and energy.
- A wide world of healthy, flavorful food awaits my exploration.
- Every time I eat well, I sip from the fountain of youth.
- Good food fuels my adventures.
- I'll risk redesigning my eating habits for the thrill of reaching my peak potential.
- The best fuel makes the best Thrill-Seeker.

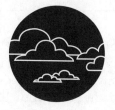

28

THE DREAMER'S PERSONAL PRESCRIPTION

Perhaps you've always dreamed of having a perfectly healthy body—fit, trim, and just the right size. But diets that deprive you in the here and now never seem like the right way to make these dreams come true. If your highest hopes for health and fitness have always seemed just out of reach, I have a happy announcement: The solution is right here, right now, in Eating By Design.

Unlike a knight in shining armor, fitness is one dream you don't have to wait for. You hold the key in your own hand. You simply have to turn your faith in the future to your advantage. Take action in the present to ensure your eternal (or at least long-lived) well-being. Eating By Design makes your dream of a happy, healthy self come true with a plan incorporating wonderfully light and nourishing versions of all the foods you've loved since childhood. Your Personal Prescription works magic on familiar food to help you eat healthily ever after.

✳

Fantasize a World Free from Fat

Imagine fat as an obstacle in your path to the streets paved with gold, like the witches, ogres, and dragons of myth. Eliminating this obstacle from your diet works magic on your body. For instance:

- Take the tablespoon of butter or margarine off your baked potato and save 100 calories.
- Have a cup of frozen nonfat yogurt instead of premium ice cream and save 200 calories.
- Top your salad with two tablespoons of fat-free dressing instead of regular ranch and save 150 calories.
- Save these 450 calories a day for about a week and lose a pound of body fat!

In a world with no easy answers, some are simpler than others. There are over five thousand new low-fat and fat-free foods on the market, in addition to the natural bounty of fruits, vegetables, and grains that have nourished mankind through the millennia. Eat of these foods to free your diet and your body from fat. Feed yourself with low-fat foods to make your dreams of a perfectly healthy self come true.

The supermarket is a modern-day wonderland of fat-free fun. Use the Master Market List in Chapter 30 to stock your kitchen and unlock the secret of a long and healthy life. Each new low-fat food you discover holds a hidden key.

One word of warning: The benefits of fat-free foods become a fairy tale if you eat too much of them. Avoid the overeating ogre by sticking to the portions appropriate to your EQ. The meal plan that follows shows you how to put your low-fat dreams into action.

✳

Fantasy Foods: Low-fat Comfort for Your Inner Child

Traditional diets seem to require every ounce of your adult discipline. They always demand that you deny the inner voice that says, "Feed me something warm and smooth and creamy—now!"

Eating By Design to the rescue! My Rx for your hungry inner child includes all these comforting foods—in slimmed-down versions that will miraculously make a slim and beautiful you:

✓ Hot Cream of Wheat with raisins and maple sugar
✓ Lentil soup
✓ Macaroni and cheese
✓ Crispy oven-fried chicken
✓ Steak
✓ Sloppy Joes
✓ Turkey pot pie
✓ Mashed potatoes and gravy
✓ Corn on the cob
✓ Chocolate mousse
✓ Rice pudding
✓ Brownies

Are you feeling happy yet? Dream about your beautiful body, and read on to the meal plan that will take you there.

✳

The Dreamer Meal Plan*

EQ 1 (Low)

BREAKFAST

Choose from:
✓ ½ c. orange juice; hot oatmeal or Cream of Wheat (1 oz. dry) with 2 t. raisins and 1 t. maple sugar; 1 c. skim milk
✓ 1 low-fat frozen waffle with ½ c. nonfat yogurt and ¾ c. fruit

LUNCH

Assorted raw vegetables
Choose from:
✓ 1 serving Macaroni & Cheese 📑
✓ 1 c. Lentil Soup 📑 (homemade or canned fat-free) with a sourdough or whole grain roll
✓ Large salad (mixed greens, assorted vegetables, and fat-free dressing) with a sourdough or whole grain roll

SNACK

1 piece fresh fruit

DINNER

Choose from:
✓ 1 serving Crispy Chicken with Apricot Dipping Sauce 📑
✓ 3 oz. grilled or broiled lean steak (sirloin, tenderloin, filet mignon, or round)
✓ 1 serving Turkey Pot Pie 📑 (no rice or potato side dish)

Choose from (if having chicken or steak):
✓ ½ c. Mashed Potatoes 📑 with ¼ c. Gravy 📑
✓ ½ baked potato with 2 T. fat-free sour cream
✓ ½ c. rice

Choose from:
✓ ½ ear corn on the cob
✓ Steamed spinach

Choose from:
✓ ½ c. Chocolate Mousse 📑
✓ ½ c. Rice Pudding 📑
✓ 1 Fudge Brownie 📑
✓ 2 fat-free cookies

---

* 📑 =See recipe in Chapter 33.

EQ 2 (Low-Medium)

BREAKFAST

Choose from:
✓ ½ c. orange juice; hot oatmeal or Cream of Wheat (1 oz. dry) with 2 t. raisins and 1 t. maple sugar; 1 c. skim milk
✓ 1 low-fat frozen waffle with ½ c. nonfat yogurt and ¾ c. fruit

SNACK

1 piece fresh fruit

LUNCH

Assorted raw vegetables
Choose from:
✓ 1 serving Macaroni & Cheese 📄
✓ 1 c. Lentil Soup 📄 with a sourdough or whole grain roll
✓ 1 can low-fat chicken noodle soup
✓ ¾ c. Sloppy Joes 📄 on a light hamburger bun
✓ Salad (mixed greens, assorted vegetables, 3 oz. chicken or turkey breast or shrimp, and fat-free dressing) with a sourdough or whole grain roll

SNACK 1

4 oz. nonfat frozen yogurt

SNACK 2

Choose from:
✓ 1 oz. fat-free chips
✓ 1 soft pretzel

DINNER

Choose from:
✓ 1 serving Crispy Chicken with Apricot Dipping Sauce 📄
✓ 3 oz. grilled or broiled lean steak (sirloin, tenderloin, filet mignon, or round)
✓ 1 serving Turkey Pot Pie 📄 (no rice or potato side dish)

Choose from (if having chicken or steak):
✓ ½ c. Mashed Potatoes 📄 with ¼ c. Gravy 📄
✓ ½ baked potato with 2 T. fat-free sour cream
✓ ½ c. rice

Choose from:
✓ ½ ear corn on the cob
✓ Steamed spinach

Choose from:
✓ ½ c. Chocolate Mousse 📄
✓ ½ c. Rice Pudding 📄
✓ 1 Fudge Brownie 📄
✓ 2 fat-free cookies

EQ 3 (Medium-High)

BREAKFAST

Choose from:
✓ ½ c. orange juice; hot oatmeal or Cream of Wheat (1 oz. dry) with 2 t. raisins and 1 t. maple sugar; 1 c. skim milk
✓ 1 low-fat frozen waffle with ½ c. nonfat yogurt and ¾ c. fruit

SNACK

1 piece fresh fruit

LUNCH

Assorted raw vegetables
Choose from:
✓ 1 serving Macaroni & Cheese 🗒
✓ 1½ c. Lentil Soup 🗒 with a sourdough or whole grain roll
✓ 1 can low-fat chicken noodle soup
✓ 1½ c. Sloppy Joes 🗒 on a light hamburger bun
✓ Salad (mixed greens, assorted vegetables, 6 oz. chicken or turkey breast or shrimp, and fat-free dressing) with a sourdough or whole grain roll

SNACK 1

4 oz. nonfat frozen yogurt

SNACK 2

Choose from:
✓ 1 oz. fat-free chips
✓ 1 soft pretzel

DINNER

Choose from:
✓ 1 serving Crispy Chicken with Apricot Dipping Sauce 🗒
✓ 3 oz. grilled or broiled lean steak (sirloin, tenderloin, filet mignon, or round)
✓ 1 serving Turkey Pot Pie 🗒 (no rice or potato side dish)

Choose from (if having chicken or steak):
✓ 1 c. Mashed Potatoes 🗒 with ¼ c. Gravy 🗒
✓ 1 baked potato with 4 T. fat-free sour cream
✓ 1 c. rice

Choose from:
✓ ½ ear corn on the cob
✓ Steamed spinach

Choose from:
✓ ½ c. Chocolate Mousse 🗒
✓ ½ c. Rice Pudding 🗒
✓ 1 Fudge Brownie 🗒
✓ 2 fat-free cookies (or save for bedtime snack)

BEDTIME SNACK

Choose from:
✓ Hot cocoa (nonfat milk with unsweetened cocoa powder and NutraSweet or sugar to taste)
✓ 1 c. skim milk with 2 fat-free cookies (if saved from dessert)

EQ 4 (High)

BREAKFAST

Choose from:
✓ 1 c. orange juice; hot oatmeal or Cream of Wheat (2 oz. dry) with 2 t. raisins and 1 t. maple sugar; 1 c. skim milk
✓ 2 low-fat frozen waffles with ½ c. nonfat yogurt and 1½ c. fruit

SNACK

1 piece fresh fruit

LUNCH

Assorted raw vegetables
Choose from:
✓ 1 serving Macaroni & Cheese 📄
✓ 1½ c. Lentil Soup 📄 with a sourdough or whole grain roll
✓ 1 can low-fat chicken noodle soup
✓ 1½ c. Sloppy Joes 📄 on a light hamburger bun
✓ Salad (mixed greens, assorted vegetables, 6 oz. chicken or turkey breast or shrimp, and fat-free dressing) with a sourdough or whole grain roll

SNACK 1

4 oz. nonfat frozen yogurt

SNACK 2

Choose from:
✓ 1 oz. fat-free chips
✓ 1 soft pretzel

DINNER

Choose from:
✓ 1 serving Crispy Chicken with Apricot Dipping Sauce 📄
✓ 3 oz. grilled or broiled lean steak (sirloin, tenderloin, filet mignon, or round)
✓ 1 serving Turkey Pot Pie 📄 (no rice or potato side dish)

Choose from (if having chicken or steak):
✓ 1½ c. Mashed Potatoes 📄 with ¼ c. Gravy 📄
✓ 1 baked potato with 4 T. fat-free sour cream
✓ 1½ c. rice

Choose from:
✓ ½ ear corn on the cob
✓ Steamed spinach

Choose from:
✓ ½ c. Chocolate Mousse 📄
✓ ½ c. Rice Pudding 📄
✓ 1 Fudge Brownie 📄
✓ 2 fat-free cookies (or save for bedtime snack)

BEDTIME SNACK

Choose from:
✓ Hot cocoa (nonfat milk with unsweetened cocoa powder and NutraSweet or sugar to taste)
✓ 1 c. skim milk with 2 fat-free cookies (if saved from dessert)

Fun Foods for Festive Events

Remember going to the fair, the carnival, or other fun and festive events? Fanciful snacks were always part of the experience. There's no reason you can't have special snacks for special occasions when you're Eating By Design.

Look for these fun foods next time you're at a street fair, movie, or sporting event, and choose one wherever your meal plan calls for a snack:

✓ Roasted chestnuts
✓ Soft pretzel (with mustard)
✓ Frozen fruit bar
✓ Frozen nonfat yogurt
✓ Cappuccino with nonfat milk
✓ Fat-free muffin
✓ Popcorn (no butter)
✓ Cotton candy
✓ Snow-cone, slush, or shaved ice
✓ Biscotti (no chocolate coating or nuts)

SUPPLEMENT YOURSELF

- DO save yourself from deficiency with a good vitamin and mineral supplement specially formulated for women, such as Optivite.
- DON'T fall for other unsubstantiated supplement claims.

Build Your Castle Block by Block

Now that you have your meal plan, where to begin? It's always easier to dream of a completed structure than it is to pick up the first building block and put it into place. But once you lay the foundation, the excitement of watching your structure grow will motivate and reward you, until your castle in the air becomes a healthy lifestyle grounded in reality.

Break ground *today* on your new resolutions, then build gradually. Start at the bottom and work your way up. Follow this general blueprint, or design a more specific one of your own:

The Tower
Reward yourself with a grand prize for successfully completing your castle—a new outfit, a trip, collection of CDs, day at the spa. Now prepare yourself and enlist the help of others to defend your castle against all unhealthy invaders.

Second Floor
Take your healthy eating plan out with you, to restaurants, parties, movies, holiday meals. Give up your excuses to stray.

First Floor
Start to exercise every day, anything from a walk, to tennis, to an aerobics class—any activity that challenges you and makes you feel good.

The Ground Floor
Begin to follow the meal plan for your EQ at home, experimenting with the recipes and measuring all your portions.

The Foundation
Use the Master Market List to clean out your kitchen of bad foods and stock it with good ones. Buy some new cookware and storage containers to inspire your healthy efforts.

START HERE

WORK YOURSELF OUT

- Take long walks with a friend or partner.
- Hire a personal trainer to help you with a workout program one-on-one.

✳

Follow Through!—Don't Follow the Leader

You've built your castle in the air—now the trick is living in it. After three months on the Diet Designs program Luella was accustomed, through careful training, to making her own eating choices. But on a first date with a very attractive man—one of her first since her lover left—she found herself in a fancy restaurant with the menu written only in French. Her date charmed her by offering to order for both of them, then doing so in fluent French, leaving her completely in the dark about what was in store for their meal. Luella was awed and impressed, but increasingly distressed as she faced courses of fois gras, snails in butter, tournedos of beef in cream sauce, and crème brulée for dessert. Much as she loved the worldly *savoir faire* of her companion, she went to sleep unhappy that her hopes for health had been, at least temporarily, compromised. She resolved that next time she would let her date know her desires.

You can *follow through* on your dream by *following these guidelines:*

- Refer to your EQ and the Eating By Design Mosaic for how much to eat of which foods. The preceding meal plan for your EQ helps you map out an entire day. Stick to your designated portion size. This might be very different from that of your friends.
- Eat like royalty on public display: Take tiny bites. Chew and swallow carefully. Put your fork down often. Attend to the conversation. Find a role model at the table, someone who looks like your vision of perfection, and make sure you eat no more than that person.
- Don't wait for someone to tell you "no" as you hover over the cheese dip or debate the dessert menu. Even the most attentive friend or lover might fail to rescue you.

Make Your Prince a Partner

Often, the leader you're following into dietary disaster is the very friend who can help make your Personal Prescription work for you. Here are some ways to get healthy eating help from your partner:

- Photocopy your Personal Prescription, along with lists such as the Eating By Design Mosaic, Master Market and Snack List, and Restaurant and Fast Food Guidelines. Give them to your partner, explaining that these are the basics of your new healthy eating plan and that you would really appreciate his or her help in sticking to the program.

- Ask your partner to shop, cook, or order for you according to the Eating By Design principles. Make gentle suggestions and requests that will make your partner feel needed and appreciated. This will help you take care of *yourself* even as you let someone else take care of you.
- Ask your partner to buy you nutrition books, low-fat cookbooks, nonstick cookware, exercise equipment and clothing, and subscriptions to healthy lifestyle magazines as gifts on your birthday or holidays. Let him or her know that this will make you feel well taken care of.
- Ignore lapses on the part of your prince like offering you inappropriate foods, encouraging you to skip your workout to go to a movie, questioning the importance of your healthy lifestyle, or assuring you that you already are or never will be fit and should abandon your efforts. Soon your prince will reward you for staying true to your resolutions.

Take a Healthy Honeymoon

When newcomers embrace the Eating By Design lifestyle it's often something like a honeymoon—they fall in love with the good feelings of living a healthy life. The infatuation is even more intense when they share their new knowledge with someone they love, adding freshness to their relationship with a fresh approach to food and nutrition.

For a healthy honeymoon, try a romantic dinner à deux, Eating By Design style. Eating healthfully with your partner ensures a long life together. Like any good honeymoon, I bet that this one will leave you hooked.

A ROMANTIC RESTAURANT DINNER À DEUX

Depend on your dinner companion to keep your portions in line by sharing plates. Here's how one couple I know dines at their favorite romantic Italian restaurant. Because they share everything, it feels like a splurge. And because they leave feeling light and energized, this restaurant meal never fails to renew their romance.

To start:

A salad of fresh Roma tomatoes drizzled with balsamic vinegar, sprinkled with basil and a few shavings of Parmesan cheese.

A bowl of house minestrone soup.

Entree:

A glass of red wine.

One plate of fettuccine with marinara sauce and mixed seafood.

Steamed spinach with garlic.

He adds a slice of crusty Italian bread.

They skip the cappuccinos and stop at the frozen yogurt store on the way home.

Home for the Holidays

Dreamers tend to have strong emotional ties to their childhood homes that can make visits there both a comfort and a healthy eating challenge. Mature adults suddenly find themselves reduced to impressionable children at the family table, eating willy-nilly without planning or portioning. Many mothers collude in this process by fixing childhood favorites for their returning children, getting great satisfaction when their offering is eaten with youthful enthusiasm. When you're homeward bound, try to follow a few pointers:

- Watch your portions! You're not a child anymore, and you *can't* just eat as much as you want.
- Beware that the emotional ups and downs of family reunions can make you vulnerable to overeating. Look for more constructive ways to express your feelings.
- Suggest that the family share some low-fat traditional favorites from your meal plan or the Eating By Design Recipes in Part Four.
- If high-fat or heavy foods are starting to get you down, offer to cook a meal, or suggest going out to a restaurant.

✳

Let Health Fulfill You

Good health is a physical, mental, and emotional feeling of happiness. When you're healthy you are beautiful, radiant, strong, and full of an irresistible personal energy.

Try this exercise to experience the fulfillment of feeling healthy:

After a healthy, low-fat meal, sit still and think about the nutritive, healing powers of the food you've eaten. Feel the energy flowing to your cells, feeding them and flushing them clean. Feel your inner flame kindle and ignite, spreading a sensation of warmth and well-being through your body and into your head. This is a happiness all your own.

Now focus on your heart. This metaphorical center of your being, where you feel love and joy, is also your literal life force. Would you starve this force by lining your arteries with fatty deposits, or deny it the deep breaths of oxygen that a brisk walk delivers? A happy heart is both physically and emotionally sound, pumping power and joy into your body and soul.

Set Yourself Free

Remember: You've come as far as you have under your own horsepower. No matter how much help or how many advantages you've enjoyed, your accomplishments belong to *you.* Allowing yourself to take joy in your own achievements—like following your Personal Prescription for Eating By Design—is the first step toward empowering a healthy mind, body, and spirit.

You can extend your self-empowerment efforts beyond your eating plan by enrolling in assertiveness training, self-awareness seminars, or classes in anything that interests you—art, political science, literature, physics. Developing your autonomy will help you make healthy decisions in all aspects of your life.

Weight loss can free your body of fat, rescuing you from poor health and self-image. But this rescue, no matter how welcome and dramatic, is just the beginning of the rest of your life. Remember, to rescue really means to liberate, to set free. Once rescued, what you do with your freedom is even more important than how you attain it. When your prince shows up with that glass slipper, fill it up with sparkling mineral water and toast a happy, *healthy* future.

Sweet Dreams for Sleeping Beauties

Say these phrases every night before bed to plant the seeds of your dreams. Or, make a tape and play it while you sleep, for subliminal suggestion.

- My happy future begins in the present.
- I envision a fit and beautiful me, and live my life accordingly.
- I eat right today so that I'll be ready for happiness and love tomorrow.
- I take small steps to build my castle in the air.
- I can live in the body I want.
- There are no limits to my dreams of health and fitness.
- I pay attention to myself.
- I will eat healthy foods happily ever after.

29

EATING BY GENDER: Men Eat from Their Stomachs, Women Eat from Their Hormones

Only recently has nutrition become a coeducational concern. "Diet" has gone from a watchword of women's magazines to a national health care issue for both sexes. As men and women seek ways to eat well together (doesn't that shared plate of pasta beat the old days of a steak at his place and a salad at hers?) the question arises: Do nutritional needs vary by gender? The answer is yes, in certain areas and at certain times. Furthermore, many people have been socially conditioned to eat in a gendered way. The PMS chocolate bar and the postgame steak are both ways of experiencing gender identity.

Certain sex differences cut across all the food personality types. The subtle differences between men's and women's bodies that allow us to reproduce (and keep life interesting), and the psychological attributes that go along with those differences, bring up some eating issues that you should be aware of, for your own sake and that of your partner, date, brother or sister, or other mysterious member of the opposite sex. A little insight into the gender gap will help you Eat By Design in accordance with your sex.

The Psychology of Gendered Eating

From infancy on, we associate food with female nurturing. The result is that many girls grow up associating food with their female role, while boys are more likely to view eating as a "natural" act, a simple response to physiological need. To simplify and extend this concept, man eats because nature and his mother tell him to; woman feeds others, and, by extension, herself, to nurture and care for them. Another way of saying this is that for women, food is love; for men, food is fuel.

319

In reality, these conceptions probably overlap. Women do indeed eat for fuel, and men, to feel cared for. But it may be possible to say that, in general, women's relationship with food tends to be more emotional, and men's, more physical. Socially, this contrast plays itself out in the concept that a man who eats a lot has a "healthy appetite," while a woman who offers a lot of food has a lot of love. Boys are often coached to believe that food is inherently good for them, and more is better and healthier (we know different now, but old habits die hard). Leftovers tend to go to the man at the table, whether or not his weight and caloric needs warrant it. When a man eats, he's doing what comes naturally.

Women, on the other hand, are encouraged from girlhood on to sacrifice other activities to cook for and feed others—but when it comes to their own plate, less is better and healthier, an indicator of self-sacrifice and self-control. A woman who eats too hungrily or with too much enjoyment might be suspected of having an emotional problem with food. But eating "forbidden" food with other women can be an act of female bonding, a sign of caring for each other through shared indulgence. Taken a step further, a private binge might seem like a way of caring for yourself.

These gendered expectations can sabotage the physical and psychological health of either sex. The healthiest diet is based on *your own* particular needs. Your Personal Prescription tackles this topic for both sexes; this chapter describes how some Eating By Design principles break down by gender.

✳

Feeding Your Feminine Self

Women in America have long been haunted by complicated relationships with food and their own bodies. The reasons are physical, social, and psychological, and are thoroughly explored in the literature on dieting. In recent years, the nation as a whole has become increasingly overweight. The bad news is that women are leading this trend; despite all the attention lavished on the female diet, more women than men are currently becoming overweight. This section briefly focuses on some of the life situations that being female presents, and their implications for Eating By Design.

Women are genetically programmed to have more body fat than men (18–25% body fat is fit for women, versus 12–19% for men), to assist in the reproduction of the species by providing energy stores for the growing fetus and nursing infant. To add insult to the injury of extra fat cells, women are subject to strict social norms for body image; undergo a pubescent reshaping of their bodies just when that image is becoming important; experience a major body transformation with each baby; and constantly live with hormonal cycles that directly affect moods and food cravings. All these biological disturbances make it particularly important that you know how to nourish yourself well.

PLUSES AND PITFALLS OF FEEDING YOUR FEMININE SELF

PLUSES	PITFALLS
+ Women have more body fat than men—it's biologically unavoidable!	− Media images of women often portray hard, muscular bodies composed more like men than women.
+ Before menopause, less likely than men to store abdominal fat, which is linked with increased risk of heart disease (not to mention unsightly).	− After menopause, equal risk of heart disease as men; higher risk of breast cancer, also associated with a high-fat diet; equal risk of colon cancer, another diet-related killer. Likely to concentrate fat in hips and thighs, resulting in the dreaded (but better-than-a-spare-tire) "pear shape."
+ Lots of societal support and approval for efforts to be thin.	− Preoccupation with appearance leads to poor self-esteem and body image, even among thin women.
+ Women socially "allowed" to enjoy food, cooking, and the associated rituals.	− Women pressured to plan and cook food whether they want to or not.
+ Pregnancy and lactation increase nutritional requirements, allowing for higher caloric intake.	− The 25–35 pound weight gain and subsequent loss associated with pregnancy can be physically and psychologically challenging.
+ Hormonally driven food cravings might be physiologically justified.	− Hormonal food cravings can lead to eating excess quantities and unhealthful foods.

Premenstrual Syndrome

Elise, a Shooting Star, had an excuse for poor eating related to her menstrual cycle for every week of the month. I had to gently remind her that this was going to be a fact of life all the way up to menopause, and did she really want to postpone losing weight until then? When she said "no," we worked out a strategy to deal with each of her hormonally induced obstacles. But I never invalidated Elise's excuses. The hormonal cycles of womanhood can certainly challenge your commitment to Eating By Design.

"Premenstrual syndrome" generally refers to an assortment of symptoms experienced by some women in the two weeks prior to their period. Ranging from irritability, anxiety, and depression to breast tenderness and food cravings, these symptoms seem to be related to hormonal fluctuations, but no one knows quite how.

Though doctors are experimenting with a range of treatments for PMS, including hormone therapy and antidepressant medication, diet and exercise remain crucial factors in your premenstrual well-being. This is kind of a catch-22, since the mood swings and cravings of PMS often prompt you to abandon your healthy eating and exercise habits. Do you have a monthly craving for chocolate bars? The caffeine and sugar in chocolate are likely to aggravate your mood swings and make you feel worse than before. Do preperiod days find you quaffing an extra cup of coffee to get out of the doldrums, or a glass of wine to alleviate anxiety? The first tactic can make you anxious, the second, depressed. The days before your period seem to be one time when your body gives you all the wrong messages for how to make it feel better.

PMS PERSONALITIES

Certain personality types are especially prone to PMS upsets.

- The **Nurturer** is already overworked and underpaid, and a case of PMS nasties can send you running to the Chips Ahoy as you stifle a scream at the kids.
- The **Artful Dodger** is expert at using the mysteries of the feminine hormonal cycle as an excuse to neglect your health and fitness goals.
- The **Blue Rose** should be sure to avert PMS sadness with a steady stream of serotonin snacks.
- The **Shooting Star** feels *everything*, including hormonal fluctuations, deeply. PMS sweeps through you like a tornado, leaving only chocolate bar wrappers in its wake.
- The **Lotus Eater** is highly pain-averse, and may turn to food and alcohol to wipe out premenstrual discomfort—only to end up feeling worse.
- The **Power Player** is under too much pressure to lose a minute to PMS—so you might "self-medicate" with bad snacks in the rush of a high-stress day.
- The **Dreamer** is a tender and vulnerable sort, and unexpected bad feelings upset your happy world and eating habits.

Since many women experience PMS differently, it's useful to know which nutritional treatments will match your symptoms. Experiment with these prescriptions to tame your hormonal upheaval.

No matter what your symptoms, follow your healthy eating plan with the following guidelines:

- Eat your complex carbohydrates without fat and separately from your protein. This will stimulate the neurotransmitter serotonin to smooth out mood swings and lift depression.
- Supplement yourself with vitamins B2, B6, and magnesium, all of which are likely to be deficient during this time. Some women also find that supple-

Personal Prescriptions for PMS	
Symptom	*Prescription*
Mood swings	■ Eliminate or reduce sugar.
	■ Emphasize complex carbohydrates.
	■ Take a magnesium supplement.
Anxiety and irritability	■ Eliminate or reduce sugar.
	■ Eliminate or reduce caffeine.
	■ Emphasize complex carbohydrates.
Depression, fatigue	■ Emphasize complex carbohydrates.
	■ Avoid alcohol.
Water retention, breast tenderness	■ Eliminate or reduce sodium.
	■ Eliminate or reduce caffeine.

ments of evening primrose oil alleviate PMS symptoms—take 4–6 capsules a day in the two weeks before your period, 1–3 capsules a day for the rest of the month.

■ Drink lots of water.
■ Exercise.

Like many ailments, the symptoms of PMS can be significantly reduced with a healthy lifestyle. If you suffer from severe PMS despite these practices, consult your doctor for alternate treatments.

PMS PICKS

What to pick up when you're hungry and your hormones are raging.	
YES (high carb, low salt and sugar):	*NO:*
✓ Bagel or bread, plain or with fruit-sweetened preserves	✓ Chocolate
✓ Baked potato	✓ Sugary sweets (including fat-free)
✓ Rice, pasta, grains, or legumes	✓ Coffee
✓ Unsalted baked tortilla chips with fat-free bean dip	✓ Tea
✓ Fruit-sweetened fat-free muffin, cookies, granola, or granola bar	✓ Alcohol
✓ Plain rice cake with fruit-sweetened preserves	✓ All the other fatty, unhealthy things you don't normally eat but might be tempted by now.
✓ Unsalted, unbuttered popcorn	

Maternity

Good nutrition is crucial to healthy babies and mothers. Most women know that no matter what, this is one time in your life that you have to eat right. As a result, many clients come to me to perfect their pregnancy, lactation, and postpartum weight loss diets—only to stay with the Diet Designs way of life once they realize that healthy eating enhances the quality of everyday life too. The same basic principles of good nutrition apply whether or not you're creating new life—but any new life deserves extra attention.

I'm happiest when a client with pregnancy plans comes to me before she even conceives. Women who are significantly overweight (35% over ideal weight) at conception are at increased risk for complications during and after pregnancy including gestational diabetes and high blood pressure. Furthermore, obesity can lead to infertility. The best way to make a healthy baby and a safe return to a fit physique yourself is to begin with a healthy body.

If you're fit when you conceive, you should expect to gain 25–35 pounds over the next nine months, eating about 300 extra calories a day and paying special attention to getting enough protein, vitamins, and minerals. The importance of eating and gaining weight in a controlled and nutritionally balanced plan are dramatized by the risks poor eating habits can present to your baby (see sidebar).

WHY EAT WELL FOR YOUR BABY?

Poor eating habits can increase your baby's risk of:

- Premature birth
- Low birth weight
- Low Apgar score
- Toxemia
- Neural tube defects
- Learning disabilities

It takes about 80,000 total extra calories to produce a baby. Ideally, those additional calories supply all the nutritional requirements outlined on the facing page. In practice, most obstetricians recommend supplements to insure adequate vitamin and mineral intake, with a diet emphasizing protein and calcium-rich foods.

Postpartum

The first cry I hear from most of my new mothers is "Give me back my body!" My first response is, take heart. Statistics indicate that the majority of mothers who gain the recommended weight (25–35 pounds) take off most or all of it within ten to eighteen months. With the focused effort and low-fat emphasis of the Diet Designs program, I have most of my clients back to their pre-

HOW TO EAT WELL FOR YOUR BABY

Nutrient:	Additional requirement:	Sources:
Protein To build the baby's tissues	**+66%** 74 g versus RDA of 44 g	Each of the following supplies about 15 grams of protein (1/5th of your daily requirement): ✓ 2 oz. of cooked poultry, lean meat, or seafood ✓ 1 c. cooked legumes ✓ ½ c. nonfat cottage cheese ✓ 2 c. nonfat yogurt ✓ ¾ c. cooked soybeans
Calcium For baby's bones and teeth, blood clotting, and muscle contracton, and to prevent hypertension in Mom	**+50%** 1,500 mg versus RDA of 1,000 mg	Each of the following supplies about 300 mg of calcium (1/5th of your daily requirement) ✓ 1 c. nonfat milk or yogurt ✓ 1 c. collard or turnip greens ✓ 3 oz. firm tofu ✓ 3 oz. canned salmon with bones
Iron To prevent anemia as your blood volume doubles	**+100–300%** 30–60 mg versus RDA of 15 mg	✓ Raisins, apricots, dried beans Because you absorb only a small percentage of the iron in foods, most doctors recommend a supplement
Folic acid To support the growth of the baby's nervous system	**+100–300%** 400–800 mcg versus RDA of 180 mcg	✓ Green leafy vegetables, broccoli, asparagus, brussels sprouts, orange juice, wheat germ Most doctors recommend a supplement of 400 mcg before and 800 mcg during pregnancy
Vitamin C	**+33%** 80 mg versus RDA of 60 mg	✓ Citrus fruits, strawberries, melon, tomatoes, peppers, cabbage
Vitamin A	**+25%** 5,000 IU versus RDA of 4,000 IU	✓ Milk, orange fruits and vegetables
Vitamin D	**+100%** 400 IU, versus RDA of 200 IU	✓ Fortified skim milk
Vitamin E	**+25%** 15 IU versus RDA of 12 IU	✓ Whole grains, wheat germ, sweet potatoes

pregnancy weight within four to eight months. But like all weight loss, your postpartum paring down should be gradual and controlled.

If you choose to breast-feed your baby, you must continue to exercise particular nutritional care. Though your body will produce nutritious milk for your baby, any deficiency in your diet will shortchange *you*. In addition to insuring adequate protein and calcium intake, you should avoid any food that aggravates the baby (see sidebar), continue with a vitamin and mineral supplement, and drink plenty of water. A nursing mother requires at least three quarts of fluids per day to keep her milk supply up; remember to drink at least eight ounces of milk or water every hour.

FOODS THAT MUDDLE MOM'S MILK

Some babies would prefer that you abstain from certain foods while breast-feeding. Every mom and baby is different; following are some frequent offenders:

- Gas-producing vegetables: broccoli, cauliflower, cabbage, brussels sprouts, onions.
- Acidic fruits and vegetables: tomatoes, citrus fruits.
- Chocolate.
- Caffeine.
- Excessive fruits or juices.
- Excessive sugars.

Nursing burns an extra 500–1,000 calories a day (40 calories per ounce of milk produced), so you generally need to eat up to 500 calories more than your usual daily intake—even higher than during pregnancy! On the Diet Designs program, I provide 1,800–2,500 calories to nursing mothers, depending upon body composition, for safe and controlled weight loss. Whether or not you are

POSTPARTUM PERSONALITIES

Some personality types face particular obstacles in taking off that baby weight.

- The **Nurturer** is often going on to another pregnancy before you have time to trim down. The cumulative effect of multiple pregnancies and the demands of caring for others tend to push weight loss down the list of priorities.
- Maternity weight has a way of permanently lodging on the **Artful Dodger.** Who has time to diet with this new person on the planet? And what did I do to deserve this?
- The **Shooting Star** can be so desperate to re-create your former glamorous self that you crash-diet—disastrous to your health and the energy levels you need for baby care.
- The **Dreamer** and the **Blue Rose** can get overwhelmed by the enormity of postpartum weight loss. Remember, you can lose it just as you gained it—gradually and joyfully.

breast-feeding, you should reduce your caloric intake gradually after giving birth.

For tips on feeding yourself and your family well, see Chapter 1, The Nurturer.

Menopause

As if puberty and maternity were not enough, women have to endure another major biological change with implications for their body composition and nutritional needs: menopause. The good news is that good behavior in your youth and middle age can lessen the undesirable effects of aging. A healthy, balanced diet and exercise program before menopause sets you up for healthier golden years and may actually delay the onset of menopause. And getting at least 1,000 milligrams of calcium a day, in foods and/or supplements, *from childhood onward*, reduces the risk of postmenopausal osteoporosis.

The most dramatic physiological change during menopause is that the body stops producing estrogen. This hormonal change has several threatening effects:

- Increased risk of heart disease—the number one killer of women—requiring increased attention to your fat intake (especially saturated fat), monitoring of your serum cholesterol levels, and a regular cardiovascular conditioning program. See the following section for what every woman should know about heart disease.
- Possible redistribution of body fat away from breasts and buttocks and toward the abdomen. Such fat distribution is also correlated with increased risk of heart disease.
- Increased risk of osteoporosis, a potentially debilitating weakening of the bones. Nearly 25% of women over age 65 suffer from spontaneous bone fractures. Postmenopausal women should get at least 1,200 milligrams of calcium a day (most people require a supplement to reach that level) and engage in weight-bearing exercise to maintain bone mass. You can also have a bone density analysis to determine your risk of osteoporosis.

Some women choose to counter these risks with estrogen replacement therapy, a somewhat controversial treatment linked with higher risk of breast, uterine, and endometrial cancer. You should discuss any treatment for menopause thoroughly with your doctor.

There might be a natural dietary alternative to hormone replacement. Recent research indicates that the phytoestrogens in soy products such as tofu, tempeh, and miso may provide an estrogen "lift" to alleviate menopausal hot flashes and mood swings without increasing the risk of breast cancer. In fact, phytoestrogens in the diet might actually *reduce* the risk of breast cancer in pre- and post-menopausal women. Asian countries with high soy intake have much lower breast cancer rates and fewer reported menopausal symptoms than in the U.S.

The other unfortunate side effect of menopause is a decrease in metabolic rate of up to 20%—requiring, in the absence of increased activity, a corresponding cut in caloric intake. However, a good deal of this metabolic slowdown is due to declining muscle mass, which you can prevent with strength-training exercise. The more muscle you have, the higher your resting metabolic rate. A consistent cardiovascular and strength training regimen will both boost your metabolism and burn extra calories. Combined with the beneficial effects of bone strengthening and prevention of heart disease, exercise is undeniably the single best thing you can do for your postmenopausal health.

PERSONALITIES AND THE PAUSE

- The **Nurturer** might see menopause as signaling the end of family life; you might have to go through some serious soul-searching to find your next role in life. Unfortunately, soul-searching and excess snacking can go together.
- The **Artful Dodger** perceives menopause as the final blow in a lifelong string of female disadvantages. But buck up—we're still living longer than men, especially when we eat right!
- The **Shooting Star** can be so traumatized at this reconfiguration of your sexual identity that you surrender all hope of physical beauty and let loose with food. But what about those statistics on heart disease?
- The **Perfectionist** can have a hard time readjusting portions to your decreased caloric needs. Time to start pumping iron and make a new Menopausal Meal Map!
- The **Lotus Eater** is likely to dull the uncomfortable sensations of menopause with substances, including food.

Feeding the Feminine Heart

The widespread myth that women don't have heart disease is untrue, dangerous, and loaded with the politics of gender. Rather than addressing the complex social roots of the myth here, I'd like to cut to the heart of the matter: Heart disease is the number one killer of women, and it is strongly correlated with obesity, hypertension, and high cholesterol levels—all associated with poor eating and exercise habits, and thus, all preventable to some degree. Here are the facts proving the imperative to feed the feminine heart with healthy, low-fat foods:

- About 1 in 30 women under age 45 suffer from some form of heart disease. The greatest risk factors among premenopausal women are:
  —Obesity. One study found that 40% of heart attacks in this group are directly or indirectly caused by obesity.

—Hypertension and high cholesterol levels, both directly related to diet. Women who have had more than 5 children tend to have lower HDL "good" cholesterol levels, increasing their risk of heart disease unless corrected with diet and exercise.

—Smoking.

—Family history.

- Women of any age who are 20–30% over their ideal weight increase their cardiac risk.
- Yo-yo dieters are at greater risk of heart attack than those who maintain a steady weight.
- Women who have premenopausal hysterectomies are three times more likely to develop heart disease.
- Within 10–15 years after menopause, a woman's risk of dying from a heart attack equals that of a man.

Despite the prevalence of female heart disease, research on appropriate treatment for women lags behind that for men. The medical profession is only now playing catch-up to test drugs, therapies, and hormone replacement on women. The jury remains out on the efficacy, safety, and side effects of many potential lifesavers in the female population—so in the meantime, protect your heart the way you know how, with a low-fat, low-sodium, high-fiber diet like Eating By Design and a regular exercise program. Feminine fitness is far more than a point of vanity. It's a matter of life itself.

Feeding the Feminine Future

At Diet Designs, I've watched women live through two decades of changing gender roles, leaving many of them confused about the role of dieting and weight management in their busy professional lives. I like to think that greater opportunity for women is whittling away at the bad reasons to diet—to please others, punish yourself, or become unnaturally thin—while making the health and longevity benefits of weight management all the more essential. As scientific evidence mounts on the relationship between diet and health, women have a tremendous advantage over men: We have been taught to watch what we eat. Women's challenge in the coming century is to be sure that we watch what we eat for all the right reasons—and that we teach our daughters to do likewise.

✳

Masculine Meals

Weight management is traditionally women's territory. Men aren't supposed to "diet"; they are supposed to be naturally hale and hearty, self-regulating, inhaling generous quantities of whatever they like, miraculously maintaining the trim fitness of youth.

The high incidence of heart disease, hypertension, and obesity in men reveals the essential untruth of this cultural myth. A recent study showed that of 19,000 Harvard graduates, the death rate of the heaviest men was two and a half times that of the leanest. Trained since birth to subscribe to the clean plate club and the "see food, eat food" diet, most male adults need to reassess their body's nutritional needs, and use portion control and low-fat foods to match intake with expenditure now that football is only a weekend activity. Men need to manage their weight just as much as women; they need a comprehensive, long-term eating plan like Eating By Design to keep their arteries clear and their weight loss permanent.

MASCULINE PLUSES AND PITFALLS

Pluses	Pitfalls
+ Men are naturally leaner than women.	− Hormonal balance, tendency to store fat in abdomen, and other factors put men at greater risk of heart disease than premenopausal women. Also at risk for prostate and colon cancer.
+ High metabolic rate, especially during youth and adolescence.	− Most men don't have to face the issue of weight management until after adult eating habits are well established.
+ Little social pressure regarding appearance.	− Little social support for weight management and healthy eating.
+ Able to lose weight fairly quickly.	− Tendency to lose too quickly and competitively, resulting in weight regain.
+ Generally not required to cook and provide food to others.	− Generally undereducated in basic nutrition and cooking techniques.
+ No-nonsense, sensible attitude toward food.	− Often expected to eat "macho" foods like red meat, skip fruits and vegetables, and drink lots of alcohol.

Competitive Dieting

Men in America are culturally conditioned to be competitive and goal-oriented in all their undertakings. Bruce, a Thrill-Seeker, was accustomed to removing extra pounds by the most extreme, goal-directed method there is: fasting. But he found he always put a few pounds back on as soon as he resumed eating.

The weight got harder and harder to take off, it always eventually came back, and deep down inside, he knew it couldn't be good for him.

I challenged Bruce to redirect his competitive urge to help him find the lowest-fat, highest-flavor versions of his favorite foods, engage in a comprehensive workout program, and watch the notches on his belt. Since men are most likely to store fat in the gut, you can easily gauge your progress by the fit of your pants or your belt. A small reduction there can make you feel a thousand pounds lighter.

And small reductions are the best goal for men to aim for—no more than one to two pounds a week. Faster weight loss will slow down your metabolism, which means you have to work extra hard to achieve the same results. And even a small weight reduction has big health payoffs, including lower blood pressure, cholesterol, and insulin levels, and reduced risk of heart disease, prostate and colon cancer, and gallbladder and gastrointestinal problems.

The single most important issue that my male clients face is what to do when they reach their weight loss goal. Many are inclined to tick "weight loss" off their to-do list and return to their former eating habits the minute they reach their goal. *Fait accompli* in the food department, you might say to yourself.

But if you annul your achievement by regaining your weight and returning to risky high-fat foods, you stand to be even less healthy than before the initial weight loss, have a harder time taking off the weight again, and face the bother of another bout of dieting. It's far more efficient and healthy to incorporate low-fat eating habits into your lifestyle. If you race to the dieting finish line too fast and too frequently, you might hasten your progress to the final finish line: death.

FIERCELY COMPETITIVE DIETERS

Perfectionists and **Power Players** are particularly prone to yo-yo dieting. Highly goal-oriented, you're likely to lose weight too fast, then move on to the next project with such concentration and force that you don't notice the encroaching return of body fat. Beware! With each cycle, your chance of losing the weight again decreases even as your risk of heart disease increases. You won't stay perfect or powerful for long if you compromise your health on the yo-yo track.

Manly Minerals

Certain minerals are particularly important to masculine health. Anyone who doesn't eat a carefully balanced, healthful diet is susceptible to mineral deficiency, and that includes a lot of men: fast-food junkies, meal skippers, hardcore meat-and-potatoes guys, prowlers of packages and cans—anyone who doesn't dine consistently on fresh, unprocessed, whole foods. The chart below shows compelling reasons to do so, or to take a balanced mineral supplement. By activating protein-based enzymes that run the body in various way, minerals make the man.

Mineral	Function	RDA	Food Sources
■ Zinc	Potency, fertility, sex drive, immunity. You lose zinc through manly activities such as sweating and ejaculation. The **Passionflower** especially needs his daily dose!	15 mg	Lean beef, turkey, oysters, cereals, beans.
■ Calcium	Seems to control high blood pressure, from which 1 in 4 men suffer. Also builds bones and maintains blood, muscles, and nerves. The **Power Player** particularly needs calcium's stress relief.	800 mg	Milk, canned salmon or sardines with bones, collard and turnip greens.
■ Chromium	Regulates blood sugar levels to help prevent those with diabetes indicators (3 million American men) from developing full-blown diabetes. Steady blood sugar helps to keep the **Lotus Eater** on track. And the **Power Player** likes evidence that chromium enhances fat metabolism—doesn't that sweeten the deal!	None; 50–200 mcg considered safe.	Fruits, vegetables, fish, chicken; most men need to supplement to reach 200 mcg.
■ Copper	Prevents heart disease (deficiency can raise cholesterol and blood pressure), and boosts immunity, which gives peace of mind to the **Yin-Yang.**	2–3 mg	Peas, beans, fruits, oysters and other shellfish.
■ Magnesium	Builds muscle tissue; prevents heart disease by dilating arteries and inhibiting blood clotting. The **Thrill-Seeker** and **Power Player** appreciate the enhanced strength gain magnesium gives to a workout.	350 mg	Spinach, bananas, seafood, meats.
■ Selenium	Fights free radicals to prevent skin, lung, and stomach cancer. The **Yin-Yang** is a big selenium subscriber.	70 mcg	Grains, fish, broccoli, cucumbers, onions, garlic, radishes, mushrooms.

A vitamin note: Along with these minerals and all the vitamins essential to a healthy diet, men should make an extra effort to get plenty of folic acid. This B vitamin currently prescribed to pregnant women to prevent birth defects also appears to prevent heart disease in men. A recent study of men with and without coronary disease found that high levels of folate in the bloodstream correlated with 60% less chance of heart disease. To take advantage of folate's fighting power, incorporate beans, lentils, spinach, wheat germ, citrus fruits, and asparagus into your diet.

Another important element of the male diet may be soy products. Evidence indicates that the phytoestrogens in soy may help block the growth of prostate tumors. Laboratory research is reinforced by demographic data: in Asia, where soy consumption is high, death from prostate cancer is rare. The average life expectancy of Japanese men is four to five years longer than men in the U.S. With prostate cancer the number two cancer killer of American men, a little tofu and tempeh might go a long way.

✳

Macho Menus: Meat and Malt

It seems that when men get to feeling like men, the meat gets red and the drink strong. There may be good reason for associating red meat and machismo: Beef is rich in zinc, the potency-boosting mineral, and magnesium, a muscle-builder. Our evolutionary subconscious might sense that meat's nutritional content helps make a man a real man.

Many men are raised with the message that meat is masculine, necessary to the cultivation of muscles, red blood, and a manly approach to life. To a certain extent, eating meat makes physiological sense. Its high protein content provides mental alertness, prolonged energy, and psychological satisfaction, along with performing all kinds of vital cellular functions. But red meat tends to come with a very high saturated-fat price tag attached, bringing bad LDL cholesterol and body fat along with its toothsome bite. Frequent and/or large-scale consumption of fatty meats simply has no place in a healthy diet.

Carl, a Shooting Star client, told me he couldn't imagine going out with the crew after finishing up a movie shoot without downing a couple of Scotches, a few beers, and a juicy sixteen-ounce steak. That's what they *did*, he said. This was no place to be asking for broiled fish and lemon, or pasta with an oil-free tomato sauce, or sparkling mineral water. Besides, said Carl, too many meals of pasta and salad made him feel kind of hollow and deprived, the very state that tended to send him to the fast-food drive-up.

Deprivation is high on my list of dietary errors, so I told Carl to try ordering the filet mignon and eating a piece no bigger than the palm of his hand, skipping the fried potatoes and limiting himself to one cocktail and one beer. Success! Carl went home feeling like a virtuous Iron John.

A bit of moderation and exploration of lower-fat meat options can keep meat in your menus. In addition to choosing the leanest cuts of beef, from the loin and the round, you now have the alternative of beef specially bred for low fat content. Another choice is the fascinating hybrid of three-eighths bison and five-eighths beef cow, producing beefalo. Both specially bred lean beef and beefalo have approximately the same nutritional profile as skinless chicken breast. And all game meats are naturally lean—running from the hunter's gun keeps these specimens fit and trim.

The Moderate Meat-Eater's Diet

Use these guidelines to regulate your meat-eating meals.
No more than once a month:
- Semilean cuts of beef: tenderloin (including filet mignon), top loin, and sirloin.
No more than once a week:
- Leaner cuts of beef: top round, eye of round, round tip.
Use interchangeably with poultry:
- Specially bred leanest beef (available in some supermarkets and by mail order from Covington Ranch, 800-365-2333).
- Beefalo.
- Game meats and birds: venison, ostrich, pheasant, quail, Cornish game hen.

Other meat-eating musts:
- Prime beef is prohibited!—it gets about half its calories from fat. Look for Select, the lowest-fat grade.
- Trim off all visible fat, and broil, grill, or roast without added fat.

As for washing down your lean meat with copious quantities of alcohol: In addition to endangering your liver and brain cells, there is evidence that alcohol may encourage you to store fat rather than burn it—and worse, it may contribute to the storage of abdominal fat, which is associated with increased risk of heart disease. A source of empty calories and mental haze, alcohol is not your ally in health. If you choose to drink, limit your drinks to 3–4 times a week and count each one as a snack.

The Carbohydrate Commitment

For some of my male clients accustomed to high-protein diets, the amount of carbohydrates called for in the Eating By Design program is something of a shock. "But bread (bagels, pasta, potatoes, etc.) makes you fat!" they protest. "It's filler food! It adds extra calories, but it won't make me *run!*" Speaking of running, **Thrill-Seeking** runners stoking up for a burst of activity often register this complaint as they reach for the steak.

My answer to this carb concern is, "*Au contraire,* Pierre." Carbohydrates are the most efficient source of energy, breaking down into glucose—immediate fuel—and glycogen, the energy stores in your muscles that power you through athletic activity. They also provide fiber, vitamins, and minerals, are virtually fat-free, and fill up your hungry stomach. And the **Blue Rose** knows that they release a medicinal burst of feel-good neurotransmitters. Carbohydrates are true power food. So dig into granola instead of bacon and eggs, or pasta instead of prime rib, and enjoy the health and energy benefits of continual carb loading. (Check the Eating By Design Mosaic for your daily carbohydrate quota.)

No matter what your machismo factor, eating well will give you an indispensable edge on present performance and long-term mortality. Weight management is definitely men's work.

❋

Though it may seem that the sexes speak d fferent languages when it comes to food, we do share most aspects of our physiology. We run fairly equal risks of excess body fat and diet-related disease from poor eating habits. We all need to eat healthful foods in proper portions on a regular basis. No matter what snags you encounter as you share meals across the gender line, keep this in mind: Don't let the battle between the sexes sabotage the battle with the bulge.

30

MASTER LISTS AND GUIDELINES

❋

Master Market List

Use this list to stock your healthy kitchen with the building blocks of the Eating By Design program. These are my name-brand choices; feel free to substitute other fat-free or lowfat products available in your local market.

DAIRY/FRESH FOOD

NONFAT MILK

NONFAT YOGURT

    FRUIT-SWEETENED (ALTA DENA EUROPEAN STYLE, MOUNTAIN HIGH, CONTINENTAL, BROWN COW)

    PLAIN (DANNON)

LOW-FAT BUTTERMILK

NONFAT OR LIGHT SOUR CREAM (KNUDSEN FREE, LAND-O-LAKES, REAL DAIRY)

FAT-FREE CHEESES (ALPINE LACE, LIFELINE, SONOMA, FRIGO, POLLY-O, HEALTHY CHOICE)

FAT-FREE SOY CHEESE (SOYA KAAS)

PART-SKIM MOZZARELLA CHEESE (GARDENA, PRECIOUS)

STRING CHEESE (GARDENA, CALIFORNIA GOLD, PRECIOUS)

NONFAT RICOTTA CHEESE (FRIGO, POLLY-O, PRECIOUS)

NONFAT OR LIGHT CREAM CHEESE (PHILADELPHIA, HEALTHY CHOICE)

NONFAT COTTAGE CHEESE (KNUDSEN FREE)

PARMESAN CHEESE

GOAT CHEESE

EGGS

FAT-FREE OR LIGHT TOFU

FAT-FREE FRESH MARINARA SAUCE (HUXTABLE'S)

FRESH SALSA

JELL-O OR SWISS MISS FAT-FREE PUDDING

LOW-FAT CRUMPETS (WOLFERMAN'S)

CORN AND WHOLE WHEAT TORTILLAS (MISSION)

336

BREADS/CEREALS

RICE, CORN, OR WHEAT CEREAL WITHOUT ADDED FAT OR SUGAR (SHREDDED WHEAT, GRAPE
    NUTS, HEALTH VALLEY FRUIT LITES, KASHI, PUFFED WHEAT, RICE, OR CORN, BACK TO
    NATURE BRAN FLAKES, GRAINFIELD'S)

FAT-FREE GRANOLA (HEALTH VALLEY)

HOT CEREALS: OATMEAL (PLAIN OR FLAVORED), CREAM OF WHEAT OR RICE, WHEATENA,
    MALT-O-MEAL, ROMAN MEAL ORIGINAL OR CREAM OF RYE, MOTHER'S WHOLE WHEAT)

FAT-FREE BAGELS OR BIALYS (INTERNATIONAL)

FAT-FREE OR LIGHT WHOLE GRAIN BREAD (OROWHEAT LIGHT, COUNTRY HEARTH,
    BROWNBERRY, PEPPERIDGE FARM, WEBER'S)

SOURDOUGH BREAD (PIONEER, WEBER'S)

SOURDOUGH OR WHOLE WHEAT BREAD CRUMBS

ENGLISH MUFFINS (SARA LEE, THOMAS')

FAT-FREE TOASTER PASTRIES (TOAST-N-JAMMERS)

GRAINS/LEGUMES/PASTAS

EGG- & OIL-FREE PASTA (DE CECCO, RONZONI, AMERICAN BEAUTY, NAPOLINA)

RICE—WHITE, BROWN, WILD, ARBORIO, BASMATI, JASMINE

BULGHUR

COUSCOUS

BARLEY

QUINOA

LENTILS

BEANS

LOW-FAT DRIED SOUPS, PASTA, RAMEN NOODLE, OR COUSCOUS CUPS (UNDER 200 CALORIES,
    3 G FAT, AND 550 MG SODIUM; FANTASTIC FOODS, NILE SPICE, SPICE HUNTER)

DRIED BEAN SOUP MIXES (AUNT PATSY'S PANTRY, JUST DELICIOUS GOURMET FOODS)

VEGETARIAN BURGER MIX (FANTASTIC FOODS NATURE'S BURGER)

CANNED GOODS

FAT-FREE SOUP (HEALTH VALLEY, PRITIKIN, PROGRESSO HEALTHY CLASSICS, BEARITOS,
    HEALTHY CHOICE, CAMPBELL'S HEALTHY REQUEST, ANDERSON'S NO-FAT)

FAT-FREE VEGETARIAN CHILI (HEALTH VALLEY)

LOW-FAT TURKEY CHILI

DEFATTED CANNED CHICKEN, BEEF, OR VEGETABLE BROTH

FAT-FREE BEANS: BLACK, KIDNEY, PINTO, GARBANZO, CANNELLINI (BEARITOS "REFRIED,"
    ROSARITA, S&W, PROGRESSO)

FAT-FREE PASTA SAUCE (HEALTH VALLEY, MILLINA'S FINEST, ENRICO'S, CI BELLA)

LOW-SODIUM TOMATO SAUCE (HUNT'S)

LOW-SODIUM CANNED TOMATOES (HUNT'S, POMI, CONTADINA)

LOW-SODIUM TOMATO PASTE (HUNT'S, CONTADINA)

EVAPORATED SKIM MILK (CARNATION, BORDEN LIGHT)

CLAM JUICE

WATER PACKED ALBACORE TUNA, SALMON, SARDINES (STARKIST, BUMBLE BEE, GEISHA)

WATER CHESTNUTS
ARTICHOKE HEARTS
HEARTS OF PALM
JALAPEÑO PEPPERS

BAKING STAPLES
UNBLEACHED ALL-PURPOSE FLOUR
WHOLE WHEAT PASTRY FLOUR
CORNMEAL
WHEAT GERM
BAKING POWDER
BAKING SODA
CORNSTARCH
ARROWROOT
GRANULATED SUGAR
BROWN SUGAR
MAPLE SUGAR
POWDERED FRUCTOSE
HONEY
MAPLE SYRUP
CORN SYRUP
COCOA POWDER
SHREDDED COCONUT
WALNUTS OR PINE NUTS
CHOCOLATE CHIPS (REGULAR OR MINI)
DRIED HERBS AND SPICES
PAUL PRUDHOMME'S POULTRY SEASONING
SEASONING BLENDS (MRS. DASH, NILE, SPICE ISLANDS SALT-FREE)
POPPYSEEDS
VANILLA EXTRACT
LEMON EXTRACT
SANS SUCRE MOUSSE
SUGAR-FREE JELL-O INSTANT PUDDING

CONDIMENTS/SAUCES
NATURAL PEANUT BUTTER (LAURA SCUDDER'S, HOLLYWOOD HAIN)
APPLE BUTTER (L & A, TAP & APPLE, KOZLOWSKI FARMS)
FAT-FREE FUDGE SAUCE (WAX ORCHARDS, SMUCKERS, MRS. RICHARDSON'S)
PURE FRUIT SYRUPS (WAX ORCHARDS, KNUDSEN'S, S&W)
FRUIT-SWEETENED JAM (SIMPLY FRUIT, SORREL RIDGE, DICKINSON'S)
FAT-FREE LOW-SODIUM BARBEQUE SAUCE (LEA & PERRINS)
LOW-SODIUM SOY SAUCE (KIKKOMAN, CHUN KING)
LOW-SODIUM WORCESTERSHIRE SAUCE (LEA & PERRINS)
HORSERADISH

HOT SAUCE (TABASCO)

CHILI SAUCE

KETCHUP (HUNT'S NO SALT)

VINEGARS: BALSAMIC, WINE, RICE, APPLE CIDER

MUSTARDS: DIJON, 3-GRAIN, HONEY, ETC.

FAT-FREE MAYONNAISE (KRAFT FREE, MIRACLE WHIP FREE, SMART BEAT)

SALAD DRESSINGS (FAT-FREE WITH LESS THAN 150 MG OF SODIUM PER 2-T. SERVING: WALDEN FARMS, PAULA'S NO-OIL, PRITIKIN FAT-FREE, WEIGHT WATCHERS, HAINS)

OLIVE OIL

SESAME OIL

VEGETABLE COOKING SPRAY (CORN, CANOLA, OR OLIVE OIL)

SHERRY AND COOKING WINE

SUNDRIED TOMATOES (NOT PACKED IN OIL)

BLACK OLIVES

CAPERS

POULTRY/MEATS/SEAFOOD

GROUND TURKEY BREAST

WHOLE TURKEY BREAST

GROUND CHICKEN BREAST

SKINLESS CHICKEN BREAST

FRESH SEAFOOD: WHITE FISH, SALMON, SWORDFISH, TUNA, SHRIMP, SCALLOPS, CRAB, ETC.

LEAN BEEF: TENDERLOIN, TOP LOIN, SIRLOIN, TOP ROUND, EYE OF ROUND, OR ROUND TIP

BEVERAGES

SPRING WATER (ANY BRAND)

SPARKLING MINERAL WATER WITHOUT FRUIT JUICE OR SODIUM

DECAFFEINATED OR HERBAL TEA (PARADISE, CELESTIAL SEASONINGS, STASH, GOOD EARTH, BIGELOW, LIPTON)

SUGAR-FREE COCOA MIX (SWISS MISS, CARNATION)

POSTUM

SOY BEVERAGE (WEST SOY LITE, VITA SOY, EDEN SOY)

FROZEN

LOW-FAT OR FAT-FREE WAFFLES (NUTRIGRAIN, VAN'S, SPECIAL K, DOWNEYFLAKE CRISP AND HEALTHY)

NONFAT EGG SUBSTITUTE (EGG BEATERS, BETTER 'N EGGS)

LOW-FAT ENTREES AND PIZZAS (NO MORE THAN 400 CALORIES, 10 GRAMS OF FAT, 15 GRAMS OF SUGAR, AND 550 MG OF SODIUM PER SERVING; NO HYDROGENATED, COTTONSEED, COCONUT, OR PALM OILS: JACKLYN'S, AMY'S, SHELTON FARMS, HEALTHY CHOICE, WEIGHT WATCHERS SMART ONES)

VEGETARIAN BURGERS (NO MORE THAN 250 CALORIES AND 3 GRAMS FAT APIECE: MORNINGSTAR FARMS MEATLESS GARDEN VEGE PATTIES, GREEN GIANT HARVEST BURGERS)

FROZEN JUICE CONCENTRATES
FROZEN VEGETABLES AND FRUITS
FROZEN FRUIT BARS (FRUIT A FREEZE, DOLE)
FROZEN YOGURT BARS (HAAGEN DAZS, STARBURST)
NONFAT FROZEN YOGURT OR ICE CREAM (DREYER'S, DANNON)
FUDGESICLES (REGULAR OR SUGAR-FREE)
FRESH FRUIT SORBET
COOL WHIP LITE
FROZEN RICE DREAM

PRODUCE
FRESH FRUITS
FRESH VEGETABLES
FRESH FRUIT JUICES
FRESH LEMON JUICE
LETTUCE AND SALAD GREENS (READYPAK)
POTATOES—BAKING, BOILING, SWEET
GARLIC, ONIONS, SHALLOTS, GINGER
FRESH HERBS

SNACKS
FAT-FREE PRETZELS (AUNT BARBARA'S WHOLE WHEAT MINIS, EAGLE, KEEBLER PRETZEL
    KNOTS, SNYDER'S SOURDOUGH, ZAIDY'S)
LIGHT CHEESE PUFFS (AUNT BARBARA'S, HEALTH VALLEY CHEDDAR LITES)
RICE CAKES, MINI OR REGULAR (QUAKER, CHICO SAN, HAINS)
FAT-FREE CHIPS:
    POLENTA CHIPS (AMERICAN GRAIN)
    RISOTTO CHIPS
    POTATO CHIPS (AMERICAN GRAIN POPSTERS, LOUISE'S)
    PASTA CHIPS
    BAGEL CHIPS (BURNS & RICKER)
    BAKED TORTILLA CHIPS (GUILTLESS GOURMET)
    APPLE CHIPS (TREE TOP)
    "NO FRIES" (PACIFIC GRAIN)
FAT-FREE PARTY MIX (BURNS & RICKER)
FAT-FREE CRACKERS (SNACKWELLS, HEALTH VALLEY, RYE CRISPS, MELBA TOAST, WASA
    CRISPBREAD, DEVONSHEER MELBA ROUNDS, VENUS, FINN CRISP, AUBURN FARMS,
    HEALTH VALLEY, ZESTA FAT-FREE SALTINES, AK MAK SESAME, MATZO)
BROWN RICE SNAPS (EDWARD & SONS)
FAT-FREE BEAN DIPS (GUILTLESS GOURMET, SAGUARO)
LOW-FAT POPCORN (ORVILLE REDENBOCKER SMARTPOP, POP SECRET)
FAT-FREE CARAMEL CORN (LOUISE'S)
FAT-FREE GRANOLA BARS (HEALTH VALLEY, AUNT BARBARA'S, QUAKER)
LOW-FAT GRANOLA BARS (KELLOGG'S, QUAKER CHEWY, FIBAR BERRY BEST)

FAT-FREE BREAKFAST BARS (HEALTH VALLEY, FAMOUS AMOS)
GRAHAM CRACKERS (SUNSHINE, NABISCO, HEALTH VALLEY, KEEBLER GRAHAM SELECTS LOWFAT)
FAT-FREE OR LOW-FAT COOKIES (HEALTH VALLEY, BAKERY WAGON FRUIT COBBLER, WEIGHT WATCHER'S SMART SNACKERS, STELLA D'ORO BREAKFAST TREATS, FROOKIES' FRUITINS, SUNSHINE OH! BERRY, KEEBLER ELFIN DELIGHTS DEVIL'S FOOD, BARBARA'S, SNACKWELL'S)
FAT-FREE FIG NEWTONS (NABISCO, MOTHER'S)
GINGER SNAPS (NABISCO)
ANIMAL CRACKERS
TEA BISCUITS
VANILLA WAFERS (SUNSHINE, NABISCO)
BISCOTTI (NO NUTS OR CHOCOLATE COATING)
SOKEN FRUCTOSE-SWEETENED HARD CANDIES
DRIED FRUIT (RAISINS, APRICOTS, PITTED DATES, CRANBERRIES, CHERRIES, PEARS)
FRUIT LEATHER
TURKEY JERKY (SNACK MASTER'S)

※

Master Snack List

I am strictly pro-snack. It's a healthy habit that boosts your energy, gets you to your next meal, and gives you another opportunity to eat fun, nutritious food. Snacks give the **Nurturer** energy for one more round of carpooling. They give the **Artful Dodger** a chance for fun that feels like a cheat. They de-stress the **Power Player** and cheer the **Blue Rose. Lotus Eaters** use snacks to stay satisfied, **Dreamers** and **Shooting Stars** for sweet treats, **Thrill-Seekers** for rocket fuel, **Perfectionists** as a regularly scheduled treat.

Your Personal Prescription makes snack and dessert recommendations that work for your food personality type, but all the following options fit Eating By Design principles. You can choose from them whenever your meal plan calls for a snack or dessert. Remember to count each snack as a serving from the appropriate group of the Eating By Design Mosaic.

The Master Market List gives brand-name suggestions. When selecting other brands, look for snacks that are approximately 100 calories and less than 3 grams of fat per serving.

Complex Carbohydrate Group
1 serving from the Eating By Design Mosaic
10 mini flavored rice cakes
1 large rice cake with 1 T. nonfat ricotta or cream cheese and 1 t. fruit preserves
2 graham crackers

4 c. unbuttered air- or microwave-popped popcorn
1 oz. fat-free potato chips
1 oz. baked tortilla chips
1 oz. fat-free bagel, pita, pasta, or risotto chips
1 oz. fat-free party mix
1 oz. brown rice snaps
1 oz. fat-free bean dip with ½ oz baked tortilla chips or vegetables
1 oz. fat-free pretzels or 1 large
1 oz. fat-free crackers
1 oz. baked cheese or corn puffs
1 low-fat or fat-free granola bar
½ c. fat-free granola
1 oz. (2 medium) low-fat or fat-free cookies (includes biscotti, tea biscuits, vanilla wafers, ginger snaps, animal crackers, or any cookie labeled low-fat or fat-free)
10 Snackwells mini cookies
1 small fat-free muffin
½ bagel or bialy with 1 T. nonfat cream or ricotta cheese or 2 t. fruit preserves
1 cup fat-free or low-fat soup
½ cup low-fat grain, legume, or pasta cup-of-soup
4 oz. red or white wine or light beer
1 frozen fruit bar
1 Fudgesicle
½ c. fruit sorbet

Vegetable Group
FREE SNACKS! Dip them in salsa or fat-free dressing if you like (check the Extras Group for dressing limits).

Fruit Group
1 serving from the Eating By Design Mosaic
1 oz. dried fruit or fruit leather
1 c. pure fruit juice

Dairy Group
1 serving from the Eating By Design Mosaic
½ c. fruit-sweetened nonfat yogurt with 2 T. fat-free granola
½ c. frozen nonfat yogurt with 2 t. fat-free fudge sauce or fruit syrup
1 frozen yogurt bar
4 oz. fat-free pudding
1½ oz. nonfat or 1 oz. low-fat cheese
1 cappuccino or latte with nonfat milk, hot or blended frozen (no yogurt or ice cream)

✳

Restaurant Guidelines

Eating By Design doesn't end at your own front door. You take your eating style with you everywhere you go. Here are some pointers on making your Personal Prescription mobile.

These tips are useful for all personality types, but they will be particularly helpful for the frequent restaurant habits of **Power Players** and **Passionflowers.** Bon appétit!

- Start with uncreamed soup, or salad with fat-free dressing, or half of an appetizer.
- Bring your own homemade fat-free salad dressing, or ask the kitchen to mix you one from balsamic vinegar, Dijon mustard, lemon juice, and black pepper.
- Remove the bread basket from the table.
- Order everything without butter, oil, or cream. Specify your restrictions with every order, and remember:
  - ✓ No cream-based soups or sauces.
  - ✓ No fried food.
  - ✓ No added butter or oil at the table.
- Eat half an entree. Share with a companion, or send the rest back to the kitchen.
- Order seafood, skinless white meat poultry, pork tenderloin, and lean cuts of steak including top sirloin, tenderloin, round, or flank. Smother with grilled onions and mushrooms (no oil) for added flavor.
- Ask the kitchen to top your pasta with an oil-free sauce of tomato, basil, and garlic, or any other sauce they can prepare without oil. Watch your pasta portion!—ask for an appetizer-sized serving.
- Order pizzas without cheese or with a light topping of part-skim mozzarella. Share individual pizzas with a friend.
- Remember to balance your order with your EQ—for instance, you probably don't need a protein dish for both appetizer and entree.
- Request all the condiments you need: mustard, Tabasco, lemon, vinegar, herbs, garlic, low-sodium soy sauce.
- If you choose to have a glass of wine or beer, limit it to one and count it as a snack.
- Finish with a cappuccino or mixed berries and count either as a snack.

✳

Fast Food Guidelines

These tips on dining in the fast lane are indispensable for **Nurturers, Shooting Stars, Thrill-Seekers, Soloists,** and **Artful Dodgers.** Many other personality styles will find themselves needing fast fuel from time to time. **Yin-Yangs** and **Lotus Eaters** don't like to compromise their inner purity with fast food; try baked potatoes and salads for a reasonably clean compromise.

Use the following guidelines to translate your fast food order into the Eating By Design Proportions:

Cereal or muffin	= 1 serving from the Complex Carbohydrate Group
Small sandwich, burger, or 2 tacos	= 2 servings from the Complex Carbohydrate Group and 1 serving from the Protein Group
Entree salad with fat-free dressing	= 1 serving from the Vegetable Group and 1 serving from the Protein Group
Side salad with fat-free dressing	= 1 serving from the Vegetable Group
Baked potato	= 2 servings from the Complex Carbohydrate Group
Frozen nonfat yogurt	= 1 snack from the Dairy Group

✓ Order skim milk with your breakfast cereal.
✓ Choose fat-free muffins.
✓ Burgers may be turkey, chicken, vegetarian, or low-fat beef.
✓ Order skinless breast meat chicken; remove the skin yourself if necessary.
✓ Order all dishes without cheese or cheese sauce.
✓ Top sandwiches or burgers with lettuce, tomato, onion, and mustard. No mayonnaise or Secret Sauce!
✓ Order Mexican dishes without sour cream or guacamole. Choose soft (not fried) corn tortillas instead of flour. Use as much salsa as you like.
✓ Top salads and baked potatoes with salsa, fat-free dressing, or vinegar with mustard.
✓ Look for fat-free frozen yogurt with 15–18 calories per ounce. Have a 4-ounce serving with 2 t. fat-free syrup or 2 T. fresh fruit or granola.

Order from the following "redesigned" fast food menus:

Arby's

LUNCH OR DINNER

Choose from:
Baked Potato
Chicken Fajita Pita
Grilled Chicken Barbeque
Chef Salad with Turkey
Roast Chicken Salad

SIDES
Choose one of the following to accompany any entree:
Garden Salad
Small Soup:
Beef and Vegetable
Mixed Vegetable
Chicken Noodle
Tomato Florentine

✳

Burger King

LUNCH OR DINNER
Choose from:
Chef Salad with Turkey
BK Broiler Chicken Sandwich

✳

Carl's Jr.

BREAKFAST
Choose from:
English Muffin with Jam and Small Orange Juice
Bran Muffin and Small Orange Juice

LUNCH OR DINNER
Choose from:
Charbroiler BBQ Chicken Sandwich
Lite Baked Potato

SIDES
May accompany lunch or dinner entree:
Garden Salad

✳

Hardee's

BREAKFAST
3 Pancakes with Jam (no syrup) and Small Orange Juice

LUNCH OR DINNER
Choose from:
Chicken Filet
Grilled Chicken Sandwich
Chef Salad with Turkey
Chicken Fiesta Salad

✳

Kentucky Fried Chicken

LUNCH OR DINNER
Colonel's Rotisserie Gold

SIDES
Choose one of the following to accompany any entree:
Baked Beans
Corn on the Cob (no butter)
Mashed Potatoes (no gravy)

✳

Long John Silver's

LUNCH OR DINNER
Choose from:
Light Portion Baked Fish (Paprika or Lemon Crumb) with Rice Pilaf and
Salad
Baked Chicken Sandwich (no sauce)
Chicken Plank
Seafood Salad

✳

McDonald's

BREAKFAST
Choose from:
Apple Bran Muffin and Small Juice
Blueberry Muffin and Small Juice
Cheerios with ½ cup Skim Milk and Small Juice
Wheaties with ½ cup Skim Milk and Small Juice

LUNCH OR DINNER
Choose from:
Chunky Chicken Salad
Chef Salad with Turkey
Chicken Fajitas
Grilled Chicken Breast Sandwich
McLean Deluxe

SIDES

Choose one of the following to accompany any entree:
Garden Salad
Low-Fat Frozen Yogurt
Orange Sorbet

✳

Pizza Hut

LUNCH OR DINNER
1 Slice Thin 'n Crispy Cheese Pizza

SIDES

May accompany pizza:
Mixed Green Salad

✳

Subway

LUNCH OR DINNER
Choose from:
Small Turkey Sandwich
Chef Salad with Turkey

SIDES

May accompany sandwich:
Garden Salad

✳

Taco Bell

LUNCH OR DINNER
Choose from:
Border Light Taco
Burrito
Taco Salad

✳

Wendy's

LUNCH OR DINNER
Choose from:
Chef Salad with Turkey
Grilled Chicken Sandwich
Baked Potato with Broccoli (no cheese sauce)

SIDES
Choose one of the following to accompany any entree:
Garden Salad
Applesauce
Honeydew Melon
Pineapple Chunks
Strawberries

✳

National Restaurant Chains

National restaurant chains offer a little more variety and relaxation than fast food outlets, and often make convenient dining options for **Soloists** and for **Nurturers** with their families. Remember to follow the restaurant guidelines in placing your order, account for your meal in your EQ, and always watch your portions!

✳

Coco's

STARTER
Choose from:
Soup of the Day (uncreamed)
Green Garden Salad (no croutons)

LUNCH/DINNER
Choose from:
Fresh Steamed Vegetable Plate
Vegetable Omelette with Eggstraordinaire
Fresh Fish
Stir-Fry Chicken
Thai Chicken Salad (no peanuts)
Oriental Chicken Salad (no wontons)
Turkey Sandwich (no bacon)
Albacore Tuna Salad
Honey Dijon Chicken
Teriyaki Chicken

DESSERTS
Choose from:
Mixed Berries or Fruit
Cappuccino with Skim Milk

✳

El Torito

ENTREES

Choose from:

Sizzling Chicken Fajitas Salad (no avocado, cheese)
Grilled Chicken Soft Tacos (no guacamole)
Vegetable Enchiladas (no cheese, cream)
Vegetable Fajitas (no guacamole)
Vegetable Enchiladas

DESSERTS

Choose from:

Mixed Berries or Fruit
Cappuccino with Skim Milk

✳

Houston's

STARTERS

Choose from:

Field Greens
Soup of the Day (uncreamed)

ENTREES

Choose from:

Biltmore Special (no cheese, mayonnaise)
Turkey Burger
Grilled Chicken Salad (dressing on the side)
Pizza Marguerita (½ as entree)
Pizza Caponata (½ as entree)
Sashimi Tuna Salad
Fish of the Day with Couscous
Roasted Chicken with Couscous
Barbeque Chicken with Couscous
Baked Potato with Salsa or Fat-Free Salad Dressing

DESSERTS

Choose from:

Mixed Berries or Fruit
Cappuccino with Skim Milk

*

TGIF

STARTERS

Choose from:

Soup of the Day (uncreamed)

Peel and Eat Shrimp

Friday's House Salad (no garlic bread)

LUNCH/DINNER

Choose from:

Soup (uncreamed) and Sandwich

Fresh Vegetable Medley (no cheese, garlic bread)

Grilled Chicken Caesar

Friday's Thai Chicken Salad (no Chinese noodles)

Chinese Chicken Salad (no Chinese noodles)

Fresh Vegetable Baguette

Pacific Coast Tuna

Pacific Coast Chicken

Friday's Garden Burger

California Charbroiled Turkey (no avocado)

Charbroiled Chicken (no butter, mayonnaise)

Chicken Fajitas (no guacamole, sour cream)

Broken Noodles (no mozzarella)

Herb Grilled Chicken

Fish of the Day

DESSERTS

Choose from:

Mixed Berries or Fruit

Cappuccino with Skim Milk

*

31

MOVING BY DESIGN: Master Exercise Plan

Now that you know everything there is to know about fueling your body, let's talk about burning that fuel off. Exercise is eating's natural partner in health and weight management; it burns fat and calories, conditions your cardiovascular system, and boosts your metabolism. A regular exercise program is a crucial complement to Eating By Design, balancing the metabolic equation in your favor. Exercise makes your body work, at any level and any age.

✳

The Exercise Equation

Exercise in the Health Equation

In addition to its power against obesity and related diseases, a regular exercise program protects against killer illnesses by lowering serum cholesterol and blood pressure, conditioning the heart muscle, enhancing the body's ability to dissolve blood clots, and boosting the immune system. Other rewards of an active lifestyle include:

✓ Muscle tone, strength, and flexibility.
✓ Stronger bones with higher calcium content, reducing the risk of osteoporosis.
✓ Reduced stress and anxiety.
✓ Enhanced relaxation ability.
✓ Increased energy and self-esteem.
✓ Decreased hunger.
✓ Enjoyable diversion for body and mind.

351

Exercise in the Metabolic Equation

Exercise burns calories for as long and hard as you work out, and it raises your resting metabolic rate, so that after a vigorous workout, you expend more energy even sitting still. This metabolic boost is particularly important if you're trying to lose body fat by cutting calories. Increased activity will both burn fat and help convince your metabolism not to slow down to low-fuel starvation mode.

How effective is exercise in encouraging weight loss? Consider this: A daily half-hour jog (about 300 calories expended) can burn 30 pounds of body fat in one year. Add strength training to increase your proportion of metabolically active tissue, and your healthy eating efforts are doubly enhanced.

Once you lose body fat, exercise is crucial to maintenance. Surprisingly, there is a better than one-to-one calorie relationship between exercise and weight maintenance. Some evidence suggests that the psychological benefits of exercise help maintainers stick to their healthy eating plan.

✳

Prescription for a Fit Physique

The basic components of fitness are simple and common to every body. My prescription provides a framework to allow you to work at your own level and progress toward a perfectly fit physique.

A complete workout program should improve and maintain your fitness level in four basic areas:

1. Cardiovascular efficiency and endurance.
2. Muscular strength and endurance.
3. Flexibility.
4. Body composition.

If you're embarking on exercise for the first time or beginning from a low level of fitness, remember that anything is better than nothing. A brief walk is better than sitting still. Jogging, aerobics, or jumping rope can be interspersed with walking or strength training to give you a chance to catch your breath. A leisurely swim might feel like pure relaxation, but it burns calories, strengthens your muscles, and conditions your heart nevertheless.

Just as you need to tailor your caloric intake to your body's needs, it's important that you exercise at your own level of fitness. To estimate your fitness level, refer to the Activity Level you calculated to determine your Eating Quotient in Chapter 13. Use that number to choose a workout level on the facing page.

Your Activity Level (from EQ quiz):	Your Workout Level for Weight Loss or Progressive Training Benefits:
1–2	Level 1, Beginner
3	Level 2, Intermediate
4	Level 3 or 4, Advanced or Maintenance

You should aim to progress upward through the levels as you master them, to either the Advanced or Maintenance Level. The Advanced workout will take you into the upper echelon of fitness and conditioning. If this kind of commitment to training is out of step with your lifestyle or fitness goals, you can proceed directly from the Intermediate to the Maintenance workout. **Thrill-Seekers, Power Players,** and **Perfectionists** will probably jump at the Advanced challenge. **Nurturers, Shooting Stars,** and **Artful Dodgers** might be happy to manage Maintenance-level work.

Note that at every level, the frequency of your workout determines its effect in providing training benefits and stimulating weight loss. Use these guidelines to determine the frequency of your workout:

- **3 times a week** is the minimum frequency required for training results and maintenance of a fit body.
- **4–5 times a week** is optimal for accelerating weight loss and achieving significant training results. For the most efficient weight loss, opt for five times per week, focusing on aerobic training for two of those sessions.
- **More than 5 times a week** is not recommended for intensive workout sessions; your body needs some time to rest and repair muscle tissues. But there's nothing wrong with being active every day of the week. In fact, daily activity is the healthiest way to live. Use your days off to walk, bike, swim, garden, or play sports. Any extra activity will burn calories and boost your metabolism!

CALCULATING YOUR TARGET HEART RATE

Take your heart rate by finding your pulse, either on the side of your neck below your jawbone or on your wrist below the base of your thumb. Count the beats for 15 seconds, then multiply this number by 4 for your "beats per minute" (BPM). Use your resting heart rate in the calculations below.

Resting heart rate
You need to exceed this rate
to realize training benefits.

Your resting pulse   = ___BPM

Maximum heart rate
You should never exceed this
rate while training.

220 − (your age) ___   = ___BPM

Target training rate
See the workout plan for your
fitness level for the percentage of your
capacity at which you should work.

Maximum heart rate ___ × Target % ___   = ___BPM

Heart rate range
Generally, the more fit you are,
the wider this range will be.

Maximum heart rate ___ − resting heart rate ___   = ___BPM

For instance, if you are 30 years old with a resting heart rate of 80 beats per minute and want to work out at 60% of your capacity, your calculations would be as follows:

Maximum heart rate   220 − 30   = 190 BPM
Target training rate at 60%   190 × .60 = 114 BPM
Heart rate range   190 − 80   = 110 BPM

You should check your heart rate periodically during exercise to make sure you're below your maximum and close to your target training rate.

Master Exercise Program

	Activity	Duration	Intensity*
LEVEL 1	Warm-up	10 minutes	30–50% of max
BEGINNER	Aerobics	20 minutes	55–65% of max
1 hour	Strength training	20 minutes	—
	Cool-down and flexibility	10 minutes	30–50% of max to resting
LEVEL 2	Warm-up	10 minutes	30–50% of max
INTERMEDIATE	Aerobics	30–40 minutes	65–70% of max
1 hour 10 minutes to 1½ hours	Strength training	20–30 minutes	—
	Cool-down and flexibility	10 minutes	30–50% of max to resting

*The percentages in this column refer to your maximum heart rate; see the sidebar Calculating Your Target Heart Rate for instructions on measuring the intensity of your workout.

LEVEL 3	Warm-up	10 minutes	30–50% of max
ADVANCED	Aerobics	40–60 minutes	70–85% of max
1½ to 2 hours	Strength training	30–40 minutes	—
	Cool-down and flexibility	10 minutes	30–50% of max to resting
LEVEL 4	Warm-up	10 minutes	30–50% of max
MAINTENANCE	Aerobics	30 minutes	60–85% of max
1 hour 10 minutes to 1 hour 20 minutes	Strength training	20–30 minutes	—
	Cool-down and flexibility	10 minutes	30–50% of max to resting

BURNING BODY FAT

Your body burns a greater percentage of calories from body fat during moderate than intense aerobic activity. A brisk walk at 60–70% of your maximum heart rate, for instance, will draw 70% of its calories from fat, versus the 60% from fat used by jogging at 75–85% of your maximum. The remaining calories come from glycogen, the temporary carbohydrate stores in your muscles that either get burned by your metabolism or stored as body fat.

But because intense aerobics burn more calories overall than moderate activity, you're still likely to burn more body fat in an intense than a moderate aerobic workout—along with the muffin you had for breakfast, now lurking in your glycogen stores wondering whether it will be burned when you hit the health club tonight, or laid down as fat when you hit the couch instead. That walk will burn 280 fat calories and 120 glycogen calories in an hour; the jog eats up 300 fat calories and 200 glycogen calories in just 45 minutes. Better for busy schedules!

When is intense aerobic exercise *not* recommended for burning body fat?

1. If your cardiovascular fitness level is insufficient to safely stress the heart at peak levels, or
2. If your physical or mental condition is such that you'll happily walk for an hour, but give up after fifteen minutes of jogging.

In either of these cases, go for more moderate activities on a regular basis. The fat will eventually surrender to fitness.

Ways to Work Out

What makes a workout? Any activity that works or stretches your heart or other muscles. Here's a collection of some of the most effective ways to work out, classified by activity type. Use the suggestions here and in your Personal Prescription to choose the movement forms that work for you.

Aerobic	Strength	Flexibility
Jogging	Floor exercises	Stretching
Power walking or hiking	Free weights	Yoga
Aerobics	Nautilus or other weight	Dance exercises
Step aerobics	machines	T'ai chi
StairMaster or stepper	Rubber bands	
Treadmill	Boxing	
Bicycling	Martial arts	
Stationary bicycling or		
spinning		
Swimming		
Skiing or ski machine		
Rollerblading		
Rowing or rowing machine		
Aerobic boxing		

Personality and Physique

Like an eating plan, the best way to stick to a workout program is to tailor it to your personality type. Here are some general tips:

- **Nurturer:** Aim to work out three times a week, while the kids are in school. Emphasize aerobics to get maximum fat-burning benefits in the limited time you have to yourself.
- **Shooting Star:** Find exercise everywhere you go. Walk to the party, go dancing instead of out to dinner, and make sure you're donning your spandex at least three times a week.
- **Dreamer:** Think of exercise as a fun hobby. Whether it's swimming, walking, or a home video, make it a special time for yourself that you look forward to, three times weekly or more.
- **Power Player:** Start every day with the surge of adrenaline that exercise brings. You burn more fat by working out on an empty stomach and set the stage for power performance all day long. Emphasize cardiovascular activities and aim to work out every workday for stress control.
- **Blue Rose:** Less is more than nothing! Do something every other day, no matter how small.

- **Perfectionist:** Pick a workout time and stick to it every day, with one day off a week. Rotate systematically between aerobic, strength, and flexibility training. Once you find a pattern you like, settle in.
- **Lotus Eater:** Get hooked on the healthy habit of daily exercise. Make sure you vary your activities for cross-training, and never overwork any single part of your body.
- **Yin-Yang:** Explore low-impact, meditative forms of exercise, like yoga and t'ai chi, which can be done every day. But don't neglect aerobics; your heart needs a workout at least three times a week.
- **Soloist:** Make your workout a low-stress time by picking off-hours at the health club or on the jogging trail. If you're prone to nighttime eating, try an evening exercise program.
- **Thrill-Seeker:** Keep up your workout routine no matter how hectic your schedule. If you're on the go, pack a jump rope and rubber bands; use hotel gyms; and schedule physical adventures into your travels.
- **Artful Dodger:** Use excuse-busters like hiring a personal trainer, making dates for biking or tennis, or exercising at the same time every day. Start each session with a "just do it" mentality—the first ten minutes are always the worst.
- **Passionflower:** You need lots of fat-burning to counter your food-loving ways. Consider taking up marathon running, or at least a daily aerobic workout. It feels so good!

Whatever activities you choose for your workout program, be sure to vary them to prevent burnout and insure all-around conditioning. Change your routines consistently, at least every few months and as often as every few weeks. For maximum flexibility in your workouts and your muscles, cross-train by varying your activities every time you exercise. Use the treadmill one day, the bicycle the next, and a jog on the beach or in the park on the third day. Use the tips in your Personal Prescription to individualize your workouts, and enjoy the experience of letting your body do what it was designed for: MOVE!

Exercising Through Weight Loss Plateaus

Plateaus are a frustrating but very natural hitch in the weight loss process, generally caused by your body trying to "hold on" to its current shape by slowing down your metabolism. Cutting calories further can send even more threatening messages of impending starvation to your body and leave you stuck even more firmly on your plateau. Your best bet for jumping off to a new level of fat burning is exercise.

Exercise stimulates your entire fat burning machinery, reassuring your metabolism that it's okay to convert those stubborn body fat deposits to energy.

It's the only way your mind can tell your body that you know what you're doing, and starvation doesn't wait just around the bend. It mobilizes your inner ability to alter your body composition for the better.

If you hit a weight loss plateau, add an exercise session to your week, or extend each of your aerobic workouts by fifteen minutes. Movement is the completely organic way to put mind over matter and press ahead toward fitness.

Recalculating Your EQ to Account for Exercise

Because activity level is an important component of your Eating Quotient, you may need to recalculate your EQ if you dramatically change your workout lifestyle.

I hope that you enthusiastically embrace this exercise program to speed your progress in the Eating By Design program and enhance your overall health. Every calorie you expend in your workouts tips your metabolic equation toward fat loss. If you're working out much more intensely and frequently than before beginning the Eating By Design program (remember to go gradually!), your caloric needs might be higher than they were when you calculated your EQ. Retake the quiz to properly align your caloric input with your increased output.

Conversely, if a busy schedule, illness, or injury interferes with your normal workout schedule, you might need to recalculate your EQ to account for decreased output.

You can retake the EQ quiz any time you feel uncertain that your calories match your fitness goals. Your EQ is a dynamic tool to make the metabolic equation work for *you*.

THE DIET
DESIGNS KITCHEN

The Diet Designs kitchen has always been a warm and welcoming place of heady aromas and intense low-fat flavors. Even now that my food is prepared by a professional staff in a commercial kitchen, the room is always full of the smell of chicken on the grill and caramelized onions, the gentle bubbling of simmering stock and marinara sauce, and the warm feeling of creating top-notch cuisine for appreciative eaters. Though you don't have to be a slave to the stove to eat healthfully and well, I hope that you take the opportunity to experience the joy, personal satisfaction, and aesthetic reward of cooking and sharing your own fresh, healthy food.

This section contains the basic principles underlying the cooking at Diet Designs. Get to know your healthy kitchen, then let your personal eating style run wild with creative acts of cookery.

32

COOKING BY DESIGN

✳

Low-Fat Cooking Techniques

Sautéeing in Liquid

Eliminate the fat used in traditional sautés by substituting flavorful liquids for butter, margarine, or oil. Depending on the elements of your dish, choose from chicken or vegetable stock, dry sherry, red or white wine, fruit juice, vinegar, soy sauce, or a combination of two or more.

1. Heat 2 tablespoons of liquid in a sauté pan over medium-high heat.
2. When the liquid begins to steam, add vegetables, meat, or poultry and stir.
3. Continue to sauté, stirring frequently, until the liquid in the pan evaporates. Quickly add 2 more tablespoons of liquid, stirring to scrape up the glaze formed at the bottom of the pan.
4. Continue to cook in this manner, adding liquid as necessary, until done. Meats and poultry should be browned on the outside and cooked through; onions should be very soft and a deep, caramelized brown; other vegetables should be tender and succulent.

Naked Pasta

■ Always select pasta made without oil or eggs. All the quantities called for in Eating By Design recipes are for dry, not fresh, pasta.

- Many pasta boxes instruct you to add oil and salt to the cooking water. There's no need for the extra fat and sodium; your sauce will provide plenty of flavor and moisture.
- Pasta should always be cooked in a large pot of boiling water. If you have a hot drinking water faucet, use the preheated water to jump-start the boiling process. Add pasta to the pot gradually, so that the water continues to boil.
- In pasta dishes requiring assembly, rinse the cooked pasta, arrange in a single layer on a baking sheet, and cover with plastic. This will prevent the pasta from sticking together or drying out.
- 2 ounces of dry pasta yields 1 to 1½ cups cooked, depending on the type.
- Saucing rule of thumb: Use ¾ cup of sauce per serving of cooked pasta. Remember to account for pasta sauce in your EQ!

Grilling, Baking, and Poaching

Poultry, meats, and seafood all contain natural fats, and should be cooked without any additional oils. Grilling, baking and poaching are the most versatile fat-free methods.

- **Grilling** is the fastest cooking method, best suited to thicker cuts. Begin with a preheated grill or broiler, turning when the grilled side is done (fish should flake; poultry should begin to brown). Flip and cook the other side; the second side will probably require less time. Depending on thickness, grill 5–7 minutes per side.
- **Baking** is a slower cooking method. Bake most cuts 20–30 minutes at 350°.
- **Poaching** involves a slow simmer in liquid—water, stock, or wine—that can be flavored with herbs, onions, shallots, or garlic. In a wide saucepan, heat to a very slow simmer enough liquid to just cover the food. Add the food in a single layer and cook, uncovered, 7–10 minutes. If desired, remove food and reduce the cooking liquid to 2 tablespoons, adding it to your sauce for extra flavor. Poaching is a good choice for delicate cuts like chicken breast, fish fillets, and shellfish.
- **For added flavor and moisture,** brush seafood, meat, or poultry with fresh citrus juice, mustard, Worcestershire sauce, soy sauce, or fresh herbs before grilling or roasting. Or use an oil-free marinade; for best flavor, marinate at least 2 hours, or overnight in the refrigerator. Boil leftover marinade to use as a sauce.
- **Saucing** seafood, meat, or poultry with an Eating By Design or other fat-free sauce makes for an easy and elegant meal. Saucing rule of thumb: Use 2 tablespoons per serving.

Baking Basics

- Fruit purees can substitute for butter, margarine, shortening, or oil in many baking recipes. Dried fruits, mashed bananas, and applesauce all work well for fat-free baking. For dried fruit, cook first with water to reconstitute, drain, and puree. Substitute one-to-one for shortening in recipes.
- Separate eggs; their parts are not equal. Egg yolks are laden with fat (60 calories and 5 grams of fat per yolk) while an egg white has a mere 15 calories and no fat. Most cakes and cookies are just fine yolk-free. You can compensate for a missing yolk with an additional egg white, or add a tablespoon of liquid, such as fruit juice concentrate.
- Top desserts with an improved version of whipped cream by chilling evaporated skim milk in the freezer and whipping until thickened. Sweeten lightly, if you like. Or, drain nonfat vanilla yogurt overnight in the refrigerator, in a yogurt strainer or a colander lined with cheesecloth. Discard the water, and dollop the thickened, calcium-packed "cream" without guilt.

Thickening Sauces

- For roux-based sauces, substitute stock for the butter, cooking it into a paste with the flour before whisking in hot liquid.
- Substitute skim milk (regular or evaporated), buttermilk, or yogurt for cream. To prevent curdling, add 1 teaspoon cornstarch per cup of liquid.
- Finish sauces with arrowroot instead of butter: Dissolve about 1 tablespoon of arrowroot per cup of sauce in cold stock, milk, or water. Whisk into sauce and cook over low to medium heat until desired consistency.

Salad Dressings

Eliminate oil, mayonnaise, and sour cream; mix and match from the following ingredients:

- Vinegar (all types and flavors)
- Mustard (all types and flavors)
- Fruit juices and concentrates
- Fresh and dried herbs and spices
- Garlic, onions, and shallots
- Chicken or vegetable stock
- Honey
- Fat-free mayonnaise, ricotta cheese, buttermilk

Roasting Garlic

Roasted garlic is soft and sweet, a gentle seasoning, a rich spread for bread, or a thick and tasty addition to sauces and soups.

1. Preheat the oven to 450°.
2. Place the whole, unpeeled heads of garlic in a small baking dish and roast until they give lightly when squeezed, about one hour. Cool.
3. Slice off the root (bottom) ends of the heads with kitchen scissors or a sharp knife and squeeze the garlic out from the top down.

✳

The Low-Fat Gadget List

A variety of kitchenware makes low-fat cooking a breeze, and who doesn't love a good gadget? Here are my personal picks:

✓ Measuring cups and spoons
✓ Kitchen scale
✓ Nonstick sauté pans, casseroles, baking pans, and cookie sheets
✓ Dripping-release loaf pan
✓ Wok
✓ Juicer
✓ Immersion (hand) blender
✓ Air popper
✓ Water smoker
✓ Electric steamer
✓ Crockpot
✓ Food dehydrator
✓ Pressure cooker
✓ Fish poacher
✓ Stovetop grill
✓ Cast iron skillet grill
✓ Salad spinner
✓ Yogurt strainer
✓ Vertical roasting rack
✓ Fat-skimming ladle
✓ Zester

33

EATING BY DESIGN RECIPES FOR YOUR FOOD PERSONALITY TYPE

✳

Eating By Design Basics

All personality types will want to take advantage of these classic and versatile basics: a quartet of sauces and a salad vinaigrette to dress up Eating By Design.

Marinara Sauce

¾ cup fat-free chicken broth
4 cups diced onions
2½ teaspoons minced garlic
1 cup dry red wine
3½ pounds Pomi tomatoes, chopped
3½ pounds Pomi tomatoes, strained
¼ cup maple sugar
¾ cup chopped fresh Italian parsley
⅓ cup chopped fresh basil
2½ tablespoons chopped fresh oregano
1 tablespoon chopped fresh thyme
½ teaspoon salt

MARINARA,
PUTTANESCA, AND
PRIMAVERA SAUCE

Portion
¾ c

Calories, 79
(average)

Fat 0.9 g (10% of
calories)

Protein 2.2 g

Carb 14.7 g

Chol. 0 mg

Sodium 105 mg

1. In a large stockpot, heat 2 tablespoons of the chicken broth over medium-high heat. Add the onions and sauté, stirring and adding broth as necessary, until caramelized, about 15 minutes. Add the garlic and cook 5 minutes more.

2. Add the red wine and reduce by one half. Add all the tomatoes and the maple sugar and simmer for 30 minutes. Remove from the heat and stir in the parsley, basil, oregano, thyme, and salt. Serve ¾ cup over pasta or a baked potato, ¼ cup over chicken or fish, or use in recipes.

Yields 13½ cups.

2 servings from the Vegetable Group

Variations:

Puttanesca Sauce: Add ½ cup chopped pitted black olives, 4 teaspoons drained capers, and crushed red pepper or cayenne to taste to 4 cups Marinara Sauce.

Primavera Sauce: Sauté assorted julienned vegetables (peppers, mushrooms, zucchini, carrots, broccoli, etc.) in fat-free chicken broth until tender and add to Marinara Sauce.

BOLOGNESE SAUCE

Portion ¾ c
Calories 150
Fat 2.8 g (17% of
calories)
Protein 20.6 g
Carb. 9.6 g
Chol. 45 mg
Sodium 90 mg

Bolognese Sauce: Sauté 1 pound ground turkey breast meat, 2 diced carrots, and 2 stalks diced celery together over medium-high heat, adding chicken broth as necessary to prevent mixture from sticking, until turkey is cooked through. Drain off fat. Add 4 cups Marinara Sauce, bring to a simmer, and cook for 20 minutes.

1 serving from the Protein Group

Eating By Design "House" Dressing

¾ cup balsamic vinegar
1 tablespoon fresh lemon juice
3 tablespoons Dijon mustard
2 teaspoons chopped shallots
2 teaspoons chopped fresh basil
Freshly ground black pepper to taste

Portion 2 T

Calories 4

Fat 0 g (0% of calories)

Protein 0 g

Carb. 1.8 g

Chol. 0 mg

Sodium 49 mg

1. Whisk together all ingredients in a small bowl. Store, covered, in a nonreactive container in the refrigerator.

Yields 1 cup

Free Condiment

✳

The Nurturer

Orange-Bran Muffins

12 ounces seedless raisins
¾ cup water
½ teaspoon vanilla
2 cups wheat bran
½ cup low-fat buttermilk
½ cup frozen orange juice concentrate, thawed
⅓ cup powdered fructose
¾ cup all-purpose flour
¼ cup whole wheat pastry flour
1 teaspoon baking soda
1 teaspoon baking powder
6 egg whites, beaten
1 teaspoon grated orange zest

Portion 1 large muffin
Calories 196
Fat 0.8 g (4% of calories)
Protein 5.8 g
Carb. 47.2 g
Chol. 0 mg
Sodium 144 mg

1. Preheat the oven to 375°. Line 24 mini-muffin or 12 regular muffin tins with papers.

2. Combine the raisins and water in a microwave-safe dish and cook on high, covered, until raisins are very soft (2–3 minutes; check and stir every minute). Reserve 1 tablespoon liquid and drain off the rest. Put the raisins, reserved liquid, and vanilla in the food processor and puree until very smooth. Set aside.

3. Spread the bran on a cookie sheet and toast until golden brown, about 8 minutes. In a large mixing bowl, combine the toasted bran, buttermilk, orange juice concentrate, and fructose. Stir in the raisin puree and let stand for 20 minutes (or leave overnight in the refrigerator; return to room temperature before proceeding).

4. In a separate bowl, sift together the flours, baking soda, and baking powder. Stir the egg whites and orange zest into the bran mixture, then add the flour mixture. Stir just until combined.

5. Spoon the batter into the muffin tins, mounding slightly. Bake for 28 minutes, or until crusty on top. Cool the muffins for 5 minutes in the pan before removing to a rack.

Yields 12 large muffins or 24 mini muffins.

2 servings from the Complex Carbohydrate Group

Pizza Crust

¼ cup warm water
1 tablespoon sugar
¼ ounce (1 package) dry yeast
2 tablespoons plain nonfat yogurt
½ teaspoon salt
¾ cup water
3 cups all-purpose flour

1. Combine ¼ cup warm water, sugar, and yeast in bowl of an electric mixer fitted with a dough hook and mix to combine. Let stand until foamy (about 10 minutes). Add yogurt, salt, and ¾ cup water. Mix with dough hook at medium speed and gradually add flour. Continue mixing, adding flour as needed, until dough pulls from side of bowl and has a velvety texture.

2. Turn dough into a clean bowl and lightly spray surface with vegetable cooking spray. Cover and let rise in a warm spot until doubled in volume, about 2 hours.

3. For individual pizzas, divide dough into 8 equal balls and stretch or roll into rounds. Or, roll whole dough into one large round and place on prepared pizza pan. Spray surface lightly with vegetable spray.

4. Preheat oven to 400°. Partially prebake crust by pricking all over with a fork and baking 5–8 minutes. Remove to add toppings and continue baking 5–8 minutes until crust is golden brown.

Note: Dough may be frozen before or after rolling or stretching. Stretched dough can be baked directly from the freezer. Thaw unrolled dough 24 hours in the refrigerator.

Serves 8.

Barbecued Chicken Pizza

Pizza Crust for one individual pizza, partially prebaked (page 368)
2 tablespoons julienned red onion
2 teaspoons fat-free chicken broth
2 tablespoons Marinara Sauce (page 365)
2 tablespoons Barbecue Sauce (page 370)
2 ounces chicken breast, poached in water and shredded
1 ounce part-skim mozzarella cheese, shredded

Portion 1
   individual pizza

Calories 359

Fat 6.5 g (16% of
   calories)

Protein 27.1 g

Carb. 45.8 g

Chol. 47 mg

Sodium 600 mg

1. Partially prebake Pizza Crust.

2. Sauté onion in chicken broth over medium-high heat until brown and caramelized. Combine with Marinara and Barbecue Sauces.

3. Coat partially prebaked crust with the sauce mixture, then layer with chicken, onions, and mozzarella. Continue baking at 400° for 5–8 minutes or until crust is golden brown.

Serves 1.

1 serving from the Protein Group
2 servings from the Complex Carbohydrate Group

No-Cook Barbecue Sauce

¼ cup ketchup
¼ cup chili sauce
2 tablespoons Worcestershire sauce
2 tablespoons red wine vinegar
2 teaspoons stone-ground mustard
1 teaspoon dark brown sugar
Dash cayenne pepper
2½ teaspoons crushed garlic

Portion 2 T

Calories 22

Fat 0.3 g (12% of calories)

Protein 0.6 g

Carb. 4.8 g

Chol. 0 mg

Sodium 137 mg

1. Blend all ingredients together in a small bowl. Refrigerate until ready to use.

Yields 1 cup.

1 serving from the Extras Group

Turkey Roll-Ups

1½ pounds skinless turkey breast
Dash of Paul Prudhomme Poultry Seasoning
½ cup sun-dried tomatoes
4 ounces light cream cheese (Neufchatel), softened
½ teaspoon salt
½ teaspoon black pepper
8 whole wheat tortillas
16 fresh basil leaves

Portion 1 roll

Calories 286

Fat 8.7 g (27% of calories)

Protein 26.1 g

Carb. 27.4 g

Chol. 62 mg

Sodium 570 mg

1. Preheat the oven to 400°. Wrap the turkey breast tightly in microwaveable plastic wrap, then loosely in aluminum foil. Place in a roasting dish and bake until the juices run clear, about 1 hour. Season to taste with Paul Prudhomme poultry seasoning. Set aside to cool.

2. Soak the sun-dried tomatoes in boiling water to cover until soft, about 10 minutes. Drain, reserving liquid. Cut the tomatoes into julienne strips. Put half in the bowl of a food processor and reserve the remainder.

3. Puree half the tomatoes, adding just enough of the reserved soaking liquid to form a smooth paste. Add the cream cheese, salt, and pepper and process until smooth.

4. To assemble, thinly slice the cooled turkey breast. Spread each tortilla with 2 tablespoons of the cream cheese mixture, then top with 3 ounces sliced turkey, 2–3 sun-dried tomato strips, and 2 basil leaves. Roll up tightly. If desired, slice rolls into pieces on the diagonal to serve.

Serves 8.

2 servings from the Extras Group
1 serving from the Protein Group
1 serving from the Complex Carbohydrate Group

Tuna or Chicken Salad

24 ounces (4 cans) tuna packed in water
or 24 ounces boneless, skinless chicken breast
¾ cup fat-free mayonnaise
¼ cup plain nonfat yogurt
¼ lemon, juiced
1 tablespoon lemon zest
½ bunch fresh dill weed, chopped
2 teaspoons celery seed
½ teaspoon black pepper
1 cup chopped red onions
1 cup peeled, grated carrots
1 cup diced celery

Portion ¾ c

Calories 167

Fat 1.1 g (6% of calories)

Protein 31.0 g

Carb. 8.5 g

Chol. 48 mg

Sodium 681 mg

1. Drain tuna or poach and dice chicken breast.

2. In a medium bowl, combine the mayonnaise, yogurt, lemon juice and zest, dill, celery seed, and pepper. Add the tuna or chicken, onion, carrots, and celery and stir well to combine. Chill until ready to serve.

Yields 6 cups

Variation: For **Curried Chicken Salad,** add ½ cup chopped green apple, ¼ cup currants, and 1 teaspoon curry powder.

1 serving from the Protein Group
1 serving from the Vegetable Group

Italian Meatloaf

½ cup diced onions
2 tablespoons fat-free chicken broth
1 teaspoon minced garlic
1½ pounds ground turkey breast meat
½ cup sourdough bread crumbs
½ cup plus 2 tablespoons Marinara Sauce (page 365)
2 tablespoons chopped fresh basil
2 tablespoons chopped fresh Italian parsley

Portion 1 slice

Calories 169

Fat 3.4 g (18% of calories)

Protein 26.2 g

Carb. 6.5 g

Chol. 59 mg

Sodium 105 mg

1. Preheat the oven to 350°.

2. Sauté the onions in the chicken broth until lightly browned. Add the garlic and cook 5 minutes more. Remove from heat and cool slightly.

3. In a large mixing bowl, combine the onions with the ground turkey, bread crumbs, ½ cup Marinara Sauce, basil, and parsley. Form mixture into a loaf shape and place in an ungreased loaf pan. Brush with the remaining 2 tablespoons Marinara Sauce and bake until cooked through, 30–45 minutes. Drain off fat and let cool 20 minutes before cutting into 8 slices.

Serves 8.

1 serving from the Protein Group

Cajun Meatloaf

½ cup diced onion
½ cup diced yellow bell peppers
½ cup diced celery
1 clove minced garlic
¼ cup fat-free chicken broth
1 tablespoon Cajun Spice Mix (page 373)
½ cup plus 2 tablespoons tomato puree
1½ pounds ground turkey breast meat
½ cup sourdough bread crumbs
2 tablespoons Worcestershire sauce

Portion 1 slice
Calories 179
Fat 3.8 g (19% of calories)
Protein 26.7 g
Carb. 8.5 g
Chol. 59 mg
Sodium 159 mg

1. Preheat the oven to 350°.

2. Sauté the onion, peppers, celery, and garlic in 2 tablespoons chicken broth until soft. Stir in Cajun Spice Mix and ½ cup of tomato puree. Reduce heat to low and cook 10 minutes more. Remove from heat and cool slightly.

3. In a large mixing bowl, combine the sautéed vegetables with the ground turkey, bread crumbs, remaining 2 tablespoons chicken broth, and Worcestershire sauce. Form mixture into a loaf shape and place in an ungreased loaf pan. Brush with the remaining 2 tablespoons tomato puree and bake until cooked through, 30–45 minutes. Drain off fat and let cool 20 minutes before cutting into 8 slices.

Serves 8.

1 serving from the Extras Group
1 serving from the Protein Group

Cajun Spice Mix

1 teaspoon fennel seed
1 teaspoon dried oregano
1 teaspoon dried thyme
¼ teaspoon ground cumin
1 teaspoon paprika
2 teaspoons onion powder
2 teaspoons garlic powder
1 teaspoon ground black pepper
1 teaspoon ground white pepper
½ t. cayenne pepper, or to taste

1. Combine all ingredients in a small bowl.

Yields 3 tablespoons.

Country Meatloaf

½ cup diced onions
2 tablespoons fat-free chicken broth
1½ pounds ground turkey breast meat
½ cup sourdough bread crumbs
½ cup plus 2 tablespoons Barbecue Sauce (page 370)
2 tablespoons Worcestershire sauce
½ teaspoon Dijon mustard
1 teaspoon minced garlic
½ teaspoon dried thyme

Portion 1 slice

Calories 177

Fat 3.3 g (17% of calories)

Protein 26.1 g

Carb. 8.2 g

Chol. 59 mg

Sodium 271 mg

1. Preheat the oven to 350°.

2. Sauté the onions in the chicken broth until lightly browned. Remove from heat and cool slightly.

3. In a large mixing bowl, combine the onions with the ground turkey, bread crumbs, ½ cup Barbecue Sauce, Worcestershire, mustard, garlic, and thyme. Form mixture into a loaf shape and place in an ungreased loaf pan. Brush with the remaining 2 tablespoons Barbecue Sauce and bake until cooked through, 30–45 minutes. Drain off fat and let cool 20 minutes before cutting into 8 slices.

Serves 8.

1 serving from the Extras Group
1 serving from the Protein Group

Cheese Lasagna

1 pound lasagna noodles
15 ounces nonfat ricotta cheese
½ pound part-skim mozzarella cheese, shredded
½ bunch fresh basil, chopped
½ bunch fresh [Italian] parsley, chopped
1½ quarts Marinara Sauce (page 365)
1 ounce Parmesan cheese, grated

Portion 1 piece

Calories 337

Fat 6.7 g (18% of calories)

Protein 21.9 g

Carb. 44.1 g

Chol. 21 mg

Sodium 257 mg

1. Preheat oven to 350°. Cook lasagna noodles according to package directions. Drain, rinse, and set aside.

2. Mix the ricotta and mozzarella cheeses with the basil and parsley. Set aside.

3. Spray a 13-by-9-inch baking dish with cooking spray and add enough Marinara Sauce to cover the bottom of the pan. Cover with half the noodles, half the cheese mixture, and half the remaining Marinara Sauce. Repeat the layers. Sprinkle the Parmesan over the top layer of sauce.

4. Bake uncovered, 30 to 40 minutes, until bubbling and brown. Let stand for a few minutes, then cut into 10 pieces and serve.

Serves 10.

1 serving from the Dairy Group
1 serving from the Vegetable Group
2 servings from the Complex Carbohydrate Group

Southwest Casserole

1½ cups dried black beans or 3 cups canned
3 tablespoons minced garlic
1 pound ground turkey breast meat
½ onion, diced small
1 tablespoon chili powder
12 corn tortillas
4 cups Enchilada Sauce (page 377)
5 ounces low-fat or fat-free cheddar cheese, shredded
2 tablespoons chopped fresh cilantro
Tomato salsa for garnish

Portion 1 piece

Calories 341

Fat 5.9 g (16% of
   calories)

Protein 27.6 g

Carb. 45.9 g

Chol. 42 mg

Sodium 484 mg

1. If using dried beans, cover with 6 cups of water in a large pot, adding 1 tablespoon of the garlic. Bring to a boil, reduce to a simmer, and cook for 1 hour or until the beans are tender. Drain cooked or canned beans and lightly mash. Set aside.

2. In a large frying pan, sauté the ground turkey with the onions and remaining garlic until cooked through. Drain off the fat, stir in the chili powder, and set aside.

3. Preheat the oven to 350°. Lightly spray a 13-by-9-inch baking pan with cooking spray. Line the bottom with half the tortillas, then layer with ½ the turkey mixture, ½ the beans, ⅓ of the Enchilada Sauce and ½ the cheese. Repeat, finishing with a final layer of Enchilada Sauce.

4. Cover and bake until melted and bubbling, about 20 minutes. Remove from the oven, sprinkle with the cilantro, and let set a few minutes before cutting into 10 pieces. Serve with salsa on the side.

Variation: For a **vegetarian version,** omit the ground turkey and sauté the garlic and onions in broth.

Serves 10.

1 serving from the Protein Group
2 servings from the Complex Carbohydrate Group

Enchilada Sauce

1 26-ounce box Pomi tomatoes
2 cups water
1 onion, coarsely chopped
1 serrano pepper, coarsely chopped
¼ cup chopped fresh cilantro
2 teaspoons ground cumin
2 teaspoons ground coriander
1 teaspoon chili powder
¼ teaspoon salt

Portion ¼ c

Calories 18

Fat 0.4 g (18% of calories)

Protein 0.7 g

Carb. 3.4 g

Chol. 0 mg

Sodium 48 mg

1. Combine all ingredients except the salt in a saucepan and bring to a boil over high heat.

2. Reduce heat and simmer the sauce until the vegetables are soft, about 15 minutes. Add salt.

3. Puree the sauce in a food processor.

Yields 3½ cups.

1 serving from the Vegetable Group

Apricot Chicken

Sauce:
½ cup fruit-sweetened apricot preserves
½ cup dried apricots
1½ cups fresh orange juice
2 tablespoons fresh lemon juice
1 cup fat-free chicken broth
2 tablespoons cider vinegar
2 tablespoons Dijon mustard
1 teaspoon minced garlic
1 teaspoon minced ginger
1½ tablespoons grated orange zest

8 boneless, skinless chicken breast halves

Portion 1 breast
half

Calories 208

Fat 1.7 g (7% of
calories)

Protein 27.2 g

Carb. 20.1 g

Chol. 64 mg

Sodium 126 mg

1. Combine sauce ingredients in a small, nonreactive saucepan. Bring to a boil, reduce heat, and simmer for 5 minutes. Remove from heat and cool.

2. Preheat oven to 350°. Place chicken in a baking dish. Reserve ½ cup sauce and pour the remainder over the chicken. Bake, uncovered, for 30 minutes or until the juices run clear.

3. Turn the oven to broil. Baste the chicken with the cooking juices and broil for 3 to 4 minutes per side, or until lightly browned. Meanwhile, reheat the reserved sauce. Spoon the sauce over the chicken and serve at once.

Serves 8.

| 1 serving from the Protein Group |
| 1 serving from the Fruit Group |

Spinach Dip

2 tablespoons minced garlic
2 teaspoons fat-free chicken or vegetable broth
1 10-ounce package frozen spinach, thawed
½ cup plain nonfat yogurt
⅓ cup grated Parmesan cheese
¼ teaspoon black pepper

Portion 2 T

Calories 34

Fat 1.0 g (27% of calories)

Protein 3.2 g

Carb. 3.4 g

Chol. 3 mg

Sodium 96 mg

1. In a small skillet, sauté the garlic in broth over medium heat until tender.

2. Place garlic and remaining ingredients in a food processor or blender and process until smooth. Cover and chill for several hours. Serve with vegetables, pita chips, or fat-free crackers.

Yields 1¼ cup.

> With ½ oz. fat-free crackers, 1 snack from the Complex Carbohydrate Group

Crab Dip

8 ounces fat-free cream cheese
¼ cup fat-free mayonnaise
2 teaspoons prepared horseradish
2 tablespoons skim milk
2 tablespoons fresh lemon juice
¼ cup chopped green onions
½ pound cooked lump crabmeat
Dash white pepper

Portion 2 T

Calories 36

Fat 0.3 g (7% of calories)

Protein 5.8 g

Carb. 2.1 g

Chol. 19 mg

Sodium 93 mg

1. Preheat the oven to 375°. Combine the cream cheese, mayonnaise, horseradish, milk, and lemon juice in a food processor or blender and process until smooth. Scrape into a medium bowl.

2. Stir in the green onions, crabmeat, and white pepper. Spoon mixture into a shallow 1-quart dish and bake for 20 minutes, or until heated through. Serve hot with vegetables, pita chips, or fat-free crackers.

Yields 1¾ cups.

> With ½ oz. fat-free crackers, 1 snack from the Complex Carbohydrate Group

Chocolate Chip Cookies

4 ounces pitted dates
½ cup water
¾ teaspoon vanilla extract
⅓ cup firmly packed brown sugar
⅓ cup granulated sugar
1 egg white
1 cup all-purpose flour
½ teaspoon baking soda
Dash salt
½ cup chocolate chips

Portion 2 cookies

Calories 126

Fat 1.8 g (13% of calories)

Protein 1.6 g

Carb. 26.3 g

Chol. 0 mg

Sodium 55 mg

1. Preheat oven to 375°. Combine the dates and water in a microwave-safe dish and cook on high, covered, until dates are very soft, about 5 minutes (check and stir every minute). Drain dates and puree with the vanilla in a food processor.

2. Turn the date puree into a mixing bowl and cream in the sugars with an electric mixer. Add the egg white and blend.

3. Combine the flour, baking soda, and salt in a small bowl. Stir into the puree mixture by hand, mixing until well combined. Stir in the chocolate chips. Chill the dough in the refrigerator for 10 minutes.

4. Drop the dough by level tablespoons onto cookie sheets coated with cooking spray. Bake until the edges are golden brown, about 7 minutes. Let set for a few minutes, then remove to wire rack to cool.

Yields 28 cookies.

1 snack from the Complex Carbohydrate Group

*

The Artful Dodger

Banana Chocolate Chip Muffins

1¾ cups mashed ripe bananas
2 cups wheat bran
½ cup low-fat buttermilk
⅓ cup powdered fructose
½ cup frozen apple juice concentrate, thawed
¾ cup all-purpose flour
¼ cup whole wheat pastry flour
1 teaspoon baking powder
1 teaspoon baking soda
6 egg whites, beaten
½ cup chocolate chips

Portion 1 large muffin

Calories 171

Fat 2.8 g (15% of calories)

Protein 5.2 g

Carb. 34.9 g

Chol. 0 mg

Sodium 142 mg

1. Preheat the oven to 350°. Line 24 mini-muffin or 12 regular muffin tins with papers.

2. Puree the bananas in the food processor.

3. Spread the bran on a cookie sheet and toast until golden brown, about 8 minutes. In a large mixing bowl, combine the toasted bran, buttermilk, fructose, and apple juice concentrate. Stir in the bananas and let stand for 20 minutes (or leave overnight in the refrigerator; return to room temperature before proceeding).

4. In a separate bowl, sift together the flours, baking powder, and baking soda. Stir the egg whites into the bran mixture, then add the flour mixture. Stir just until combined. Fold in the chocolate chips.

5. Spoon the batter into the muffin tins, mounding slightly. Bake for 20 minutes, or until crusty on top. Cool the muffins for 5 minutes in the pan before removing to a rack.

Yields 12 large muffins or 24 mini-muffins.

2 servings from the Complex Carbohydrate Group

Poppyseed Dressing

1 cup frozen apple juice concentrate, thawed
6 tablespoons fresh lemon juice
6 tablespoons balsamic vinegar
4 tablespoons Dijon mustard
2 tablespoons honey
1 tablespoon poppyseeds
1 teaspoon black pepper

1. Whisk together all ingredients in a small bowl. Store, covered, in the refrigerator.

Yields 1¾ cups.

Portion 2 T

Calories 51

Fat 0.3 g (5% of calories)

Protein 0.2 g

Carb. 11.6 g

Chol. 0 mg

Sodium 38 mg

| 3 servings from the Extras Group |

Vegetable Soup

10 cups fat-free chicken broth
4 red potatoes, cut into 1-inch cubes
4 cups quartered onions
1 cup carrots sliced 1 inch thick
3 cups celery sliced 1 inch thick
2 cups green bell peppers cut into 1-inch pieces
2 cups zucchini sliced 1 inch thick
1 8-ounce can tomato sauce
2 cloves garlic, minced
¼ bunch fresh parsley, chopped
¼ bunch fresh cilantro, chopped
Dash black pepper

Portion 1 c
Calories 67
Fat 0.4 g (5% of calories)
Protein 3.0 g
Carb. 7.2 g
Chol. 0 mg
Sodium 193 mg

1. In a large stockpot, combine the chicken broth, potatoes, onions, carrots, celery, and green peppers. Bring to a boil, reduce heat to medium-high, and simmer until the potatoes are tender, about 30 minutes.

2. Add the zucchini, tomato sauce, garlic, parsley, and cilantro. Reduce heat to medium-low and cook for 10–15 minutes more, or until the zucchini is just tender. Season to taste with black pepper and serve.

Yields 18 cups.

2 servings from the Vegetable Group

Fat-Free Fudge Sauce

¼ *cup unsweetened cocoa powder*
2 *tablespoons sugar*
½ *cup corn syrup*
1 *tablespoon water*

Portion 2 t
Calories 55
Fat 0.3 g (4% of calories)
Protein 0.3 g
Carb. 14.3 g
Chol. 0 mg
Sodium 19 mg

1. Whisk all ingredients together in a small saucepan and heat, stirring, just until boiling. Remove and serve warm.

Yields ⅔ cup.

3 servings from the Extras Group

✳

The Passionflower

Stuffed Blueberry French Toast

2 cups fresh or frozen blueberries, thawed if frozen
2 tablespoons frozen apple juice concentrate, thawed
½ teaspoon arrowroot
4 egg whites
½ cup skim milk
2 tablespoons fresh orange juice
2 teaspoons vanilla extract
½ teaspoon ground cinnamon
Dash ground nutmeg
8 slices sourdough bread, 1½" thick

Portion 1 slice

Calories 177

Fat 2.3 g (12% of calories)

Protein 6.3 g

Carb. 32.6 g

Chol. 0 mg

Sodium 293 mg

1. Combine the blueberries and apple juice concentrate in a medium saucepan and simmer over low-medium heat until slightly thickened, 6–7 minutes. Whisk in the arrowroot and cook until thick, about 1 minute more.

2. In a large, shallow bowl beat together with a fork the egg whites, milk, orange juice, vanilla, cinnamon, and nutmeg. Cut a pocket into the side of each slice of bread.

3. Coat a large nonstick skillet with cooking spray and warm over medium-high heat. Meanwhile, soak both sides of each bread slice in the egg mixture.

4. Reduce the heat to medium, add half the bread to the skillet in a single layer, and cook until browned on one side. Spoon 1 tablespoon blueberry mixture into the pocket of each slice, flip, and cook until browned on the other side.

5. Keep French toast warm in the oven and cook remaining slices. Serve at once with the remaining blueberry mixture and pure maple syrup.

Serves 8.

2 servings from the Complex Carbohydrate Group

Carrot Ginger Soup

4 cups julienned onions
1 gallon fat-free chicken broth
2 pounds carrots, peeled and cut into chunks
2 ounces fresh ginger root, peeled and minced, or pureed
  with a bit of the broth in the food processor
2 bay leaves
½ teaspoon salt
1 cup cooked white rice
2 tablespoons sherry

Portion 1 c

Calories 114

Fat 0.9 g (7% of calories)

Protein 7.0 g

Carb. 19.8 g

Chol. 0 mg

Sodium 396 mg

1. Combine the onions and 2 tablespoons of the chicken broth in a large stockpot and cook over low heat, covered, until onions are tender, stirring occasionally and adding broth if they start to stick. Add the carrots, ginger, and bay leaves, and continue to cook, covered, for 5 minutes more.

2. Add the remaining broth and the salt, and bring to a simmer uncovered. Cook until carrots are very tender. Remove from the heat.

3. Combine the soup with the cooked rice in a food processor or blender and process until smooth. Return soup to pot, stir in sherry, and bring to a simmer on medium heat, before serving.

Yields 10 cups soup.

1 serving from the Complex Carbohydrate Group

Cilantro Pesto Vegetable Torte

2¾ cups water
1½ cups long-grain basmati rice
1½ cups plus ½ cup Cilantro Pesto Sauce (page 387)
3 large red bell peppers, roasted, seeded, and sliced in strips
3 large yellow bell peppers, roasted, seeded, and sliced in strips
3 medium zucchini, sliced thin and roasted on grill
3 medium yellow squash, sliced thin and roasted on grill
4 teaspoons balsamic vinegar
¼–½ teaspoon salt, to taste

Portion 1 square
Calories 314
Fat 11.4 g (33% of calories)
Protein 13.7 g
Carb. 41.6 g
Chol. 6 mg
Sodium 339 mg

1. In medium saucepan, bring water to a boil. Add rice, reduce heat to low, cover, and cook 25 minutes or until tender.

2. Toss rice with 1½ cups of the pesto sauce.

3. Toss each roasted vegetable separately with a dash of salt and a teaspoon of balsamic vinegar.

4. Lightly coat an 8-inch square baking pan with cooking spray.

5. Assemble the torte in the following order in the dish: ½ rice mixture, zucchini, red peppers, ½ cup pesto sauce, yellow squash, remaining ½ rice mixture, and the yellow peppers.

5. Press the top down slightly, chill, and cut into 8 squares.

Serves 8.

3 servings from the Extras Group
2 servings from the Vegetable Group
2 servings from the Complex Carbohydrate Group

Cilantro Pesto Sauce

1 cup pine nuts or walnuts
4 cups fresh cilantro leaves, packed
2 tablespoons chopped garlic
1 cup grated Parmesan cheese
⅓ cup white wine
⅓ cup fresh lemon juice
½ cup fat-free chicken broth
½ teaspoon salt or to taste

Portion 2 t

Calories 29

Fat 2.0 g (62% of calories)

Protein 1.8 g

Carb. 1.5 g

Chol. 1 mg

Sodium 50 mg

1. Heat skillet over medium-high heat and toast the nuts, stirring, about 5–6 minutes until golden brown.

2. In food processor, puree cilantro, toasted nuts, and garlic. Add Parmesan cheese, wine, lemon juice, and broth. Process well to blend. Add salt to taste and blend. Store, covered, in the refrigerator.

Yields 2½ cups sauce.

2 servings from the Extras Group

Spring Salmon Salad

24 ounces poached, grilled, or baked salmon filets
¼ cup nonfat mayonnaise
¼ cup plain nonfat yogurt
2 tablespoons fresh lemon juice
2 teaspoons minced fresh ginger
1 teaspoon lemon-pepper seasoning
¼ teaspoon cayenne pepper
2½ cups julienned carrots
1 cup julienned red bell peppers
1½ tablespoons dried currants
1 honeydew melon, cut into balls
1 cantaloupe, cut into balls
1 red onion, cut into 8 slices
6 radishes, sliced thin
32 whole spinach leaves, well washed and dried
16 rose or orchid petals
8 whole fresh basil leaves
8 sprigs fresh dill weed

Portion 1 salad

Calories 309

Fat 5.4 g (16% of calories)

Protein 29.9 g

Carb. 43.7 g

Chol. 33 mg

Sodium 323 mg

1. Cook salmon filets as desired and flake.

2. Combine the mayonnaise, yogurt, lemon juice, ginger, lemon-pepper seasoning, and cayenne pepper in a medium bowl. Add the salmon and gently combine. Set aside in the refrigerator.

3. Bring a large pot of water to a boil. Add the carrots and peppers and blanch for 30 seconds. Drain and cool in the refrigerator.

4. When ready to assemble the salads, toss the peppers and carrots with the currants. Mix together the honeydew and cantaloupe balls. On each of 8 plates, place ½ cup of salmon mixture. Top with the onion and radish slices. To one side, place a medley of melon balls. Next to that, arrange a bed of 4 spinach leaves and top with the carrot mixture. Garnish each salad with 2 flower petals, 1 basil leaf, and 1 sprig of dill.

Serves 8.

| 1 serving from the Extras Group |
| 1 serving from the Protein Group |
| 1 serving from the Fruit Group |
| 2 servings from the Vegetable Group |

Artichoke and Sun-Dried Tomato Pizza

*Pizza Crust for one individual pizza, partially prebaked (page
  368)*
1 canned artichoke heart, sliced
*3 sun-dried tomatoes, soaked in boiling water until soft and
  sliced thin*
1 teaspoon chopped fresh basil
½ teaspoon chopped fresh oregano
2 ounces part-skim mozzarella cheese, shredded

Portion 1 pizza

Calories 365

**Fat 11.0 g (27% of
 calories)**

Protein 23.0 g

Carb. 44.6 g

Chol. 30 mg

Sodium 574 mg

1. Prepare Pizza Crust.

2. In a small bowl, toss together the artichoke, tomatoes, and herbs. Spread on the partially prebaked crust and top with cheese. Continue baking at 400° for 5–8 minutes or until crust is golden brown.

Serves 1.

| 1 serving from the Dairy Group |
| 2 servings from the Vegetable Group |
| 2 servings from the Complex Carbohydrate Group |

Shrimp and Goat Cheese Pizza

Pizza Crust for one individual pizza, partially prebaked (page 368)
3 jumbo shrimp, peeled and deveined
1 teaspoon garlic, minced
1 ounce goat cheese
3 leaves fresh basil, chopped
3 sun-dried tomatoes, soaked in boiling water until soft and sliced thin
1 ounce part skim mozzarella cheese, shredded

Portion 1 pizza

Calories 383

Fat 12.2 g (29% of calories)

Protein 24.3 g

Carb. 44.3 g

Chol. 61 mg

Sodium 552 mg

1. Prepare Pizza Crust.

2. Spray a nonstick pan with vegetable spray. Add shrimp and garlic and briefly sauté (shrimp does not need to be fully cooked). Remove from pan, cut shrimp in half lengthwise and toss with goat cheese, basil, and tomatoes. Spread over partially prebaked crust, top with mozzarella cheese, and continue baking at 400° for 5–8 minutes or until the crust is golden brown.

Serves 1.

1 serving from the Dairy Group
1 serving from the Protein Group
2 servings from the Complex Carbohydrate Group

Vegetable Risotto

1 cup chopped yellow squash
1 cup diced carrots
1½ cups leeks, washed well and sliced
2 cups sliced mushrooms
4 cups plus 4 tablespoons fat-free chicken broth
1 tablespoon minced garlic
2 cups arborio rice
1½ cups canned cannellini beans, drained
2 tablespoons chopped fresh basil
¼ cup chopped fresh parsley
¼ teaspoon black pepper
1½ cups chopped tomatoes
1 cup grated Parmesan cheese

Portion ½ c

Calories 131

Fat 2.3 g (16% of calories)

Protein 6.0 g

Carb. 21.8 g

Chol. 4 mg

Sodium 135 mg

1. In a large pan, sauté squash, carrots, leeks, and mushrooms in 4 tablespoons of the broth until soft. Bring the 4 cups of broth to a boil in a separate saucepan.

2. Add garlic and rice to vegetable mixture. Add ¼ cup of boiling broth and stir. Continue adding broth in small amounts while cooking and stirring until rice is tender, about 30 minutes. Remove from heat.

3. Add beans, basil, parsley, pepper, tomatoes, and cheese and serve immediately.

Yields 10 cups.

1 serving from the Vegetable Group
1 serving from the Complex Carbohydrate Group

Double portion may serve as entree. Remember to double the servings from the Eating By Design Mosaic!

Tiramisu

24 ladyfingers
Filling:
¼ cup fat-free ricotta cheese
2 ounces fat-free cream cheese
¼ cup fat-free sour cream
¼ cup nonfat vanilla yogurt
2 tablespoons sugar
1 tablespoon dark rum
Soaking Liquid:
2½ tablespoons instant espresso powder
1½ tablespoons unsweetened cocoa powder
1½ tablespoons sugar
2 cups hot water
Garnish:
1 teaspoon unsweetened cocoa powder

Portion 1 square

Calories 116

Fat 1.7 g (13% of calories)

Protein 3.7 g

Carb. 19.5 g

Chol. 1 mg

Sodium 32 mg

1. Split the ladyfingers in half lengthwise.

2. Combine filling ingredients in a food processor and blend until smooth. Set aside.

3. Combine soaking liquid ingredients in a small bowl.

4. Quickly dip 24 of the ladyfinger halves, cut side down, in the expresso mixture. Arrange dipped side down in an 8-by-8-inch baking pan. Spread half of the filling evenly on top. Dip the remaining 24 halves and arrange on top of the first layer. Top with the remaining filling.

5. Place a toothpick in each corner of the pan and drape with plastic wrap (don't allow it to touch the filling). Refrigerate for 3–8 hours. Sprinkle with the remaining teaspoon of cocoa powder, cut into 12 squares, and serve.

Serves 12.

1 snack from the Complex Carbohydrate Group

Chocolate Cheesecake

4 ounces plain or chocolate graham crackers or chocolate
wafer cookies, crushed
2 pounds fat-free cream cheese, softened
1½ cups sugar
1 cup frozen nonfat egg substitute, thawed
4 teaspoons vanilla extract
¼ cup unsweetened cocoa powder
2 teaspoons cornstarch

Portion 1 slice

Calories 173

Fat 0.6 g (3% of
  calories)

Protein 10.0 g

Carb. 27.6 g

Chol. 10 mg

Sodium 104 mg

1. Preheat oven to 375°. Coat a 9-inch springform pan with cooking spray. Press the graham cracker or chocolate wafer crumbs firmly into the bottom of the pan, packing tightly. Bake for 3 minutes. Remove and reduce oven temperature to 350°.

2. Beat together the cream cheese and sugar with an electric mixer until completely smooth. Turn mixer to low and gradually add the egg substitute. Add the vanilla, cocoa, and cornstarch and blend well.

3. Pour the cheese mixture over the crust. Bake for 1 hour 5 minutes, or until firm and set. Cool on a rack at room temperature, then chill for several hours before serving.

Serves 16.

1 serving from the Dairy Group
1 serving from the Complex Carbohydrate Group

✳

The Blue Rose

Winter Squash Soup

1 onion, diced
10 cups fat-free chicken broth
1 teaspoon ground nutmeg
1 teaspoon ground allspice
1 large butternut squash (3 pounds), peeled and cubed
2 large sweet potatoes (2 pounds total), peeled and cubed
2 bay leaves
1½ teaspoons salt
1 cup evaporated skim milk
2 tablespoons dry sherry
2 teaspoons fresh lemon juice

Portion 1 c

Calories 126

Fat 0.7 g (5% of calories)

Protein 4.7 g

Carb. 27.4 g

Chol. 1 mg

Sodium 317 mg

1. In a large stockpot, caramelize the onion in 2 tablespoons of the chicken stock. Add the nutmeg and allspice and cook 5 minutes more.

2. Add the squash and sweet potatoes, remaining chicken broth, bay leaves, and salt to the pot. Bring to a boil, reduce heat, and simmer for 25 minutes or until the squash and yams are very tender. Remove from heat and puree with the evaporated skim milk in a food processor or blender. Return soup to the pot over low heat and stir in the sherry and lemon juice. Serve immediately.

Yields 16 cups.

1 serving from the Vegetable Group
1 serving from the Complex Carbohydrate Group

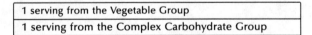

Tuscan Bean Salad

Tapenade:
¾ cup pitted black olives
2 tablespoons fat-free Italian dressing
1 teaspoon minced garlic
2 teaspoons chopped fresh thyme
2 teaspoons chopped fresh oregano
Salad:
¾ pound green beans, trimmed
2 cups cooked white beans (⅔ cup raw)
½ pound red potatoes, diced and steamed until tender
¾ cup peeled, grated carrots
1¾ cups quartered cherry tomatoes
½ lemon, juiced
2 tablespoons chopped fresh parsley
1 teaspoon salt
Dash black pepper

Portion 1 c

Calories 162

Fat 5.3 g (29% of calories)

Protein 6.0 g

Carb. 21.0 g

Chol. 0 mg

Sodium 483 mg

1. To make tapenade, puree the olives, Italian dressing, garlic, thyme, and oregano together in a food processor.

2. In a large bowl, toss the green beans, white beans, potatoes, carrots, tomatoes, lemon juice, and parsley with the tapenade.

3. Season with salt and pepper and serve.

Serves 8.

2 servings from the Extras Group
1 serving from the Vegetable Group
1 serving from the Complex Carbohydrate Group

✳

The Shooting Star

Blender Gazpacho

1 28-ounce can low-sodium tomatoes
3 cups low-sodium tomato juice or V-8
2½ cups peeled, grated hothouse cucumbers
½ cup peeled, grated carrots
¾ cup seeded and diced green bell pepper
¾ cup seeded and diced red bell pepper
½ red onion, diced
2 shallots, chopped
2 cloves garlic, minced
⅓ cup red wine vinegar
⅓ cup fresh lemon juice
1 teaspoon paprika
¼ cup chopped fresh oregano
¼ cup chopped fresh basil
¼ cup chopped fresh [Italian] parsley
¼ teaspoon white pepper
¼ teaspoon Tabasco sauce, or to taste

Portion 1 c

Calories 58

Fat 0.5 g (8% of calories)

Protein 2.5 g

Carb. 45.0 g

Chol. 0 mg

Sodium 287 mg

1. Place the tomatoes, tomato juice, cucumbers, carrots, green and red peppers, onion, shallots, and garlic in a food processor or blender and process until smooth. Add the vinegar, lemon juice, paprika, oregano, basil, parsley, and white pepper. Add Tabasco sauce to taste and blend. Chill for several hours before serving.

Serves 10.

2 servings from the Vegetable Group

Penne with Turkey and Chile Pepper Cream Sauce

1 pound penne pasta
¾ cup onions, chopped
2 cups fat-free chicken broth
2 teaspoons minced garlic
1 large red bell pepper, roasted and chopped
1 medium poblano or pasilla chile pepper, roasted and chopped
1 teaspoon chopped fresh serrano chile pepper
1 pound ground turkey breast meat
10 ounces raw spinach, chopped
Juice of half a lime
1 cup evaporated skim milk
¼ cup unbleached all-purpose flour
¾ teaspoon Paul Prudhomme Poultry Seasoning
¾ teaspoon salt
½ low-fat sour cream

Portion 1 cup

Calories 278

Fat 4.2 g (14% of calories)

Protein 21.4 g

Carb. 36.9 g

Chol. 32 mg

Sodium 238 mg

1. Cook pasta according to package directions and keep warm over steaming water in covered pot.

2. Caramelize onions in a large sauté pan by stirring with 2 tablespoons of the chicken broth over medium-high heat, adding broth as needed, until golden brown.

3. Add garlic, ¼ cup of broth, all the peppers and stir until cooked. Add ground turkey to mixture and sauté until done.

4. Add spinach and lime juice; cook until wilted. Remove from heat.

5. In small saucepan heat evaporated skim milk and one cup of broth over medium heat. In separate bowl, combine flour with ¼ cup chicken broth. Slowly whisk into hot milk mixture. Cook, stirring, until thickened. Do not let boil. Add poultry seasoning and salt.

6. Remove sauce from heat and whisk in sour cream. Add turkey mixture and stir to combine.

7. Toss with pasta and serve immediately.

Serves 12.

| 1 serving from the Protein Group |
| 1 serving from the Vegetable Group |
| 1 serving from the Complex Carbohydrate Group |

Shrimp or Chicken Fajitas

Marinade:
1 cup fresh orange juice
Juice of 1 lime
1 tablespoon Worcestershire sauce
8 cloves garlic, minced
½ teaspoon ground cumin
½ teaspoon ground coriander
½ teaspoon dried oregano
½ teaspoon dried thyme
½ teaspoon black pepper

*1½ pounds shrimp, peeled and deveined, or boneless, skinless
   chicken breast*
12 Roma tomatoes, quartered
½ cup fat-free chicken broth
4 red bell peppers, julienned
4 yellow bell peppers, julienned
4 pasilla chile peppers, julienned
4 onions, sliced lengthwise
8 whole wheat tortillas
¼ cup chopped fresh cilantro
Salsa

Portion 1 fajita

Calories 346

**Fat 6.3 g (16% of
  calories)**

Protein 25.6 g

Carb. 50.7 g

Chol. 131 mg

Sodium 435 mg

1. Combine the marinade ingredients in a nonreactive, shallow dish. Add the shrimp or chicken and stir to coat well. Cover, refrigerate, and marinate shrimp for 30 minutes, chicken for several hours.

2. Preheat grill or broiler. Remove shrimp or chicken, reserving marinade, and grill or broil until cooked through. Cut chicken into strips. Set aside.

3. Pour the reserved marinade into a skillet and bring to a boil. Add 6 of the quartered Roma tomatoes and reduce liquid by one third. Transfer to a food processor or blender and puree until smooth. Set aside.

4. Heat 2 tablespoons of the chicken broth in a large skillet over medium-high heat. Add the peppers and onions and sauté, stirring and adding broth as necessary, until onions are slightly

browned and tender. Add the remaining tomatoes and the pureed marinade mixture. Simmer until the tomatoes are soft but still intact. Add the chicken or shrimp and toss until heated through.

5. To serve, heat the tortillas for 30 seconds under the broiler or wrapped, in the microwave. Fill tortillas with fajitas mixture and garnish with the cilantro. Serve with salsa on the side.

Serves 8.

| 1 serving from the Protein Group |
| 3 servings from the Vegetable Group |
| 1 serving from the Complex Carbohydrate Group |

Mocha Mousse

1½ cups skim milk
1 1-ounce package sugar-free chocolate pudding mix
1 cup nonfat coffee or cappuccino yogurt
6 ounces Cool Whip Lite, thawed
2 tablespoons unsweetened cocoa powder

Portion ½ cup

Calories 112

Fat 2.6 g (1% of calories)

Protein 3.2 g

Carb. 10.6 g

Chol. 2 mg

Sodium 334 mg

1. Pour milk and pudding mix into food processor and puree until thick; pour into a large bowl (or whisk ingredients together by hand in the bowl).

2. Fold in the yogurt, Cool Whip, and cocoa powder. Spoon the mousse into 8 individual serving dishes and chill for several hours. (Mousse can also be frozen; defrost slightly before serving.)

Serves 8.

| 1 snack from the Complex Carbohydrate Group |

Lemon Mousse

1½ cups skim milk
1 1-ounce package sugar-free lemon pudding mix
1 cup nonfat lemon yogurt
6 ounces Cool Whip Lite, thawed
1 tablespoon grated lemon zest
1 teaspoon lemon extract

Portion ½ cup

Calories 100

Fat 2.6 g (23% of calories)

Protein 3.1 g

Carb. 10.6 g

Chol. 2 mg

Sodium 334 mg

1. Pour milk and pudding mix into food processor and puree until thick; pour into a large bowl (or whisk ingredients together by hand in the bowl).

2. Fold in the yogurt, Cool Whip, lemon zest, and lemon extract. Spoon the mousse into 8 individual serving dishes and chill for several hours. (Mousse can also be frozen; defrost slightly before serving.)

Serves 8.

1 snack from the Complex Carbohydrate Group

*

The Perfectionist

Tomato Fennel Sauce

1¼ pounds Roma tomatoes, stemmed and halved
3 cups trimmed, julienned fennel bulb
1 cup julienned red onion
1½ teaspoons minced garlic
¼ cup fat-free chicken broth
1 cup clam juice (to serve on fish) or fat-free chicken broth
   (to serve on chicken or pasta)
2 tablespoons fresh lemon juice

Portion ¼ c
Calories 28
Fat 0.3 g (8% of
   calories)
Protein 1.7 g
Carb. 5.2 g
Chol. 0 mg
Sodium 61 mg

1. Preheat oven to 350°. Arrange the tomatoes on a cookie sheet, cut side up. Spray lightly with cooking spray and roast in the oven until lightly browned, 30–40 minutes.

2. Combine the fennel, onion, garlic, and ¼ cup chicken broth in a medium pan with a tight-fitting lid. Cover and cook over medium heat until the vegetables are soft. Uncover, add the roasted tomatoes, and simmer for 15 minutes. Place in a food processor or blender and puree until smooth.

3. Return the sauce to the pan and add the clam juice or chicken broth. Return to a simmer. Season with the lemon juice and serve on specified portions of fish, chicken, or pasta.

Yields 3 cups.

1 serving from the Vegetable Group

Dijon Shallot Sauce

1 3-ounce package shallots, chopped
2 tablespoons Dijon mustard
¼ cup clam juice (to serve with seafood) or fat-free chicken
*   broth (to serve with chicken)*
½ bunch fresh dill weed, chopped

1. Combine all ingredients in a small bowl. Serve cold with specified portions of chicken or seafood.

Yields ¾ cup.

| 1 serving from the Extras Group |

Portion 2 T
Calories 14
Fat 0 g (0% of calories)
Protein 0.6 g
Carb. 2.5 g
Chol. 0 mg
Sodium 52 mg

Raspberry Sauce

½ cup fresh raspberries
½ jar (⅜ cup) fruit-sweetened raspberry preserves
½ cup frozen pineapple juice concentrate, thawed
¼ cup low-sodium soy sauce
2 tablespoons rice vinegar
½ cup chopped fresh basil
½ teaspoon garlic powder
½ teaspoon curry powder
½ teaspoon chili powder

1. Reserve half the raspberries for garnish. In a medium bowl, combine all the remaining ingredients and blend thoroughly to use as a marinade or sauce for chicken or fish.

Yields 1¾ cups.

| 3 servings from the Extras Group |

Portion 2 T
Calories 46
Fat 0.2 g (3% of calories)
Protein 0.4 g
Carb. 10.9 g
Chol. 0 mg
Sodium 200 mg

Marsala Cream Sauce with Currants

⅓ *cup dried currants*
3 cups Marsala wine
5½ cups fat-free chicken broth
1 cup chopped shallots
1 leek, well washed, dried, and chopped
4 ounces fresh shiitake mushrooms, sliced
2 teaspoons arrowroot
½ cup evaporated skim milk
1 teaspoon lemon juice or to taste
¼ teaspoon salt

Portion 2 T
Calories 60
Fat 0.3 g (5% of
　calories)
Protein 3.0 g
Carb. 11.5 g
Chol. 0 mg
Sodium 137 mg

1. Place the currants in a small saucepan and add enough Marsala to cover. Bring to a simmer, remove from heat, and set aside to steep.

2. In a medium saucepan, heat 2 tablespoons of the chicken broth over medium-high heat. Add the shallots and leek and sauté, stirring and adding broth as necessary, until well-browned and very soft. Add the remaining Marsala and reduce liquid until it just covers the vegetables. Reserve ½ cup of the remaining chicken broth, add the rest to the pan, and reduce by one third.

3. In another saucepan, sauté the shiitake mushrooms in 2 tablespoons of the reserved broth until tender. Reduce heat to low and stir in the arrowroot. Cook, stirring constantly, to make a roux.

4. Add the Marsala reduction to the mushroom roux and cook until thickened. Add the currants with their liquid. Cook, stirring, until thickened. Do not boil.

5. Remove sauce from the heat and stir in the evaporated milk. Season to taste with lemon juice and salt. Serve with specified portions of poultry or pork tenderloin.

Yields 1½ cups sauce.

2 servings from the Extras Group
1 serving from the Vegetable Group

Pesto Sauce

1 cup pine nuts or walnuts
4 cups packed fresh basil leaves
2 tablespoons chopped garlic
1 cup grated Parmesan cheese
⅓ cup white wine
⅓ cup fresh lemon juice
½ cup fat-free chicken broth
½ teaspoon salt

Portion 2 t

Calories 29

Fat 2.0 g (62% of
 calories)

Protein 1.8 g

Carb. 1.5 g

Chol. 1 mg

Sodium 50 mg

1. Heat skillet over medium-high heat and toast the nuts, stir-ring, about 5–6 minutes until golden brown.

2. In a food processor, puree basil, toasted nuts, and garlic. Add Parmesan cheese, wine, lemon juice, and broth. Process well to blend. Add salt to taste and blend. Store covered in the refrigerator. Serve with specified portions of pasta, chicken, or seafood.

Variation: Puree ½ cup sun-dried tomatoes, soaked in boiling water until soft, with the basil.

Yields 2½ cups. May dilute to taste with chicken or vegetable broth.

2 servings from the Extras Group

✳

The Soloist

Blueberry or Raspberry Muffins

1¾ cups whole wheat pastry flour
2½ teaspoons baking powder
1 cup powdered fructose
¾ cup low-fat buttermilk
3 egg whites
1 cup frozen blueberries or raspberries, thawed, reserving
  juice

Portion 1 large muffin
Calories 170
Fat 0.6 g (3% of calories)
Protein 4.0 g
Carb. 39.3 g
Chol. 1 mg
Sodium 117 mg

1. Preheat oven to 375°. Line 24 mini-muffin tins or 12 regular muffin tins with papers.

2. In a small bowl, combine the flour, baking powder, and fructose.

3. In a mixing bowl, whisk together the buttermilk, egg whites, and 2 tablespoons of reserved berry liquid.

4. Add the flour mixture to the wet ingredients, stirring just to combine. Stir in the berries.

5. Spoon the batter into the prepared muffin tins, mounding slightly. Bake until lightly browned, about 20 minutes.

Yields 12 large muffins or 24 mini-muffins.

2 servings from the Complex Carbohydrate Group

Chicken Caesar Salad

24 ounces boneless, skinless chicken breast, poached or
   grilled
8 slices stale white bread or 8 ounces stale sourdough bread,
   cubed
1 teaspoon grated Parmesan cheese
Garlic powder
Onion powder
Black pepper
16 cups chopped romaine lettuce
1 cup Caesar Dressing (below)

Portion 1 salad

Calories 223

Fat 4.3 g (17% of
  calories

Protein 27.5 g

Carb. 18.2 g

Chol. 53 mg

Sodium 291 mg

1. Cook chicken breast as desired and slice across the grain.

2. Preheat the oven to 350°. Spread the cubed bread in a single layer on a cookie sheet, spray lightly with cooking spray, and sprinkle with the Parmesan, garlic and onion powders, and black pepper to taste. Bake until crisp and golden, about 15 minutes. Remove from oven.

3. In a large bowl, toss the lettuce with the Caesar Dressing. Divide among 8 plates and top with the chicken and croutons.

Serves 8.

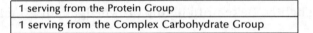

| 1 serving from the Protein Group |
| 1 serving from the Complex Carbohydrate Group |

Caesar Dressing

6 ounces nonfat ricotta cheese
¼ cup grated Parmesan cheese
1 tablespoon fat-free mayonnaise
1 tablespoon balsamic vinegar
2 tablespoons red wine vinegar
3 tablespoons fresh lemon juice
1 teaspoon olive oil
2 teaspoons anchovy paste
1½ tablespoons minced garlic
1 teaspoon black pepper
1½ teaspoons Worcestershire sauce

Portion 2 T

Calories 49

Fat 1.7 g (31% of
calories)

Protein 4.9 g

Carb. 3.3 g

Chol. 5 mg

Sodium 95 mg

1. Combine all ingredients in food processor or blender and process until combined.

Yields 1 cup.

3 servings from the Extras Group

Nachos

2 corn tortillas
1 tablespoon fresh lime juice
Salt to taste
2 tablespoons shredded fat-free cheddar cheese
2 tablespoons canned black beans, drained and rinsed
2 teaspoons chopped canned jalapeño peppers
2 tablespoons sliced scallions
2 tablespoons light sour cream
2 tablespoons salsa (fresca)

Portion Whole
recipe (2
tortillas)

Calories 327

Fat 8.4 g (23% of
calories)

Protein 20.6 g

Carb. 43.6 g

Chol. 18 mg

Sodium 330 mg

1. Preheat oven to 375°. Place the tortillas on a cookie sheet coated with cooking spray. Sprinkle with 1 teaspoon of the lime juice and salt to taste. Bake until lightly browned, about 10 minutes. Remove and cut into chip-sized wedges. Sprinkle with the remaining lime juice, return to the oven, and bake until crispy, 10–15 minutes more. Remove from oven.

2. Top the chips with the cheese, beans, jalapeños, and scallions. Return to oven and heat until the cheese melts. Top with the sour cream and salsa and serve.

Serves 1 as an entree.

3 servings from the Complex Carbohydrate Group

※

The Lotus Eater

Veggie Scramble

4 new potatoes, diced
1 cup sliced scallions
1 teaspoon minced garlic
4 Roma tomatoes, seeded and diced
3 whole eggs
18 egg whites
8 ounces fat-free cheddar cheese, shredded
Dash Hungarian paprika
Tabasco sauce to taste

Portion ⅛th pan

Calories 101

Fat 2.5 g (12% of calories)

Protein 17.9 g

Carb. 7.2 g

Chol. 105 mg

Sodium 344 mg

    1. Bring a steamer pot of water to a boil and steam the potatoes until tender but not mushy. Set aside.

    2. In a medium pan coated with vegetable cooking spray, sauté the scallions and garlic until tender, about 5 minutes. Add the potatoes and tomatoes and cook until warmed through.

    3. Meanwhile, whisk the eggs and egg whites together in a bowl. Coat another medium skillet with cooking spray and scramble the egg mixture over low heat until almost set. Add the vegetable mixture, cheese, and seasonings and cook to desired firmness. Serve at once.

Serves 8.

1 serving from the Protein Group
1 serving from the Vegetable Group

Chopped Chicken or Shrimp Salad

1½ pounds skinless chicken breast or shrimp, poached
4 cups mixed vegetables (raw cucumber, carrots, radish,
*   celery, tomatoes; canned artichoke hearts, beets, corn*
*   kernels; leftover steamed vegetables, etc.)*

2 heads iceberg lettuce
1 cup fat-free Italian salad dressing, or balsamic vinegar
mixed with lemon juice and Dijon mustard to taste

1. Chop chicken or shrimp, vegetables, and lettuce fine and place in large bowl. Toss with dressing and serve.

Serves 8.

Portion 2½ c

Calories 171

Fat 1.6 g (8% of calories)

Protein 21.4 g

Carb. 17.5 g

Chol. 48 mg

Sodium 109 mg

| 1 serving from the Protein Group |
| 1 serving from the Vegetable Group |

Turkey Burgers

1½ pounds ground turkey breast meat
½ cup sourdough bread crumbs
¼ cup low-fat buttermilk
¼ cup minced scallions
¼ cup chopped fresh parsley
½ teaspoon Dijon mustard
½ teaspoon Worcestershire sauce
Dash black pepper

1. Preheat the oven to 350°. Combine all the ingredients in a large bowl and mix gently to combine. Divide mixture into 8 equal portions and form into patties. Place on a cookie sheet.

2. Bake the burgers for 15 minutes. Turn oven to broil and brown on both sides.

Serves 8.

Portion 1 burger

Calories 166

Fat 3.4 g (18% of calories)

Protein 26.4 g

Carb. 5.6 g

Chol. 60 mg

Sodium 115 mg

| 1 serving from the Protein Group |

✳

The Power Player

Vegetable Stir-Fry

2 cups uncooked white or brown rice
2 tablespoons low-sodium soy sauce
4 teaspoons rice vinegar
1 cup fat-free chicken broth
1 teaspoon minced garlic
1 teaspoon minced ginger
4 cups red onions sliced in wedges
1½ cups broccoli florets
5 cups snow peas, trimmed
6 cups halved mushrooms
1 cup cubed yellow bell pepper
1 cup canned water chestnuts, drained

Portion 1¼ c

Calories 335

Fat 1.0 g (3% of calories)

Protein 21.8 g

Carb. 67.1 g

Chol. 0 mg

Sodium 279 mg

1. Cook rice according to package directions. Set aside.

2. Heat the soy sauce, rice vinegar, and 2 tablespoons of the chicken broth in a sauté pan over medium heat. Add the garlic and ginger and sauté until tender.

3. Add all the vegetables to the pan and continue sautéing, stirring and adding broth as necessary, until the vegetables are tender. Add the rice and stir until heated through. Serve at once.

Serves 8.

4 servings from the Vegetable Group
2 servings from the Complex Carbohydrate Group

Spaghetti Squash

1 large spaghetti squash

Portion 1½ c

Calories 80

Fat 1.0 g (11% of
  calories)

Protein 2.0 g

Carb. 18.0 g

Chol. 0 mg

Sodium 2 mg

1. Preheat the oven to 350°. Cut the squash in half and place in a baking dish. Season lightly with salt and mist with cooking spray. Cover tightly with aluminum foil and bake until squash is tender, about 1½ hours.

2. Remove squash from the oven and set aside until cool enough to handle. Using a fork, scrape spaghetti-like strands from the squash. Use like pasta, topping with Fresh Tomato, Basil, and Garlic Sauce (page 412), Marinara Sauce or a variation (page 365), or your sauce of choice.

Serves 4.

3 servings from the Vegetable Group

Fresh Tomato, Basil, and Garlic Sauce

2 cups fat-free chicken broth
4 tablespoons minced garlic
7 cups seeded and diced Roma tomatoes
½ cup chopped fresh basil
1 teaspoon salt
2 teaspoons black pepper

Portion ¾ c

Calories 80

Fat 1.1 g (12% of calories)

Protein 4.0 g

Carb. 16.6 g

Chol. 0 mg

Sodium 437 mg

1. In a medium pan, heat 2 tablespoons of the chicken broth over medium heat and sauté the garlic until browned.

2. Add the tomatoes and remaining chicken broth to the pan. Bring to a simmer and cook for 15 minutes.

3. Remove from the heat and stir in the basil, salt, and pepper. Serve at once over pasta.

Yields 4¾ cups.

2 servings from the Vegetable Group

＊

The Yin-Yang

Supersmoothie

½ banana
½ cup cubed papaya
¼ cup plain nonfat yogurt
¼ cup skim milk
2 tablespoons frozen apple juice concentrate, thawed
1 tablespoon wheat germ
½ tablespoon protein powder

Portion 1½ cups

Calories 250

Fat 1.2 g (5% of calories)

Protein 13.1 g

Carb. 48.8 g

Chol. 2 mg

Sodium 154 mg

1. Combine all ingredients in a blender and blend until smooth.

Serves 1.

1 serving from the Dairy Group
2 servings from the Fruit Group

Vegetable Roll-Ups

4 carrots, peeled and sliced on the diagonal
4 zucchini, sliced on the diagonal
4 yellow squash, sliced on the diagonal
¼ cup balsamic vinegar
1 teaspoon minced garlic
1 teaspoon dried oregano
1 teaspoon dried basil
8 whole wheat tortillas
1 cup Hummus (below)

Portion 1 roll

Calories 253

Fat 5.2 g (18% of
   calories)

Protein 10.3 g

Carb. 46.7 g

Chol. 0 mg

Sodium 308 mg

1. Preheat the grill or broiler. In a large bowl, toss the vegetables with the vinegar, garlic, oregano, and basil. Grill or broil until browned and tender on each side.

2. Warm the tortillas 30 seconds under the broiler or wrapped in plastic in the microwave.

3. To assemble, spread 2 tablespoons of Hummus on each tortilla. Top with ½ cup of the vegetables and roll up tightly. If desired, slice the rolls on the diagonal to serve.

Serves 8.

2 servings from the Vegetable Group
2 servings from the Complex Carbohydrate Group

Hummus

2 15-ounce cans garbanzo beans, drained
3 tablespoons plain nonfat yogurt
2 teaspoons minced garlic
¼ cup fresh lemon juice
1½ teaspoons chopped fresh parsley
Dash cayenne
Salt to taste

Portion 2 T

Calories 66

Fat 0.9 g (13% of calories)

Protein 3.7 g

Carb. 11.1 g

Chol. 0 mg

Sodium 20 mg

1. Combine all ingredients in a food processor and process until smooth. Store covered in the refrigerator.

Yields 2¼ cups.

With ½ oz. fat-free crackers, 1 snack from the Complex Carbohydrate Group

Black Bean Enchiladas

3½ cups Refried Black Beans (page 416)
8 ounces frozen corn kernels, thawed
16 corn tortillas
8 ounces fat-free soy cheese, shredded
1½ cups Enchilada Sauce (page 377)

Portion 2 enchiladas

Calories 343

Fat 3.0 g (8% of calories)

Protein 22.0 g

Carb. 60.6 g

Chol. 0 mg

Sodium 169 mg

1. Preheat oven to 350°.

2. In a medium bowl, mix together the refried black beans and corn.

3. Heat the tortillas for 30 seconds under the broiler or wrapped in plastic in the microwave. Spread ¼ cup of the bean mixture down the center of each tortilla, sprinkle with cheese, roll, and place in a baking dish. Pour the sauce over the enchiladas. Bake for 10 minutes, or until cheese is melted and sauce is bubbling.

Serves 8.

3 servings from the Complex Carbohydrate Group

Refried Black Beans

1 cup fat-free chicken broth
2 cups chopped onions
1 teaspoon minced garlic
2 teaspoons ground cumin
1 teaspoon chili powder
¼ teaspoon salt
2 cups drained canned black beans

Portion ¼ c

Calories 78

Fat 0.5 g (6% of calories)

Protein 4.9 g

Carb. 14.4 g

Chol. 0 mg

Sodium 92 mg

1. In a medium skillet, heat 2 tablespoons of the chicken broth over medium-high heat. Add onions and sauté until caramelized, adding broth as necessary, about 15 minutes. Add the garlic, cumin, chili powder, and salt and sauté for 5 minutes more.

2. Add the beans to the pan, mashing and adding stock until the mixture is smooth and creamy.

Yields 2 cups.

1 serving from the Complex Carbohydrate Group

Linguine with Spinach and Lentils

1½ cups dry lentils
3 quarts water
1¾ cups fat-free chicken broth
1 cup chopped onions
2 teaspoons minced garlic
4 bunches raw spinach (approx. 3 pounds), well washed
1½ cups diced ripe tomatoes
1 pound linguine (regular or whole wheat)
1 teaspoon olive oil
1 teaspoon balsamic vinegar
3 ounces Parmesan cheese, grated
2 tablespoons chopped fresh oregano
1 teaspoon salt

Portion 1½ c

Calories 397

Fat 5.2 g (12% of calories)

Protein 23.1 g

Carb. 65.1 g

Chol. 8 mg

Sodium 518 mg

1. Combine the lentils and water in a large stockpot. Bring to a boil, reduce to a simmer, and cook 25 minutes or until lentils are tender. Drain and set aside.

2. Bring a large pot of water to a boil.

3. In a large sauté pan, heat 2 tablespoons of chicken broth over medium-high heat. Add the onions and garlic and cook, stirring and adding broth as necessary, until caramelized, about 10 minutes.

4. Meanwhile, blanch the spinach in the boiling water just until wilted. Scoop from pot and drain; leave the water boiling.

5. Add the blanched spinach, tomatoes, lentils, and remaining broth to the pan with the onions. Bring to a simmer and cook for 8 minutes.

6. Meanwhile, cook the linguine in the boiling water according to package directions. Drain and place in a large bowl. Add the spinach and lentil mixture, oil, vinegar, Parmesan, oregano, and salt. Toss well and serve at once.

Serves 8.

3 servings from the Vegetable Group
3 servings from the Complex Carbohydrate Group

Asian Tuna, Salmon, or Halibut

½ teaspoon chopped garlic
1 tablespoon fresh lime juice
1 teaspoon low-sodium soy sauce
½ teaspoon sesame oil
½ teaspoon chopped fresh cilantro
½ teaspoon chopped fresh mint
4 6-ounce filets fresh tuna, salmon, or halibut
4 pieces rice paper
1 ounce enoki mushrooms

Portion 1 filet

Calories 275

Fat 2.6 g (9% of calories)

Protein 43.0 g

Carb. 18.7 g

Chol. 76 mg

Sodium 220 mg

1. Combine the garlic, lime juice, soy sauce, sesame oil, cilantro, and mint in a shallow nonreactive dish. Add the fish filets and marinate, covered and refrigerated, for several hours.

2. Preheat the oven to 350°. Dip one piece of rice paper in water to soften and place on a work surface. Place one fish filet in the center of the paper and cover with a quarter of the mushrooms. Fold paper around the filet and mushrooms like a package and place in a baking dish with the edges tucked underneath. Repeat with the remaining three filets.

3. Pour the remaining marinade into a small saucepan and bring to a boil over high heat. Pour over the fish packages. Bake for 10 minutes. Serve the fish in the rice paper, which should be translucent and soft.

Serves 4.

2 servings from the Protein Group

Note: For EQ 1, cut the serving size in half, and count as 1 serving from the Protein Group.

Three-Mushroom Sauce

½ cup white Rhine wine
½ cup sliced shallots
2½ cups sliced shiitake mushrooms
2 cups sliced oyster mushrooms
3 cups sliced cultivated mushrooms
1½ teaspoons minced garlic
Dash ground cloves
3 tablespoons balsamic vinegar
1 28-ounce box Pomi tomatoes
¾ cup fat-free chicken broth
1 teaspoon salt
3 tablespoons brandy
2 tablespoons chopped fresh [Italian] parsley
2 tablespoons chopped fresh oregano

Portion ½ c
Calories 139
Fat 0.9 g (6% of
   calories)
Protein 9.7 g
Carb. 30.4 g
Chol. 0 mg
Sodium 337 mg

1. In a large saucepan, heat 2 tablespoons of the wine over medium-high heat, add the shallots, and sauté until caramelized. Add all the mushrooms and continue cooking, stirring and adding wine as necessary, until tender. Add the garlic, cloves, and balsamic vinegar and stir well.

2. Add the tomatoes with their liquid, the broth, and the salt. Bring to a simmer and cook for 15 minutes. Meanwhile, heat the brandy in a small saucepan. Light with a match and burn until the flame dies. Add to the sauce. Remove from heat and stir in the parsley and oregano. Serve ½ cup over pasta or ¼ cup over chicken or fish.

Yields 4 cups.

4 servings from the Vegetable Group

Banana Berry Bars

⅓ cup (3 ounces) golden seedless raisins
2 tablespoons water
1¼ cups whole wheat pastry flour
¼ cup wheat germ
½ teaspoon baking soda
½ teaspoon baking powder
½ cup maple sugar
1½ large ripe bananas
1½ cups plus ½ cup fruit-sweetened berry preserves
3 egg whites
1 teaspoon vanilla
2 tablespoons lemon juice

Portion 1 bar

Calories 110

Fat 0.3 g (2% of calories)

Protein 1.7 g

Carb. 25.4 g

Chol. 0 mg

Sodium 35 mg

1. Preheat oven to 350°. Spray a 12-by-8-inch glass baking dish with nonstick spray.

2. Microwave the raisins with the water, covered, for 2 minutes on high; stir after one minute. Remove from microwave and set aside to steam.

3. In medium bowl stir together flour, wheat germ, baking soda and baking powder.

4. Drain raisins and puree in food processor or blender. Add maple sugar and process until smooth. Add bananas and blend. Add 1½ cups of the preserves, the egg whites, and vanilla and process briefly. Pour into large mixing bowl.

5. Add dry ingredients and stir just until blended.

6. Spread batter into prepared pan and bake 23–25 minutes or until a wooden pick inserted in the center comes out clean. Remove from oven.

7. Mix remaining ½ cup preserves with lemon juice. Cook in microwave, uncovered, for 1 minute on high. Pour over cake while still hot and spread evenly with knife or spatula. Cool before cutting.

Makes 24 bars.

1 snack from the Complex Carbohydrate Group

✳

The Thrill-Seeker

Mu Shu Chicken

1½ pounds boneless, skinless chicken breasts
6 tablespoons low-sodium soy sauce
¼ cup fat-free chicken broth
2 tablespoons minced garlic
1 teaspoon minced ginger
¼ teaspoon black pepper
1 cup celery cut in diagonal slices
4 carrots cut in julienne matchsticks
10 cups shredded Napa cabbage
½ jar (⅜ cup) fruit-sweetened plum preserves (or apricot)
8 whole wheat tortillas

Portion 1¼ c. mixture with 1 tortilla and sauce

Calories 350

Fat 5.4 g (14% of calories)

Protein 28.9 g

Carb. 50.2 g

Chol. 48 mg

Sodium 901 mg

1. Preheat oven to 350°. In a 13-by-9-inch baking dish, combine the chicken with 2 tablespoons soy sauce, 2 tablespoons chicken broth, and 1 teaspoon each of garlic and ginger. Bake until cooked through, about 25 minutes. Remove from oven, shred chicken, and set aside.

2. In a large sauté pan, heat 2 tablespoons chicken broth, 2 tablespoons soy sauce, remaining 5 teaspoons garlic, and black pepper over medium-high heat. Add the celery, carrots, and cabbage and sauté until the vegetables are soft. Add the chicken and toss until combined and heated through. Remove from heat.

3. Combine the plum preserves with the remaining 2 tablespoons soy sauce. Spread each tortilla with sauce, then fill with the mu shu mixture. Serve at once.

Serves 8.

2 servings from the Extras Group
1 serving from the Protein Group
2 servings from the Vegetable Group
1 serving from the Complex Carbohydrate Group

Coconut Chicken

Marinade:
½ cup plain nonfat yogurt
2 ounces shredded coconut
1 teaspoon peanut butter
1½ teaspoons minced garlic
1 teaspoon fresh lime juice
¾ teaspoon ground coriander
½ teaspoon ground cumin
Dash salt

8 boneless, skinless chicken breast halves (2 pounds)

Portion 1 breast half

Calories 164

Fat 4.4 g (24% of calories)

Protein 27.4 g

Carb. 2.7 g

Chol. 64 mg

Sodium 121 mg

1. Combine the marinade ingredients in a food processor or blender and process until smooth.

2. Place the chicken in a nonreactive dish and pour the marinade over. Cover, refrigerate, and let marinate at least 2 hours or up to overnight.

3. Preheat grill or broiler. Remove chicken and reserve marinade. Grill or broil chicken, turning once, until cooked through, about 10 minutes.

4. In a small pan, bring the reserved marinade to a boil. Reduce heat and simmer 5 minutes. Brush the cooked chicken with the sauce and serve.

Serves 8.

| 1 serving from the Extras Group |
| 1 serving from the Protein Group |

Thai Noodle Salad

Peanut Dressing:
½ cup peanut butter
⅓ cup fresh lemon juice
¼ cup fresh lime juice
¼ cup frozen apple juice concentrate, thawed

¼ cup low-sodium soy sauce
3 tablespoons rice vinegar
3 tablespoons sherry vinegar
1 tablespoon minced garlic
2 tablespoons minced ginger
1 teaspoon Tabasco sauce
2 tablespoons fat-free chicken broth
Salad:
1 pound angel hair pasta
1½ cups diced asparagus
2 tablespoons fat-free chicken broth
1 teaspoon soy sauce
½ teaspoon minced garlic
½ teaspoon minced ginger
1½ cups thinly sliced red bell pepper
1½ cups thinly sliced yellow bell pepper
½ cup chopped scallions
Garnish:
Grated carrots
Sliced cucumber
Chopped cilantro
Lime wedges

Portion 1½ c

Calories 296

Fat 7.6 g (23% of calories)

Protein 12.0 g

Carb. 47.2 g

Chol. 0 mg

Sodium 358 mg

1. Combine all the dressing ingredients in a food processor or blender and process until smooth. Set aside.

2. Bring a large pot of water to a boil. Cook the pasta according to package directions. Scoop out and drain. Add the asparagus to the pot and blanch for 1 minute. Drain and rinse under cold water. Set aside.

3. In a large sauté pan, heat 2 tablespoons broth, soy sauce, garlic, and ginger over medium-high heat. Add the peppers and scallions and sauté until tender. Remove from heat.

4. In a large bowl, toss together the pasta, vegetables, and dressing. Chill for several hours. Garnish as desired and serve.

Serves 10.

3 servings from the Extras Group
2 servings from the Vegetable Group
2 servings from the Complex Carbohydrate Group

✳

The Dreamer

Lentil Soup

1 cup chopped onions
3½ quarts fat-free chicken broth
2 cups diced celery
½ cup chopped carrots
1 teaspoon minced garlic
2 tablespoons chopped fresh parsley
2 teaspoons ground cumin
1 teaspoon dried oregano
2 bay leaves
1⅓ cups Marinara Sauce (page 365)
or 1 c. chopped fresh tomatoes
1 cup dry lentils
2 cups peeled, diced potatoes
1 teaspoon Worcestershire sauce, or to taste

Portion 1 c

Calories 110

Fat 0.8 g (7% of
  calories)

Protein 7.6 g

Carb. 12.9 g

Chol. 0 mg

Sodium 194 mg

1. In a large stockpot, caramelize onions in 2 tablespoons chicken broth over medium-high heat. Add celery, carrots, garlic, parsley, cumin, oregano, and bay leaves and sauté for 5 minutes.

2. Add the remaining 3½ quarts chicken broth and the Marinara Sauce, if using. Bring to a simmer, then add the lentils and continue to simmer until almost tender, about 45 minutes. Add the potatoes and cook until soft, about 10 minutes. Add fresh tomatoes, if using, and season to taste with Worcestershire sauce.

Yields 14 cups.

1 serving from the Complex Carbohydrate Group

Macaroni and Cheese

½ teaspoon salt
1 pound macaroni
1½ cups skim milk
1½ cups evaporated skim milk
3 tablespoons margarine
¼ cup flour
½ teaspoon paprika
Dash black pepper
12 ounces fat-free cheddar cheese, shredded
¼ cup sourdough bread crumbs
Chopped fresh parsley for garnish

Portion 1 square

Calories 388

Fat 5.6 g (13% of calories)

Protein 25.2 g

Carb. 56.9 g

Chol. 7 mg

Sodium 589 mg

1. Preheat the oven to 350°. Coat a 13-by-9-inch baking dish with cooking spray. Bring a large pot of water with ½ teaspoon salt to a boil. Add the macaroni and cook for 10 minutes, or until just barely tender. Drain and place in a large mixing bowl.

2. In a medium saucepan, combine the milk and evaporated milk over low heat.

3. Meanwhile, in another medium saucepan, melt the margarine over medium heat. Gradually whisk in flour. Reduce heat to low and whisk in ¼ cup of the hot milk, stirring constantly until smooth. Slowly whisk in the remaining milk.

4. Raise heat to medium and cook, stirring frequently, until sauce thickens, about 6 minutes. Add the paprika and pepper and remove from heat.

5. Add the white sauce and 8 ounces of the cheese to the macaroni and mix thoroughly. Turn into the prepared pan and sprinkle with the bread crumbs and the remaining cheese. Cover with microwaveable plastic wrap, then tin foil. Bake for 20 minutes, or until hot and bubbling. Remove wrap and bake for 5 minutes more to brown. Garnish with parsley and cut into 8 squares to serve.

Serves 8.

1 serving from the Dairy Group
3 servings from the Complex Carbohydrate Group

Crispy Chicken

1 cup plain nonfat yogurt
2 tablespoons minced garlic
1 tablespoon dried thyme
Dash paprika
Dash cayenne pepper
8 boneless, skinless chicken breast halves (2 pounds)
1½ cups cornmeal
1 cup Apricot Dipping Sauce (below)

Portion 1 breast half with 2 T sauce
Calories 296
Fat 2.1 g (6% of calories)
Protein 30.5 g
Carb. 36.1 g
Chol. 65 mg
Sodium 477 mg

1. In a nonreactive dish, combine yogurt, garlic, thyme, paprika, and cayenne pepper. Add chicken, turn to coat, cover, and let marinate in the refrigerator at least 2 hours or up to overnight.

2. Preheat oven to 400°. Place the cornmeal in a small bowl and dredge each chicken breast half in the cornmeal, covering completely. Place on a baking sheet and bake until the top is golden brown and crispy, about 10 minutes. Turn and cook other side. Serve at once with Apricot Dipping Sauce.

Serves 8.

3 servings from the Extras Group
1 serving from the Protein Group
1 serving from the Complex Carbohydrate Group

Apricot Dipping Sauce

½ jar (⅜ cup) fruit-sweetened apricot preserves
2 tablespoons Dijon mustard
¼ cup low-sodium soy sauce

Portion 2 T
Calories 48
Fat 0.2 g (3% of calories)
Protein 0.7 g
Carb. 10.2 g
Chol. 0 mg
Sodium 507 mg

1. Blend all ingredients in a small bowl. Serve as a dipping sauce with chicken or fish.

Yields ¾ cup.

3 servings from the Extras Group

Mashed Potatoes

2 pounds Yukon Gold potatoes, peeled and cut in chunks
½ cup skim milk
1 cup buttermilk
2 tablespoons grated Parmesan cheese
1 teaspoon salt

Portion ½ c

Calories 74

Fat 0.6 g (8% of calories)

Protein 3.2 g

Carb. 14.2 g

Chol. 2 mg

Sodium 273 mg

1. Bring a large pot of water to a boil and add the potatoes. Cook until tender and easily pierced with a fork, about 30 minutes.

2. Drain potatoes and mash over low heat with the remaining ingredients. (Do not use a food processor; it will make the potatoes gummy.) Serve at once.

Variations: Add 2 tablespoons roasted garlic for **Garlic Mashed Potatoes.**

Yields 5 cups.

1 serving from the Complex Carbohydrate Group

Gravy

5 cups fat-free chicken broth
½ cup chopped shallots
½ cup all-purpose flour
½ teaspoon salt

Portion ¼ c

Calories 29

Fat 0.2 g (7% of
 calories)

Protein 1.8 g

Carb. 5.2 g

Chol. 0 mg

Sodium 134 mg

1. In a medium saucepan, heat 2 tablespoons of the chicken broth over medium-high heat. Add the shallots and sauté until soft, stirring and adding broth as necessary.

2. Gradually whisk the flour into the shallots, adding broth as necessary to maintain a smooth paste. When the flour is incorporated, gradually whisk in the remaining broth. Continue to cook, stirring frequently, until the gravy is thickened. Stir in salt and serve.

Variation: Add 1 tablespoon chopped fresh rosemary to the finished sauce.

Yields 3½ cups.

2 servings from the Extras Group

Turkey Pot Pie

1½ pounds skinless turkey breast
6 cups fat-free chicken broth
Vegetables:
1 leek, well-rinsed and chopped
1 cup sliced mushrooms
1 teaspoon minced garlic
1 cup peeled, sliced carrots
1 cup chopped celery
1 cup peeled, diced turnips
1¼ cups diced red potatoes
1 cup frozen green peas, thawed
1 tablespoon chopped fresh rosemary
½ bunch fresh parsley, chopped
Gravy:
2 cups chopped onions
¾ cup flour
1 bay leaf
1 teaspoon salt
1 teaspoon black pepper
Biscuit topping:
1 cup flour
1 teaspoon baking powder
1 teaspoon salt
½ teaspoon sugar
1 cup skim milk
1½ teaspoons margarine, melted

Portion ⅙th pan
Calories 312
Fat 3.8 g (11% of calories)
Protein 29.5 g
Carb. 42.9 g
Chol. 52 mg
Sodium 860 mg

1. Poach the turkey breast in 2 cups of the chicken broth. Remove, reserving the broth; let turkey cool, then shred. Set aside.

2. For the vegetables: Measure out 1 cup chicken broth. In a large pan, heat 2 tablespoons of the broth over medium-high heat. Add the leek and mushrooms and sauté until soft, adding broth as necessary. Add the garlic and sauté another 10 minutes. Add the carrots, celery, turnips, potatoes, and any remaining broth. Cover and cook until potatoes are tender, about 10 minutes. Transfer mixture to a large bowl and cool slightly. Stir in the shredded turkey meat, peas, rosemary, and parsley. Set aside.

3. For the gravy: Heat 2 tablespoons of chicken broth in a medium sauté pan over medium-high heat and add the onions. Sauté until well cooked but not browned, adding broth as necessary, about 15 minutes. Gradually add ¾ flour, stirring constantly. Cook 10–15 minutes, adding broth as necessary to maintain a wet paste. Add all the remaining chicken broth, including the reserved poaching liquid. Whisk to remove lumps, then add the bay leaf. Simmer 15–20 minutes to thicken. Remove bay leaf and puree gravy in a food processor or blender. Strain gravy into the bowl with vegetables and turkey. Add the salt and pepper. Set aside.

4. For the biscuit topping: Sift 1 cup flour, the baking powder, 1 teaspoon salt, and sugar into a mixing bowl. Add the milk and margarine and mix gently, just until the dry ingredients are moistened. Set aside.

5. To assemble: Preheat the oven to 400°. Pour the turkey and vegetable mixture into a 13-by-9-inch baking dish. Spoon the biscuit dough over the top in small, dumpling-size balls. Bake for 25–30 minutes, until the biscuits are cooked through and the mixture is bubbling. Serve at once.

Serves 8.

1 serving from the Protein Group
2 servings from the Vegetable Group
1 serving from the Complex Carbohydrate Group

Sloppy Joes

1½ pounds ground turkey breast meat
1 tablespoon minced garlic
1 cup diced onions
1 cup diced celery
1 cup grated carrots
1 cup diced red or green bell peppers
3 tablespoons fat-free chicken broth
1 cup Barbecue Sauce (page 370)
1 cup low-sodium tomato juice
2 tablespoons red wine vinegar
2 tablespoons Dijon mustard
1½ tablespoons chili powder
1 teaspoon paprika
Dash Tabasco sauce

Portion ¾ c

Calories 188

Fat 3.3 g (16% of calories)

Protein 26.3 g

Carb. 11.2 g

Chol. 59 mg

Sodium 495 mg

1. In a large pan, sauté the ground turkey and garlic together over medium-high heat until thoroughly browned. Drain off fat.

2. Add the onions, celery, carrots, peppers, and chicken broth to the pan and continue to cook until the vegetables are translucent.

3. Add the remaining ingredients to the pan, reduce the heat to low, and simmer for 15 minutes or until the vegetables are completely tender. Serve with light hamburger rolls.

Serves 8.

1 serving from the Protein Group
1 serving from the Vegetable Group

Fudge Brownies

6 ounces pitted dates
½ cup water
5 teaspoons vanilla extract
1¼ cups sugar
6 egg whites
½ cup all-purpose flour
½ cup unsweetened cocoa powder

Portion 1 brownie

Calories 110

Fat 0.2 g (1% of
     calories)

Protein 1.6 g

Carb. 24.3 g

Chol. 0 mg

Sodium 19 mg

1. Preheat the oven to 375° and coat a 9-by-13-inch baking pan with cooking spray.

2. Combine the dates and water and cook in the microwave on high, covered until dates are very soft (about 5 minutes; check and stir every minute). Drain, reserving the cooking liquid, and puree the dates with the vanilla in a food processor, adding cooking liquid if necessary to make a smooth paste.

3. Turn the date puree into a large mixing bowl and cream in the sugar with an electric mixer. Blend in the egg whites one third at a time.

4. In a small bowl, stir together the flour and cocoa powder. Add to the puree and mix well by hand.

5. Spread the batter in the prepared pan and bake on the middle rack until a wooden pick inserted in the center comes out with a bit of chocolate clinging to it, approximately 15 minutes. Cool on a wire rack, chill for several hours or overnight, and cut into 18 bars.

Variation: Add ½ cup chocolate, white chocolate, or peanut butter chips for an additional 25 calories and 1.3 grams of fat per brownie.

Yields 18 brownies.

1 snack from the Complex Carbohydrate Group

Chocolate Mousse

1½ cups skim milk
1 1-ounce package sugar-free chocolate pudding mix
6 ounces Cool Whip Lite

Portion ½ c

Calories 110

Fat 3.4 g (28% of
calories)

Protein 2.0 g

Carb. 10.8 g

Chol. 0 mg

Sodium 180 mg

1. Put milk in medium mixing bowl. Slowly blend pudding mix into bowl, stir, and let stand until thick. Fold whipped topping into mixture.

2. Fill 6 individual dishes with mousse. Chill for one hour before serving. (Mousse can also be frozen; defrost slightly before serving.)

Variation: May use vanilla pudding in place of chocolate, or prepare half recipe with chocolate and half with vanilla and swirl together.

Serves 6.

1 snack from the Complex Carbohydrate Group

Rice Pudding

3 cups skim milk
¼ cup brown sugar
¼ teaspoon salt
½ cup uncooked white rice
4 egg whites, beaten
1 teaspoon vanilla extract
¼ cup raisins
2 tablespoons granulated sugar
2 teaspoons cinnamon
⅛ teaspoon nutmeg

Portion ½ c

Calories 136

Fat 0.1 g (1% of calories)

Protein 5.4 g

Carb. 27.8 g

Chol. 2 mg

Sodium 143 mg

1. Combine the milk, brown sugar, and salt in a medium saucepan. Cook over medium heat just until small bubbles form around the edge of the pan. Stir in the rice, cover, reduce heat to low, and cook for 30–45 minutes or until the rice is tender and most of the milk is absorbed.

2. Remove the pan from the heat and stir in the egg whites. Return to the heat and cook, stirring constantly, until the mixture thickens. Remove from heat and stir in the vanilla extract and raisins.

3. Combine the granulated sugar, cinnamon, and nutmeg in a small bowl. Spoon pudding into 8 individual serving dishes and sprinkle the cinnamon mixture over the top. Serve warm or cold.

Serves 8.

1 snack from the Complex Carbohydrate Group

APPENDIX
References and Recommended Reading

TEXTS AND REFERENCE BOOKS

Chopra, Deepak. *Quantum Healing.* New York: Bantam Books, 1989. *Ageless Body, Timeless Mind.* New York: Harmony Books, 1993.

Katch, Frank I., and William D. McArdle. *Introduction to Nutrition, Exercise, and Health.* Philadelphia: Lea & Febiger, 1993.

Kinder, Dr. Melvyn. *Mastering Your Moods.* New York: Simon and Schuster, 1994.

Moyers, Bill. *Healing and the Mind.* New York: Doubleday, 1993.

Netzer, Corinne. *The Corinne T. Netzer Encyclopedia of Food Values.* New York: Dell Publishing, 1992.

Wurtman, Judith. *Managing Your Mind and Mood Through Food.* New York: Harper & Row, 1986.

JOURNALS (SCHOLARLY IN APPROACH)

American Journal of Clinical Nutrition. The American Society for Clinical Nutrition, 9650 Rockville Pike, Room 3404, Bethesda, MD 20814-3998, (301) 530-7038.

Appetite. Academic Press, 24–28 Oval Rd., London, NW1 7DX, UK, (081-300-3322).

Journal of the American Dietetic Association. American Dietetic Association, 216 W. Jackson Blvd., Suite 800, Chicago, IL 60606-6995, (312) 899-0040.

The Journal of Nutrition. The American Institute of Nutrition, 9650 Rockville Pike, Bethesda, MD 20814-3998.

New England Journal of Medicine. 10 Shattuck St., Boston, MA 02115-6094.

Nutrition Reviews. USDA Human Nutrition Research Center on Aging, Tufts University, 711 Washington St., Boston, MA 02111, (617) 556-3202.

Nutrition Today. Williams and Wilkins, 428 E. Preston St., Baltimore, MD 21202, (800) 638-6423.

NEWSLETTERS (CONSUMER-ORIENTED)

Environmental Nutrition, Environmental Nutrition, Inc., 52 Riverside Drive, New York, NY 10024-6599, (800) 829-5384.

Harvard Health Letter, P.O. Box 420300, Palm Coast, FL 32142-0300, (800) 829-9045.

Nutrition Action Newsletter, Center for Science in the Public Interest, 1875 Connecticut Ave., NW, Suite 300, Washington, DC 20009-5728, (202) 332-9110.

Tufts University Diet and Nutrition Letter, 53 Park Place, New York, NY, 10007.

University of California at Berkeley Wellness Letter, Health Letter Associates, P.O. Box 412, Prince St. Station, New York, NY 10012-0007.

MAGAZINES

Cooking Light. 4929 Wilshire Blvd., Suite 690, Los Angeles, CA 90010, (213) 933-5693.

Eating Well. Telemedia Communications, Ferry Road, P.O. Box 1001, Charlotte, VT 05445-1001, (800) 678-0541.

Weight Watchers Magazine. Box 56129, Boulder, CO 80322, (800) 876-8441.

ASSOCIATIONS

American Dietetic Association, Chicago, IL, (312) 899-0040.

American Council on Science and Health, New York, NY, (212) 362-7044.

American Heart Association, Dallas, TX, (214) 373-6300.

Food and Nutrition Information Center of the National Agricultural Library, Beltsville, MD, (301) 504-5719.